Pocket Guide to the
Operating Room

Pocket Guide to the Operating Room

Second Edition

Maxine A. Goldman, BS, RN
Clinical Nurse IV
Formerly, Operating Room Clinical
 Education Instructor
Medical Center of Tarzana
Tarzana, California

 F. A. Davis Company • Philadelphia

F. A. Davis Company
1915 Arch Street
Philadelphia, PA 19103

Printed in the United States of America

Last digit indicates print number: 10 9 8 7 6

Publisher, Allied Health: Jean-François Vilain
Production Editor: Glenn L. Fechner
Cover Designer: Steven R. Morrone

As new scientific information becomes available through basic and clinical research, recommended treatments and drug therapies undergo changes. The author and publisher have done everything possible to make this book accurate, up to date, and in accord with accepted standards at the time of publication. The authors, editors, and publisher are not responsible for errors or omissions or for consequences from application of the book, and make no warranty, expressed or implied, in regard to the contents of the book. Any practice described in this book should be applied by the reader in accordance with professional standards of care used in regard to the unique circumstances that may apply in each situation. The reader is advised always to check product information (package inserts) for changes and new information regarding dose and contraindications before administering any drug. Caution is especially urged when using new or infrequently ordered drugs.

Library of Congress Cataloging in Publication Data

Goldman, Maxine A., 1947–
    Pocket guide to the operating room / Maxine A. Goldman.—2nd ed.
        p.   cm.
    ISBN 0-8036-0033-X
    1. Surgery, Operative—handbooks, manuals, etc.   2. Surgical instruments and apparatus—Handbooks, manuals, etc.   3. Operating rooms —Equipment and supplies—Handbooks, manuals, etc.   I. Title.
    [DNLM: 1. Surgery, Operative—methods—handbooks. 2. Operating Rooms—handbooks.   3. Surgical Equipment—handbooks.   WO 39 G6193p 1996]
    RD32.3.G65   1996
    617′.91—dc20
    DNLM/DLC
    for Library of Congress   95-21883
                                                                    CIP

Preface

This guide is intended for the practitioner, as well as the student surgical technologist or nurse who requires a concise, yet comprehensive reference regarding the technological aspects of the care of the patient in the operating room. The material is presented in a systematic manner to encourage the reader to follow a logical sequence of events as they actually occur when a patient enters the operating room. Background clinical information is provided in order to enhance the reader's perspective. For optimal utilization of this guide a basic understanding of anatomy, physiology, microbiology, and asepsis is presupposed.

The format for every procedure includes:

    a definition
    a discussion
    description of the procedure
    notes on preparation of the patient and draping techniques
    instrumentation equipment
    supplies
    special notes

Precise details regarding certain items (e.g., suture material), have been omitted because of the myriad of products available. Special notes particular to each surgery are provided.

Over 300 surgical procedures are described and arranged in chapters according to anatomical site and/or

surgical specialty. Chapters on psychological care of
the patient, patient and personnel safety, anesthesia,
and descriptions of certain limited access procedures
depart from the standardized format. A discussion of
laser surgery is included in the appendix.

Since the printing of the first edition of this work in
1988, there has been a veritable explosion of limited access and microinvasive surgical procedures. A general
guideline to this aspect of surgery is included, and representative procedures in the various specialities are
described as much as possible in the same detail as are
the standard comparable procedures.

The conduction of a surgical procedure varies from
institution to institution, between different sections of
the country, and according to preference of the surgeon.
Similarly, the suggested instrument trays are not
meant to imply that the instruments listed must be
used exclusively, but rather that these trays include
the basics; various instruments can be added or deleted
according to preference. This is particularly evident
noting the rapid and ongoing changes in the instrumentation for limited access surgery. Instrument
nomenclature, availability of supplies, techniques for
draping, etc. will also vary.

In an attempt to limit its physical size, this work is
confined to the operative phase of patient care; perioperative care outside of the surgical department has
been given limited attention. One must know what a
surgical procedure involves before optimal care of the
individual patient can be implemented; it is hoped that
the base of information presented herein will serve as
a generally applicable foundation upon which the reader can build.

M.A.G.

Acknowledgments

In my effort to modernize this second edition to the state of current practice, I am indebted to many persons, a recitation of whose names would be too numerous to list individually.

I wish especially to thank the knowledgeable representatives of the manufacturers of surgical instruments and equipment, particularly those whose products are used in minimal access procedures. I will always be appreciative to the physicians, nurses, and surgical technicians who imparted to me insights into the highly detailed aspects of their specialities as well as helping me to obtain pertinent reference materials.

For this current edition, I again gratefully recognize the assistance of Mrs. Francine Kubrin (medical librarian, Valley Presbyterian Hospital, Van Nuys, California) and Mrs. Francine Stockser, the transcriber of this manuscript, whose painstaking diligence was invaluable, and my editor Jean-François Vilain who with great patience appreciated the nature of the delays in accumulating the precise and diverse data involved.

I am also pleased to acknowledge the kind encouragement of my good friends and my children Laurie, Emily, Judith, and David during the preparation of this work. Finally, as always, I wish to thank my husband Harris, my partner in all endeavors, whose knowledge and love sustained me through the completion of this pocket guide.

Contents

Part 1   Perioperative
          Considerations 1
Chapter 1 Psychological Support
          of the Surgical Patient 3
Chapter 2 Protection of the Patient
          in Surgery 5
          Admission Procedure 5
          Transfer Procedure 5
          Positioning 10
          Environmental Controls..........10
          Electrical and Fire
          Hazards................................12
          Electrosurgery 12
          Operative Record 13
          Counting Procedure................14
            Sponge Counts 15
            Sharp Counts...........................15
            Instrument Counts.....................16
          Sterilization 16
            Saturated Steam Under
            Pressure 16
            Gas Chemical Sterilization 17
            Liquid Chemical Sterilization 18

               Emergencies and
               Disasters 18

Chapter 3   Safety for Operating
               Room Personnel 20
               In-Service Education 20
               Body Mechanics 20
               Fatigue Factors......................21
               Radiation Safety 21
               Infection Control....................22
               Chemical Hazards.................22

Part II   Anesthesia 25
Chapter 4   General Information 27
               General Anesthesia 29
               Conduction Anesthesia 32
                 Nerve Blocks 32
                 Local Anesthesia 34
                 Topical Anesthesia 35

Chapter 5   General Anesthesia 37

Chapter 6   Conduction
               Anesthesia 40
               Spinal, Epidural, Caudal 40
               Regional, Local, Topical 42

Part III   Surgical Procedures
               Including Minimal
               Access Procedures 45
               Technical Considerations 47

Chapter 7   Neck Surgery 48
               Thyroidectomy 48
               Parathyroidectomy 50
               Thyroglossal Duct
               Cystectomy.......................... 51

Chapter 8   Breast Procedures 53
             Breast Biopsy 53
             Mastectomy 55
Chapter 9   Abdominal Extraintestinal
             Surgery 60
             Abdominal Laparotomy 60
             Abdominal Laparoscopy 62
             Abdominal
             Herniorrhaphy 66
             Laparoscopic Groin
             Herniorrhaphy 68
             Cholecystectomy 71
             Laparoscopic
             Cholecystectomy 74
             Drainage of Pancreatic Cyst
             (Pseudocyst) 79
             Pancreaticoduodenectomy
             (Whipple Procedure) 81
             Pancreatectomy...................... 83
             Drainage of Abscess(es)
             in the Region
             of the Liver 84
             Hepatic Resection 86
             Splenectomy 89
             Laparoscopic
             Splenectomy 91
Chapter 10   Gastrointestinal
             Surgery 95
             Esophagoscopy 95
             Gastroscopy............................ 97
             Colonoscopy............................ 98
             Sigmoidoscopy........................ 98
             Esophageal Hiatal
             Herniorrhaphy 102

Laparoscopic Fundoplication
(Nissen Procedure) 103
Vagotomy and
Pyloroplasty 106
Laparoscopic Vagotomy 108
Closure of a Perforated
Peptic Ulcer 113
Laparoscopic Closure
of a Perforated Ulcer
(With Vagotomy) 113
Gastrostomy 114
Gastrectomy 116
Small-Bowel Resection 119
Cutaneous Ileostomy 120
Appendectomy 122
Laparoscopic
Appendectomy 123
Colostomy 126
Closure of Colostomy 128
Right Hemicolectomy 130
Transverse Colectomy 132
Anterior Resection
of the Sigmoid Colon
and Rectum 134
Abdominoperineal Resection
of the Rectum 135
Laparoscopic Assisted Colon
Resection 138
Transanal Endoscopic
Microsurgery 144
Hemorrhoidectomy 147
Pilonidal Cystectomy
and Sinusectomy 149
Thiersch Procedure 151

Ripstein Procedure
(Presacral Rectopexy)..........153
Perineal Resection of the
Rectum for Complete Rectal
Prolapse (Procidentia) 154

Chapter 11 Gynecologic and
Obstetric Surgery..........156
Dilation of the Cervix and
Curettage of the Uterus
(D & C) 156
Conization of the Uterine
Cervix 158
Therapeutic Abortion by
Suction Curettage 160
Marsupialization of
Bartholin's Duct Cyst..........161
Culdoscopy 163
Vaginal Hysterectomy 163
Anterior and/or Posterior
Colporrhaphy 166
Pelvic Laparoscopy/
Pelviscopy 167
Total Abdominal
Hysterectomy 170
Salpingo-Oophorectomy 172
Tubal Sterilization 174
Laparoscopic Hysterectomy
and Laparoscopic Assisted
Vaginal Hysterectomy
With or Without Salpingo-
Oophorectomy....................176
Hysteroscopy 180
Tuboplasty of the
Fallopian Tubes 183

Pelvic Exenteration 186
Shirodkar Procedure 189
Cesarean Section................190

Chapter 12   Genitourinary
Surgery 194
Hypospadias Repair............194
Epispadias Repair 196
Circumcision 197
Penile Implant 198
Marshall-Marchetti-Krantz
Procedure.........................200
Hydrocelectomy 202
Vasectomy 203
Vasovasostomy 205
Cutaneous Vasostomy 206
Spermatocelectomy 206
Orchiectomy 207
Cystoscopy 208
Cystostomy.......................210
Cystectomy.......................212
Transurethral Resection of
the Prostate (TURP) and/or
Lesions of the Bladder or
Bladder Neck (TURB) 215
Open Prostatectomy 217
Nephrectomy 221
Upper Tract Urolithotomy
(Ureterolithotomy,
Pyelolithotomy,
Nephrolithotomy) 225
Cutaneous Ureterostomy 227
Ileal Conduit 228
Adrenalectomy 230
Extracorporeal Shock Wave
Lithotripsy (ESWL) 233

Extracorporal Shock Wave
Lithotripsy Without Water
Bath 239
Ultrasonic Lithotripsy 242
Electrohydraulic
Lithotripsy 243

Chapter 13 Thoracic Procedures......246
Bronchoscopy 246
Mediastinoscopy 249
Segmental Resection
of the Lung.........................251
Wedge Resection of
the Lung 253
Pulmonary Lobectomy 254
Pneumonectomy 254
Decortication
of the Lung.........................256
Insertion of Transvenous
Endocardial Pacemaker 256
Correction of Pectus
Excavatum 259
Thymectomy.......................260
Thoracoscopy 262
Thoracscopic Wedge
Resection of the Lung..........268
Video-Assisted Thoracoscopic
Pneumonectomy 269
Video-Assisted Thoracoscopic
Esophagogastromyotomy 270

Chapter 14 Cardiovascular
Surgery 272
Carotid Endarterectomy......272
Abdominal Aortic Procedures

(Abdominal Aortic
Aneurysmectomy, Abdominal,
Aortic Endarterectomy)
With Aortoiliac Graft 274
Femoropopliteal
Bypass...............................278
Greater Saphenous Vein
Ligation and Stripping........281
Portasystemic Shunt 283
Arteriovenous Shut,
Arteriovenous Fistula 286
Cardiac Procedures 288

Chapter 15   Orthopedic Surgery 296
Open Reduction of a
Carpal Bone Fracture 296
Excision of Ganglion 298
Carpal Tunnel Release........300
Arthroscopic Carpal
Tunnel Release 301
Open Reduction of the
Humerous 301
Open Reduction of the
Radius and/or Ulna 303
Open Reduction of an
Olecranon Process
Fracture............................305
Wrist Arthroscopy 307
Repair of Recurrent
Anterior Dislocation
of the Shoulder 310
Arthroscopy of the
Shoulder 312
Open Reduction of
Fracture of the Humeral

Head (including
Humeral Head
Prosthesis) 316
Arthroscopy of the Elbow 318
Internal Fixation of
the Hip 321
Femoral Head Prosthetic
Replacement......................323
Total Hip Replacement........326
Open Reduction of the
Femoral Shaft....................330
Arthrotomy of the Knee 332
Arthroscopy of the Knee 336
Excision of Popliteal
(Baker's) Cyst 341
Total Knee Replacement......343
Open Reduction of the
Tibial Shaft 346
Open Reduction of
the Ankle 348
Arthroscopy of the Ankle
and Foot 350
Triple Arthrodesis of
the Ankle 353
Total Ankle Joint
Replacement......................354
Bunionectomy....................356
Correction of Hammer
Toe Deformity With
Interphalangeal Fusion 359
Metatarsal Head
Resection 359
Procedure for Correction
of Scoliosis 360

Amputation of Lower
Extremity...........................363
Chapter 16 Neurosurgical
Surgery 367
Craniotomy 367
Cranioplasty.....................375
Transsphenoidal
Hypophysectomy 378
Ventricular Shunts 381
Laminectomy 385
Excision of Cervical
Intervertebral Disc With
Fusion, Anterior Approach ..390
Chapter 17 Plastic Surgery.............393
Cleft Lip Repair 393
Cleft Palate Repair 395
Reduction of a Nasal
Fracture...........................397
Reduction of a Mandibular
Fracture...........................399
Reduction of a Zygomatic
Fracture...........................402
Open Reduction of an Orbital
Floor Fracture 404
Rhinoplasty 406
Mentoplasty
Augmentation....................409
Blepharoplasty 410
Rhytidectomy 412
Dermabrasion....................414
Otoplasty 416
Repair of Syndactyly 418
Digital Flexor Tendon
Repair 420
Peripheral Nerve Repair......422

Palmar Fasciectomy 425
Reduction Mammoplasty 426
Augmentation
Mammoplasty.....................428
Abdominoplasty/Abdominal
Lipectomy 430
Liposuction.......................432

Chapter 18 Otorhinolaryngological
(ENT) Surgery 435
Myringotomy 435
Mastoidectomy 437
Tympanoplasty 440
Stapedectomy 442
Submucous Resection of the
Nasal Septum (SMR) 443
Intransal Antrostomy/
Intranasal Fenestration
of the Nasoantral Wall........444
Caldwell-Luc Procedure
(Radical Drainage of the
Antrum of the Maxillary
Sinuses) 447
Nasal Polypectomy 448
Drainage of the Frontal
Sinus...............................449
Sinus Endoscopy 451
Tonsillectomy and
Adenoidectomy (T & A) 454
Laryngoscopy 456
Tracheostomy 459
Excision of the
Submaxillary (Submandibular)
Gland 461
Parotidectomy...................462
Laryngectomy...................464

Radical Neck
Dissection 467
Excision of Lesions of the
Oral Cavity (Partial
Glossectomy With
Marginal Resection
of the Mandible) 469

Chapter 19 Ophthalmic
Surgery 473
General Information 473
Excision of a
Chalazion..........................476
Canthotomy 477
Tarsorrhaphy/
Canthorrhaphy 478
Correction of Ectropion 480
Correction of Entropion 482
Blepharoptosis Repair 483
Lacrimal Duct Probing........484
Excision of Eyelid Lesions....485
Eyelid Laceration Repair 487
Dacryocystorhinostomy 488
Correction of Strabismus 490
Evisceration of the Eye........492
Enucleation of the Globe......494
Orbital Exenteration 495
Corneal Transplant/
Keratoplasty......................497
Cataract Extraction 500
Secondary Lens Implant......503
Extraction of an Intraocular
Foreign Body 505
Trabeculectomy..................507
Excision of Pterygium 509

Repair of Retinal
Detachment/Scleral
Buckling 511
Vitrectomy 513
Refractive Keratoplasty 516

Chapter 20 Pediatric Procedures 518
Pediatric General
Information 518
Pediatric Tracheostomy 520
Branchial Cleft
Sinusectomy 522
Repair of Congential
Diaphragmatic Hernia 524
Omphalocele Repair............526
Pediatric Umbilical
Herniorrhaphy 529
Pediatric Inguinal
Herniorrhaphy 530
Repair of Congenital
Atresia of the Esophagus 532
Insertion of Central Venous
Catheter (Pediatric)............535
Pyloromyotomy for
Congenital Hypertrophic
Pyloric Stenosis..................537
Pediatric Gastrostomy 539
Relief of Intestinal
Obstruction (Pediatric)........540
Reduction of Pediatric
Intussusception..................542
Pediatric Colostomy............543
Pediatric Colorectal Resection
for Aganglionic Megacolon/
Hirschsprung's Disease 546

Repair of Imperforate
Anus 550
Pediatric Limited Access
Procedures 553
Pediatric Laparoscopy 553
Pediatric Laparoscopic
Appendectomy 554
Pediatric Laparoscopic
Fundoplication/
Nissen Procedure 555
Pediatric Thoracoscopy........556
Pediatric Laparoscopic
Splenectomy 557

Part IV Instrument Trays 559
Chapter 21 General Surgery Trays 561
Major Procedures Tray........561
Basic/Minor Procedures
Tray 562
Limited Procedure Tray 563
Thyroid Tray 564
Long Instruments Tray 565
Biliary Tract Procedures
Tray 566
Choledochoscopy Tray 566
Basic Rigid Sigmoidoscopy
Tray 566
Gastrointestinal Procedures
Tray 567
Rectal Procedures Tray 566

Chapter 22 Gynecologic and Obstetric Trays..............569
Dilatation & Curettage
(D & C) Tray......................569

Cervical Cone Tray 570
Vaginal Hysterectomy
Tray 571
Abdominal Hysterectomy
Tray 572
Cesarean Section Tray 572

Chapter 23 Genitourinary Trays 574
Vasectomy Tray 574
Abdominal Prostatectomy
Tray 575
Kidney Tray 575

Chapter 24 Thoracic Trays 576
Mediastinoscopy Tray 576
Thoracotomy Tray 577
Pacemaker Tray 578

Chapter 25 Cardiovascular Trays....580
Vascular Procedures Tray....580
Vascular Shunt Tray 581
Cardiac Procedures Tray 582

Chapter 26 Orthopedic Trays 585
Basic Orthopedic Procedures
Tray 585
Minor Orthopedic Procedures
Tray 586
Bone Holding Instruments
Tray 588
Hip Retractors Tray............588
Knee Arthrotomy Tray 588

Chapter 27 Neurologic Procedures
Trays...............................589
Craniotomy Tray................589
Laminectomy Tray 591
Kerrison Rongeurs and
Pituitary Forceps Tray........592

Chapter 28   Plastic Procedures
Tray...................................594
Basic Plastic Procedures
Tray 594
Chapter 29   Otorhinolaryngologic
(ENT) Trays 596
Ear Procedures Tray 596
Nasal Procedures Tray........598
Myringotomy Tray..............599
Tonsillectomy and
Adenoidectomy Tray 600
Tracheostomy Tray 601
Chapter 30   Ophthalmic Trays 602
Basic Eye Procedures
Tray 602
Eyelid and Conjunctival
Procedures Tray 603
Basic Eye Muscle
Procedures Tray 604
Dacryocystorhinostomy
Tray 604
Globe and Orbit
Procedures Tray 605
Corneal Procedures Tray 606
Cataract Extraction and
Lens Procedure Tray 607
Glaucoma Procedures
Tray 608
Basic Eye Procedures
Microscope Tray 609
Retinal Procedures Tray......610
Chapter 31   Pediatric Trays...............612
Pediatric Major
Procedures Tray 612

Pediatric Minor
Procedures Tray 613
Pediatric Gastrointestinal
Procedures Tray 614
Pediatric Thoracotomy
Tray 615

Appendix

Laser Technology 616
Argon Beam Coagulator 624
Radiofrequency Endometrial
Ablation...........................625

Bibliography 626

Index 633

Part I

PERIOPERATIVE CONSIDERATIONS

Chapter I

Psychological Support of the Surgical Patient

Surgical procedures are classified as *major* or *minor*. These distinctions do not take into consideration the degree of anxiety the patient may experience regarding his or her surgery. The operating room personnel may allay a patient's fears by conducting themselves in a kind, reassuring, and confident manner.

Well before the patient enters the operating room suite, at the time the surgery is scheduled, the patient's physician and surgeon will have initiated the process providing psychological support for the surgical patient. The demeanor of the hospital (or surgicenter) admitting office personnel may also help to reassure the patient. The reception of the patient to the floor (or holding areas of the surgicenters) likewise must serve to reassure the patient.

In some institutions the first patient contact by the operating room staff might occur the day before surgery or, in the case of same day admissions, several hours before the procedure. An orientation (teaching) session may be offered either directly by operating room personnel or by closed-circuit television or video-cassette that describes to some extent the surgical preliminaries and immediate postoperative considerations so that fewer unanticipated events will be experienced. An opportunity may be given the patient to express anxieties or ask questions.

3

Perhaps the most significant in this chain of events occurs when the patient, although often partially sedated, is transported to the operating room suite. There the circulator will make certain of the patient's identity, the type of surgery to be performed, and the name of the surgeon. A checklist concerning the patient's fasting status, possible prosthetic devices, special physical conditions, and possible drug intolerances is again discussed with the patient and reviewed in the chart. The chart is checked with respect to consent forms and medical and laboratory data; see the Surgical Checklist, pp. 6–7. During this review the circulator will reassure the patient that every effort will be made to maintain the patient's well-being and safety during the procedure. These measures of psychological support are continued until the patient is totally anesthetized, or they may be continued throughout the procedure when there are varying degrees of consciousness.

Postoperatively these measures are continued but are now in the hands of the recovery room staff or other appropriate nursing personnel.

In no small way do these considerations affect the ultimate outcome of the patient's surgery. The importance of these measures must be anticipated by all those concerned.

Chapter 2

Protection of the Patient in Surgery

ADMISSION PROCEDURE

Upon admission of the patient to the operating room, the circulator verifies verbally with the patient and by inspection of the patient's armband and the chart the patient's name, the name of the patient's surgeon, and the surgery to be performed.

Evidence of the preoperative preparation of the patient as required by hospital protocol should be complete and recorded on the chart. Mandatory requirements include a valid signed and dated informed consent form and a record (recent) of the patient's health history and physical examination. A special permit may be required to perform operations such as sterilization, therapeutic abortion, or amputation of a body part. Other requirements may include laboratory data and a chest x-ray examination record. Most institutions have a preoperative checklist that is vital in preventing oversights in preparing the patient for surgery. An example of a Surgical Checklist is given on pp. 6–7.

TRANSFER PROCEDURE

The patient is transferred to the operating table by two persons in order to prevent injury. One person stabi-

Surgical Checklist

Patient Identification Plate
Patient's Name, Age
Hospital Number
Admitting Physician

Nursing Unit

Surgical procedure _____
Consent signed _____
Special consent signed _____
Prep done by _____
History & physical charted _____
Allergies _____
Blood ordered _____ No. units available _____
Preoperative instructions _____
NPO time _____
Height _____ Weight _____
BP _____ TPR _____
Laboratory charted
　CBC _____ PTT _____
　UA _____ K+ _____
　Other _____
Drains, catheters, intravenous lines _____
Preop medication type _____ time _____ by _____

Operating Room

Check		Comments

Prosthesis	None	Removed	Disposition	In	
Retainers, bridges, plates					
Artifical limb					
Artificial eye					
Contact lenses					
Hearing aid					
Valuables					
Glasses					
Wallet					
Jewelry					
Radio					
Electric shaver					

Identification band checked with chart _____

Special considerations (artificial joints,
    pacemaker, etc.) _____

_____   _____
Signature   date

_____   _____
Signature   date

Operative Record

Patient's Identification Plate
Patient's Name, Age
Hospital Number
Admitting Physician

Date _____ Pt. Room No. _____ O.R. No. _____
Preoperative diagnosis _____
Procedure _____
Postoperative diagnosis _____
Surgeon _____ Circulator _____
Assistant _____ Scrub person _____
Anesthetist _____ Type anesthesia _____
Drugs used _____ Intubation _____

Time patient arrived in OR _____
Anesthesia began _____ Operation began _____
Anesthesia ended _____ Operation ended _____
Position _____
Comments _____
Prep solution _____ Area prepped _____ Prep by _____
ESU Dispersive pad used _____ location _____ plate no. _____
Skin condition preop _____ Postop _____
Tourniquet used _____ Location _____
Time began _____ Ended _____

Prosthesis used _____ Manufacturer _____
   Location _____
   Type, size, serial no. _____
Irrigation solutions _____
Medications _____
Invasive lines _____
Blood given _____ No. of units _____
Blood unit(s) No. _____ No. of units _____
Cell saver used _____ Fluoroscopy _____
X-rays taken _____
Drains _____ Type _____ Location _____ Placed by _____
Packs _____ Type _____ Location _____
Specimens _____ Number _____
Cultures _____
Intraoperative notes _____
_____
_____
_____
_____

Sponge, sharps, instrument counts correct
   (1st) _____
   (2nd) _____
Signatures _____ _____
               scrub person   circulator

lizes the gurney (stretcher) as close to the operating table as possible and locks the wheels. The patient is instructed in how to move (if alert and physically capable). Care is taken to protect all catheters and tubings (e.g., intravenous lines and Foley catheter) while moving the patient. The second person stands on the opposite side of the operating room table to receive the patient and prevent falls. The restraint (safety) strap is fastened above the patient's knees. Adequate help should be obtained to safely move the patient to the operating table when the patient cannot move without assistance.

POSITIONING

The patient's position is determined according to the procedure to be performed, the physical condition of the patient, and the surgeon's preference in consultation with the anesthetist. Proper body alignment must be maintained. Adequate assistance should be obtained when lifting patients. The anesthetized patient is *never* moved without the anesthetist's permission. Care is taken to avoid interference with respiration (e.g., by use of chest rolls when patient is prone). Extremities and body prominences must be adequately padded and supported to avoid damage to the skin and nerves. There should be no interference with the circulation (e.g., crossed legs, restraints too tightly applied), and position changes (e.g., lowering the legs from lithotomy) should be made slowly to allow the circulatory system to adjust, thereby preventing a drop in blood pressure. The physical condition (e.g., arthritis) of the patient may place limitations on the desired position and should be taken into account. Special equipment and table attachments are designed to help maintain the patient's position. For descriptions of the position(s) employed and the equipment necessary, see the specific procedure.

ENVIRONMENTAL CONTROLS

The Centers for Disease Control and Prevention (CDC) asserts that all persons receiving health care are potentially infectious and therefore recommend that universal precautions be followed. All blood and body fluids are to be considered contaminated. This is particularly important in the prevention of the spreading of the human immunodeficiency virus (HIV), acquired immunodefficiency syndrome (AIDS), and hepatitis B virus (HBV). Universal precautions are directed at the control of these diseases and any others by controlling cross infection. The cleansing and disinfection of each individual operating room, including furnishings and equipment, should be performed after each procedure. In addition, the entire surgical department, including its corridors, storage rooms, and other auxiliary areas, is cleaned according to an established schedule. Traffic patterns are developed to minimize intrusion into restricted areas. Airborne contaminants are reduced by traffic restriction, air-conditioning (utilizing high-efficiency particulate air filters), and laminar airflow systems (e.g., used during joint replacement procedures). Through the use of barriers (i.e., restricting areas of the surgery department), the wearing of masks, head and shoe coverings, and specially laundered clothing, the number of microorganisms in the surgical environment is reduced. By strict attention to "scrubbing" technique by personnel involved in the sterile field, adequate skin preparation of the surgical site, and the constant implementation of aseptic technique, the number of contaminants present about the surgical field is also reduced. Careful attention to the controlled sterilization of instrumentation and proper opening of packaged sterile supplies must be observed. The disposal of waste and the removal of laundry in specially labeled plastic bags or containers is mandatory. The wearing of sterile or unsterile gloves when coming in contact with contaminated materials (e.g., instruments or sponges), frequent hand washing, and the changing of gloves when necessary (particularly when touching equipment or providing care between patients) are mandatory. The observance of restrictions regarding the changing of protective (waterproof) clothing, the use of protective head and shoe coverings, and the wearing of protective goggles when necessary is incumbent upon all members of the surgical department for all procedures.

ELECTRICAL AND FIRE HAZARDS

Electrical and fire safety precautions are set forth in hospital policy and are carried out by the operating room staff. Safety measures include the restricting of smoking to designated areas, determination of the safety of equipment before permitting its use in the operating room (by the engineering department), and the ongoing inspection of equipment prior to each use. Personnel must receive instruction for the safe operation of electrical equipment and then demonstrate their ability to use the equipment safely. All personnel should receive special instruction regarding their responsibilities in case of fire. Flammable anesthetic agents are rarely employed today. The electrosurgical unit should not be used in the mouth or pleural cavity during the administration of high concentrations of oxygen. Disposable drapes, gowns, head and shoe coverings, and so on are treated with flame-retardant chemicals. Flammable antiseptic solutions should not be used to prepare the skin when the electrosurgical unit is used.

ELECTROSURGERY

The electrosurgical unit is commonly employed in all the surgical specialties for the purpose of coagulating or cutting tissue. The current flows from the generator (electrosurgical unit) to an active electrode through tissue and returns to the unit through an inactive electrode. In the monopolar electrosurgical unit the active electrode is usually an "electrosurgical pencil" and the inactive electrode is the dispersive (grounding) pad. In the bipolar unit the active electrode is one side of the forceps and the inactive electrode is the other side of the forceps; therefore, no dispersive pad is necessary.

Precautions must be taken when employing electrosurgery in order to prevent injury to the patient. These include the following:

1. All connections must be secure.
2. The inactive electrode should cover a sufficiently large area of skin (relatively free of hair, which acts as an insulator) and be as close as possible to the site of application of the active electrode in order to minimize the pathway of the current through the body.
3. The patient's body should *not* make direct contact with metal surfaces. If the return circuit is faulty, the ground circuit could be completed through the contact area, thus creating an inadvertent burn injury.
4. Electrocardiogram electrodes should be placed as far away from the operative site as possible.

Repeated requests to increase the current should be thoroughly investigated by the circulator. Check all connections and the dispersive pad; if no problem is found, the unit may be faulty. Turn the unit off and unplug it.

Special Notes

If the patient has an implanted pacemaker, the electrosurgical unit could cause malfunction. The patient needs to be continuously monitored. The cardiac arrest cart (complete with defibrillator and paddles) should be in close proximity.

OPERATIVE RECORD

The legal rights of the patient as well as those of operating room personnel are protected by the documentation in the patient's operative record. The Joint Commission on Accreditation of Healthcare Organizations (JCAHO) requires that the operative procedure report include the preoperative diagnosis, the procedure performed, the postoperative diagnosis, specimens obtained, and the names of the surgical team providing intraoperative care. The documentation of other information such as the taking of counts (e.g., sponges, sharps, and instruments), placement of catheters, intravenous lines, wound packing, and use of equipment

(e.g., electrosurgical unit or tourniquets) is invaluable.
An example of the suggested format for the Operative
Record is shown on pp. 8–9.

In addition, the JCAHO requires an anesthesia
record for each operative procedure, completed by the
anesthetist. According to hospital policy, when an
anesthetist is not present during the procedure, the circulator documents the patient's vital signs, blood pressure, and the names and amounts of drugs and anesthetics administered by or at the direction of the
surgeon and records all pertinent times.

COUNTING PROCEDURE

Each institution should have its own written policy and
procedure regarding the counting of sponges, sharps,
and instruments. The following guidelines should be
observed when counting all objects potentially subject
to inadvertent seclusion in a wound:

1. All items are counted initially by the circulator
   and the scrub person together (aloud) as the scrub
   person touches each item.
2. The number (count) of each type of item is immediately recorded by the circulator.
3. If there is any uncertainty regarding the initial
   count, it is repeated.
4. As additional items (e.g., sponges or needles) are
   added to the sterile field during the procedure, the
   scrub person counts the item(s) with the circulator, who adds the count to the record and initials
   it.
5. Nothing (including laundry, trash, instruments,
   and sponges) may be removed from an operating
   room while a procedure is in progress until the
   final count is acknowledged to be correct.
6. Whenever there is a change of team members, a
   count is taken.
7. When an incorrectly numbered package of items
   is dispensed, the items should be bagged, labeled
   accordingly, set aside, and not recorded in the
   count.

8. Counts are taken before beginning the procedure, before wound closure begins, and when skin closure is initiated.
9. An additional count is taken prior to the closure of an organ within a cavity (e.g., uterus or bladder).

Incorrect closure counts must be repeated immediately. If the count remains incorrect, the circulator alerts the surgeon who will inspect the patient's wound for the missing item. If the item is not located, hospital policy must be followed (usually to include immediate x-ray examination), and an incident report must be filed.

Sponge Counts

All sponges, neurological sponges (cottonoids), and soft goods (e.g., umbilical tapes) are counted. Each type and size sponge is kept separate. All sponges used within the wound must be x-ray detectable. X-ray detectable sponges are never used for dressings, and dressing sponges are never used to dry the surgical field. Sponges are discarded following use in a plastic-lined receptacle. Soiled sponges are counted by the scrub person and the circulator together and then bagged in impervious plastic bags according to a predetermined number (usually in sets of 5 or 10). When the counts are taken, the scrub nurse counts the sponges according to type, beginning with the sponges on the field and proceeding to the sponges on the back table and then those off the field. The circulator informs the surgeon of the results of the counts.

Sharp Counts

All needles, knife blades, electrosurgical blades, and any other sharps are counted. Needles in multiple-suture packs may be counted according to the number on the package; some hospitals require each package to be opened and each needle counted individually. Used needles, blades, and other sharps should be retained on a needle magnet or counter pad to facilitate counting. All parts of any needle broken during a procedure must be accounted for. Closure counts for sharps follow the same format as those for sponges.

Instrument Counts

Instruments should be counted for all surgical procedures. All parts of disassembled or broken instruments must be accounted for in their entirety. Closure counts for instruments follow the format for other counts.

STERILIZATION

All items (e.g., instruments, supplies, equipment) that come in contact with the sterile field and the wound must be sterile. As soon as possible following use, soiled instruments are cleaned in the washer-sterilizer. Following terminal decontamination in the washer-sterilizer, the instruments are cleaned in an ultrasonic cleaner to remove any remaining soil.

The three most commonly used methods of sterilization employed in the operating room (or central supply) include:

1. Saturated steam under pressure
2. Gas chemical sterilization
3. Liquid chemical sterilization

Discussion of other methods of sterilization such as ionizing radiation (e.g., cobalt 60) used by manufacturers for prepackaged items is beyond the scope of this guide.

Saturated Steam Under Pressure

The *flash sterilizer* is frequently used in the operating room for urgently needed unwrapped instruments. Customarily the temperature is set at 270°F (132°C) for a 3- or 10-minute cycle. The length of the cycle is determined by the density of the item(s) to be sterilized. The recommendation of the manufacturer of the item regarding the temperature and length of exposure time at that temperature must be followed. The recording device on the sterilizer should be checked to confirm that the instrument(s) to be sterilized has (have) been exposed to the proper temperature for the desired length of time. Heat-sensitive indicators should accompany the instrument(s). Trays with mesh bottoms are recommended.

Wrapped instruments, trays, basins, and so on are usually sterilized in a prevacuum, high-temperature steam sterilizer. Proper packaging of trays and packages is mandatory, as is the proper loading of the sterilizer. The Bowie-Dick test is used to verify that there were no air pockets, which would negate the sterilizing conditions. A heat-sensitive indicator is placed within each wrapped tray (or package), and each package is secured with heat-sensitive tape.

Gas Chemical Sterilization

Ethylene oxide gas is used to sterilize items that are vulnerable to heat or moisture. Any item that can withstand sterilization by steam under pressure should not be gas-sterilized. Ethylene oxide sterilization depends on concentration of gas, temperature, humidity, and exposure time. The ethylene oxide sterilizer must be operated exactly according to the manufacturer's instructions in order to ensure that the requirements for sterilization are met. Type of item, arrangement of the load, and rate of penetration influence the amount of exposure time required. Penetration of the gas is aided by an initial vacuum within the sterilizer. Usually cycles of 3 to 7 hours are employed. An ethylene oxide chemically sensitive indicator that is placed inside the wrapped package indicates that the item was exposed to ethylene oxide but does not necessarily indicate that sterilization has occurred; therefore, the sterilization process must conform to manufacturer's specifications.

Inhalation of ethylene oxide is to be avoided, as is direct contact with the sterilized items prior to aeration. The length of aeration time required depends on the composition of the items, the type of wrapper used, the concentration of the ethylene oxide used, the airflow rate, and the temperature during aeration. When items are aerated in a mechanical aerator, the air is automatically changed a minimum of four times an hour. The temperature is controlled at 122°F (50°C) to 140°F

(60°C) for 8 to 12 hours. If a mechanical aerator is unavailable, items should be aerated in a well-ventilated room at a controlled temperature of 65°F (18°C) to 72°F (22°C) for 7 days.

Liquid Chemical Sterilization

When items cannot tolerate sterilization by saturated steam under pressure and when the time required for gas sterilization is impractical, liquid chemical sterilization is employed. A 2% activated aqueous glutaraldehyde solution (e.g., Cidex) is the agent often employed when liquid disinfection is desired. Instruments must be completely immersed in the solution for 10 hours to achieve sterilization. Disinfection is effected if the instrument is submerged for 10 minutes. All items must be thoroughly rinsed in sterile distilled water before use.

Steris 20 is a single use sterilant that employs periacetic acid as the active sterilizing agent. Periacetic acid, a highly biocidal oxidizer, maintains its efficiency even when high levels of organic soil are present. Steris 20 has a low surface tension, which makes it very effective at reaching all instrument surfaces. The sterilant is prepackaged in single use containers where dilution is automatically prepared within the environmental processing chamber. The used solution is disposed of in an ordinary drain during the processing cycle, eliminating the operator from exposure to chemicals. After use the periacetic acid decomposes into acetic acid (vinegar) and oxygen.

EMERGENCIES AND DISASTERS

Most operating rooms are equipped with a special emergency signal that can be operated from within each separate operating room to alert others to the emergency.

In the event that a patient suffers a cardiopulmonary arrest, the anesthetist and surgeon administer cardiopulmonary resuscitation (CPR). Health care providers are required to know CPR. In the absence of an anesthetist or surgeon, nursing personnel must administer CPR. An emergency cardiopulmonary arrest cart should be available in the surgery department at all times. Included on this well-stocked cart are in-date emergency drugs, needles and syringes, infusion equipment, a defibrillator, and monitoring equipment. Nursing personnel responding to the emergency signal should bring the cardiopulmonary arrest cart into the room. Documentation of all medications and procedures administered is made.

Hospitals are equipped with an alternative power source that takes over if a power failure occurs. All team members are required to know the location of high-intensity flashlights kept in the department for use during the time lapse until the alternate power source begins functioning.

Malignant hyperthermia is a rare, dangerous condition thought to be associated with the use of some general anesthetics. Proper treatment initiated immediately by administering dantrolene (Dantrium), iced intravenous solutions, and steroids, and by cooling the patient with ice packs can significantly reduce mortality. In preparation to meet this emergency situation, operating room personnel need to be informed of the protocol set up by the anesthesia department.

Should death occur in the operating room, individual state law and hospital policy must be adhered to regarding the handling of the deceased patient. An incident report is submitted detailing the events leading to the patient's death.

Chapter 3

Safety for Operating Room Personnel

The operating room staff needs to be aware of the hazards related to working in surgery. By strict adherence to departmental policy regarding safety measures, potential problems can be avoided. Many factors that apply to patient safety in the operating room also apply to personnel safety (see Chapter 2).

IN-SERVICE EDUCATION

Most hospitals have in-service orientation programs for new employees to inform them of the hospital's policies and procedures including the subjects of fire prevention and individual responsibilities in case of fire and disasters. In addition to this general orientation, most operating rooms have a departmental orientation program for new personnel and a scheduled monthly in-service education program for all personnel. These programs serve not only to keep the operating room staff abreast of new technology, procedures, instrumentation, and nursing care in general but also serve to reiterate departmental safety measures.

BODY MECHANICS

Through the application of good body mechanics, particularly when lifting or moving patients, heavy instrument trays, or equipment, strains and other injuries can be prevented. Lifting should be done by bending the knees, positioning one's body under the load, and then straightening the legs, allowing the lower extremity muscles to do the lifting. A roller (e.g., Davis) can be of significant value in preventing strains when moving unconscious or obese patients.

FATIGUE FACTORS

Fatigue can be minimized through working quickly and efficiently. Wasted motions not only increase the patient's anesthesia and operating room time but are also tiring for the staff member. Integration of individual motions and thoughtful organization of the day's total workload can greatly influence one's job performance and endurance.

RADIATION SAFETY

Operating room personnel may be exposed to radiation when intraoperative x-rays are taken and when radioactive implant procedures are performed. To reduce the deleterious effects of radiation exposure, hospital policy must be strictly followed.

The effect of radiation exposure depends on the amount of radiation, the proximity of the radiation source, and the length of time of the exposure. Hospital protective measures should include the following:

1. All nonsterile team members should leave the room (whenever possible) or wear a lead apron.
2. Sterile team members should either stand behind a lead screen or wall or wear a lead apron.
3. Monitoring devices (e.g., dosimeters) should be worn by personnel routinely exposed to radiation; readings should be computed weekly.
4. Pregnant personnel should avoid all exposure to radiation.
5. Personnel holding x-ray cassettes during radiography should wear lead gloves in addition to a lead apron.

INFECTION CONTROL

The Centers for Disease Control and Prevention recommend that all blood and body fluids of every patient be treated as though they were contaminated. Since it is impossible to determine unequivocally whether any patient has a contagious disease due to the latency inconversion period of serological tests for various communicable diseases, not the least of which are the human immunodeficiency virus (HIV) and acquired immunodeficiency syndrome (AIDS), safety precautions must be observed for every patient.

In addition to HIV positive patients and patients with AIDS, patients with other diseases, in particular blood-borne viruses such as the hepatitis B virus, also pose a threat to health care workers. Universal precautions must be observed in order to prevent the transmission of any disease to health care personnel and other patients.

AIDS, hepatitis, and pyogenic infection can be transmitted by puncture wounds. Hospital procedure must be followed regarding the disposal of sharps. A needle magnet is available encased in a flat plastic compact, the lid of which can be closed for the safe disposal of its contents. A rigid plastic container is used for the disposal of needles and plastic syringes; an attached device is employed to separate the hub and shaft of the needle and break the syringe tip prior to discarding them.

All personnel should wear gloves when handling potentially contaminated articles such as soiled sponges, instruments, and blood transfusion pouches that might cause infection through a break in the skin. Some authorities advocate double gloving when virulent infections are present or suspect.

Similarly, during endoscopy procedures or procedures in which drills or saws are employed, personnel may be spattered or sprayed by potentially contaminated tissue fragments, saliva, irrigation fluid, and so on, and safety goggles or glasses should be worn.

CHEMICAL HAZARDS

The National Institute of Occupational Safety and Health (NIOSH) has established guidelines regarding safe levels of waste anesthetic gases in the operating room. The removal of waste gases in the operating room is accomplished with scavenging systems that require careful maintenance. By employing well-maintained scavenging systems, air-conditioning systems (using high-efficiency particulate air filters), and nitrous oxide leak detectors, the exposure to hazardous gases in the operating room can be minimized.

Part II

ANESTHESIA

Chapter 4

General Information

Anesthesia is loss of sensation. In the operating room, anesthesia is administered by a physician (anesthesiologist) or a certified registered nurse anesthetist (CRNA). In addition, local or regional anesthetics may be administered by the surgeon. In this guide, the term *anesthetist* will apply to the anesthesiologist as well as the CRNA.

The most common techniques utilized in the operating room include:

1. *General anesthesia.* The patient is made unconscious.
2. *Conduction anesthesia.* Anatomical areas of the patient are anesthetized by infiltration or topical application of various agents. Nerve blocks are produced at central or peripheral sites. *Local anesthesia* and *topical anesthesia* are established immediately about the area to be treated.

The American Society of Anesthesiologists (ASA) recommends standards for basic intraoperative monitoring for care of the patient in surgery:

1. An anesthetist must be present throughout the conduction of general or regional anesthetics and monitored anesthesia care.
2. During the administration of any anesthetic, the patients oxygenation, circulation, and temperature are to be continually evaluated. This may be achieved through the use of an oxygen analyzer, pulse oximeter, ECG, and the evaluation of the patient's tem-

perature, color, and chest excursion. During general anesthesia the monitoring of the carbon dioxide content of expired gas is encouraged through the use of tidal carbon dioxide monitors ($ETCO_2$).

Prior to the administration of anesthesia, premedication, as a single drug or a combination of various drugs, is often given. The purpose of the premedication is to allay anxiety, to help the patient relax, and to diminish secretions. Premedication is usually given by intramuscular injection about 30 to 60 minutes before surgery. In emergency surgery, premedication may be given intravenously or may be omitted. These drugs are selected according to the patient's general condition and the extent and nature of the surgery to be performed. Outpatients or surgicenter patients are given less premedication or none at all.

Specialized equipment is required to implement anesthesia. For general anesthesia an anesthesia machine delivers an anesthetic gas mixture to the patient at a specific rate and concentration as determined by the anesthetist. The most simple machine might consist of a cart with attached tanks of nitrous oxide (or other agent) and oxygen with flow meters and pressure gauges. Usually expired "air" from the patient passes through a carbon dioxide absorbing tank or cartridge. In the modern operating room, a very sophisticated machine able to store and deliver several compressed gaseous and highly volatile liquid anesthetic agents is employed. In addition, the compact anesthesia cart contains a variety of monitoring devices, an oxygen depletion alarm, and special equipment that includes masks, laryngoscopes with interchangeable blades, McGill forceps, endotracheal tubes and obturators, and so on, as well as a source of suction. An additional cart of drawers is required for drugs and supplies. Equipment and prepackaged kits for various procedures (e.g., insertion of arterial and central venous catheters) must be stored nearby. A variety of intravenous fluids, administration sets, and stands for these items must be provided.

The role of the circulator with respect to anesthesia is to provide an "extra hand" for the anesthetist. In some institutions an anesthesia technologist may perform this role. Prior to the induction of anesthesia, the circulator is responsible for maintaining the patient's immediate safety, allaying anxiety, and being attentive to the special needs of the patient.

The RN assumes many roles as a perioperative nurse. Nurses act not only as the patient's advocate in the operating room, but as diligent observers and administrators of the total care of the patient. As a perioperative nurse, one identifies the needs of the patient preoperatively and passes on the information to the recovery room nurse or the floor nurse regarding the needs of the patient postoperatively. Infrequently the operating room nurse has the opportunity to intervene preoperatively beyond the preoperative visit or postoperatively when delivering the patient to the recovery room or the unit. It is fortunate when the nurse is given the time allotment that affords more perioperative care, but it is indeed rare. Of course, total perioperative care is the ultimate goal of the individual operating room nurse. At this time, perioperative care, that is, acting as the patient's advocate from the time the patient is admitted preoperatively to the moment of discharge (and sometimes even beyond as necessary, i.e., extended care facility), seems to be the responsibility of a chain of nurses who use their knowledge in a caring way to the benefit of the patient.

GENERAL ANESTHESIA

For the administration of general anesthesia, the patient is initially in the supine position. An intravenous line is inserted, and an (automatic) blood pressure cuff and oxygen sensor and electrocardiograph (ECG) monitoring electrodes are placed. Induction is usually begun by injecting a rapidly acting intravenous agent, for example, thiopental (Pentothal), Propofol (Diprovan), or methohexital (Brevital). As the patient loses consciousness, oxygen and gaseous agents are gradually introduced by mask. If an endotracheal tube is to be inserted (transnasally or transorally), a fast-acting muscle relaxant, succinylcholine chloride (Anectine), is used in adults and a rapidly acting or curare-like drug, for example, rocuronium (Zemuron), atracurium (Tracrium), or vecuronium (Norcuron), is used in children, after which the endotracheal tube is inserted under direct vision with the aid of a laryngoscope and McGill forceps, if needed. Several milliliters of lidocaine 4% solution may be instilled into the larynx prior to placing the endotracheal tube, which has been lubricated with anesthetic ointment. The tube cuff is inflated and the tube secured with tape. For the duration of the procedure, muscle relaxation is maintained with any of the several curare-like drugs, as above. Additional monitoring devices are attached, and the patient's position changed as necessary. The circulator may be required to assist the anesthetist by providing easy access to the equipment, giving additional premeasured drugs, manipulating the trachea, and so on, at the instruction of the anesthetist. A wide variety of drugs and inhalation agents are available; see Table 4–1.

Table 4–1. **General Anesthetics**

Agent	Route of Administration	Form	Comments
Nitrous oxide	Inhalation	Compressed gas	Most commonly used; not used alone for deep anesthesia; used to potentiate the effects of other agents
Thiopental (Pentothal)	Intravenous	Stable liquid	Rapid induction; short duration; respiratory depressant; can cause laryngospasm and hypotension
Metho-hexital (Brevital)	Intravenous	Stable liquid	Rapid; ultra-short-acting; for induction; maintenance; fast recovery; hiccoughs
Halothane (Fluothane)	Inhalation	Volatile liquid	Slow, smooth induction; maintenance; may cause bradycardia; increased sensitivity if used with epinephrine; good with burn patients and children; may cause liver damage

Table 4–1. **General Anesthetics** (Continued)

Agent	Route of Administration	Form	Comments
Enflurane (Ethrane)	Inhalation	Volatile liquid	Rapid induction; occasionally used for maintenance; rapid recovery; may cause hypotension; may cause convulsions in children
Desflurane (Suprano)	Inhalation	Volatile liquid	Very rapid onset and recovery; pungent odor, increased postoperative nausea
Isoflurane (Forane)	Inhalation	Volatile liquid	Maintenance; good muscular relaxation; cardiovascular stability, useful in cardiac patients
Ketamine (Ketaject, Ketalar)	Intravenous; intramuscular	Stable liquid	Induction; short-acting anesthetic; long-acting analgesic; good for children; may cause hallucinations if given in larger doses.
Propofol (Diprovan)	Intravenous	Stable liquid	Rapid induction; short duration; can be used as continuous infusion with clear-headed, rapid recovery; respiratory depressant, translent hypotension, pain on injection

To supplement the use of anesthetic agents, numerous additional drugs may be administered intravenously to balance the anesthesia. These drugs include various narcotics or morphine, miperidine, fentanyl and other muscle relaxants, amnestics, and neuroleptics.

CONDUCTION ANESTHESIA

Nerve Blocks

The term *central block* refers to spinal, epidural, or caudal anesthesia. Appropriate supplies for their administration are available in most hospitals in disposable prepackaged trays. Additional drugs may be requested. If a longer procedure is contemplated or postoperative analgesia is to be prolonged, a catheter is placed by the anesthetist to deliver increments of anesthetic agent as in continuous epidural or continuous caudal anesthesia. Postoperatively, morphine (Duramorph) specially prepared for this purpose may be similarly injected for pain relief. For these blocks, the patient, with intravenous line already established, is positioned by the anesthetist; the circulator helps the patient maintain this position while the block is administered. When an anesthetic catheter is placed, it must be secured with tape. The patient may then be placed in a temporary position to allow the block to take effect or moved to the position of surgery at the direction of the anesthetist. A central block can be supplemented by heavy sedation. Oxygen and inhalation anesthetics may be administered by mask.

To control postoperative pain, a catheter may be left in the epidural space for continuous or intermittent bolus infusion of narcotic and/or low-dosage local anesthetic. When this modality is employed, most hospitals require the concurrent use of an apnea monitor and a postoperative protocol regarding the use of additional analgesics, antinauseants, and so on, supervised by an attending anesthetist until 8 to 24 hours after the catheter is removed.

There are numerous types of *regional blocks* (Table 4–2). Often, the surgeon will administer these anesthetics. Examples include brachial plexus blocks, retrograde intravenous blocks (for surgery upon the extremities), pudendal blocks (for gynecologic surgery), perianal blocks (for anorectal surgery), and "field" blocks (as for inguinal hernia repair). These blocks may be supplemented by heavy sedation or inhalation anesthetics.

Table 4–2. **Commonly Used Conduction Anesthetics***

Method of Administration	Agent	Concentration/Dose	Comments
Spinal	Lidocaine (Xylocaine)	5%	Rapid onset; shorter acting
Spinal	Bupivicaine (Marcaine, Sensorcaine)	0.75%	Longer acting; longer lasting analgesia after return of sensation
Spinal	Tetracaine (Pontocaine)	0.5–1.0%/ 5–12 mg	Rapid onset; longer with higher dosage and/or added ephedrine or epinephrine
Epidural/ caudal	Lidocaine (Xylocaine)	1–2%/ 500 mg	Rapid onset; shorter duration
Epidural/ caudal	Bupivicaine (Marcaine, Sensorcaine)	0.25–0.75%/ 150 mg	Longer acting; obstetrics
Nerve block (regional)	Lidocaine (Xylocaine)	1–2%/ 500 mg	Rapid onset
		0.33%/100– 150 mg	Retrograde intravenous block
Nerve block (regional)	Bupivicaine (Marcaine, Sensorcaine)	0.25–0.5%	Long acting
Local	Lidocaine (Xylocaine)	0.5–2.0%/ 500 mg	Commonly used
Local	Bupivicaine (Marcaine, Sensorcaine)	0.25–5.0%/ 300 mg	Long acting; may result in less need for analgesics postoperatively
Topical	Lidocaine (Xylocaine) liquid	2–4%/ 200 mg	Low toxicity; short acting
	jelly ointment	2%/ 15–30 mL 4%/15 mL	Cystoscopy; other endoscopies

Table continued on following page

Table 4–2. **Commonly Used Conduction Anesthetics***
(Continued)

Method of Administration	Agent	Concentration/Dose	Comments
Topical	Cocaine	2–10%/200 mg	High potency; rapid absorption through mucous membranes
Topical	Tetracaine (Pontocaine)	0.5%/drops	Ophthalmic use; rapid onset

*All conduction anesthetic agents, when administered in greater than recommended dosages or if accidentally given intravenously (or by idiosyncratic reaction), may cause extreme agitation, convulsions, cardiac arrest, and death. Resuscitative equipment and drugs must be immediately available whenever these agents are employed.

This chart lists only several of the most commonly used anesthetic agents primarily for adult patients. Additional agents are employed particularly for pediatric surgeries. Numerous ancillary drugs including muscle relaxants, tranquilizers, narcotics, and amnestic agents likewise have not been listed as use of these agents varies widely between anesthetists and institutions.

Local Anesthesia

Local anesthesia is frequently used for lesser procedures and many plastic surgeries, ophthalmic procedures, anorectal procedures, and so on. The surgeon administers the anesthetic. With few exceptions an intravenous line is inserted. When "anesthesia standby" is requested, the anesthetist will monitor the patient and administer supplemental sedation or even general anesthesia as required.

When an anesthetist is not present, the circulator will insert an intravenous line (in accordance with hospital policy), place ECG electrodes and pulse oximeter, and monitor the patient's vital signs, blood pressure, and ECG. At the direction of the surgeon, the circulator may administer various drugs parenterally including narcotics (e.g., morphine, meperidine, fentanyl/Sublimaze, or Sufentanil), sedatives (e.g., diazepam/Valium, or hydroxyzine/Vistaril), and agents that have an amnestic effect (e.g., midazolam/Versed). On occasion drugs to reverse the effects of the aforementioned agents may be required such as haloxone/Narcan or flumazenil/Mazicon. The circulator also completes the anesthetic record including documenting the times of the beginning and the termination of the procedure, vital signs and blood pressure at appropriate intervals, and the times and amounts of anesthetic agents or any other drugs administered.

Topical Anesthesia

Topical anesthesia is the direct application of an anesthetic agent as a liquid solution, eyedrops, jelly, ointment, and/or spray to the site of the surgery; see Table 4–2. Local or general anesthesia may be required to supplement these anesthetics.

The preceding chart lists only several of the more commonly employed agents for adult patients. Numerous other agents can be utilized including those reserved for pediatric patients. In addition, a wide array of ancillary agents, including muscle relaxants, tranquilizers, narcotics, and amnestic agents, has not been listed because their use varies widely among anesthetists and institutions.

On completion of the surgical procedure, placement of dressings, and so on, the circulator accompanies the patient to the recovery room. While the patient is repositioned (as necessary) for movement onto the gurney (or special bed or frame), intravascular lines, urinary catheter, splinted extremities, and so on are protected. The security of the airway is the responsibility of the anesthetist. When the patient has been expeditiously transported to the recovery room, the anesthesia and operative records, special appliances, and so on are given to the recovery room nurse. The circulator reports to the recovery room nurse any significant intraoperative events as a severe fluctuation in cardiovascular or pulmonary functions, any untoward reaction to drugs, and/or the need for multiple transfusions or special medications. The chart may be temporarily retained by the surgeon to complete operative notes, postoperative orders, or dictation. If the chart is not immediately available, the circulator will advise the re-

covery room nurse of any postoperative orders requiring immediate attention such as the application of an
ice pack or the connection of drainage systems to a suction source. If significant nausea occurs, newer agents,
for example, ondansetron (Zofran), may be ordered by
the anesthetist. When the anesthetist is satisfied that
the patient has been transferred safely, the operating
room personnel resume their other assignments.

Chapter 5

General Anesthesia

Definition

Administration of agents by intravenous injection or inhalation that render the patient unconscious or extremely obtunded. Intramuscular injection and rectal instillation are rarely used.

Discussion

This anesthetic method is commonly employed. The depth and duration of the anesthetic is regulated by the type and amount of agent(s) given. In addition to numerous intravenous and inhalation anesthetics, a large number of other agents including muscle relaxants, tranquilizers, and narcotics are employed. Rarely is a single drug used, but for limited procedures, a single agent (e.g., ketamine) may be employed. During all general anesthetics the patient must be well oxygenated and the patency of the airway maintained. The anesthetist must also maintain the patient's cardiovascular system and other vital functions.

Preparation of the Patient

The patient is supine with safety strap in place. Following induction, the airway will be maintained by insertion of an endotracheal tube if the patient's position for surgery is to be other than supine or lithotomy, for a prolonged procedure in the supine position, for surgeries that affect respiration, or when profound muscular relaxation is needed. A variety of types and sizes of these tubes are available. Most often the endotracheal tube is placed transorally, but it may also be inserted transnasally or via an established tracheostomy. Prior to any change from the supine position, the anesthetist must state that the airway is secure and will then control the airway and protect the head and neck as the patient is repositioned. The patient's eyes are protected by instillation of ophthalmic ointment and/or taping the lids. For positions other than supine, refer to specific surgeries.

Draping

None.

Equipment

As selected by the anesthetist according to the needs of the individual patient. May include:
Suction source, preferably a separate unit
Laryngoscope and blades
Suction catheters
Yankauer suction tip (or as requested); McGill forceps
Facemask, headstrap, variety of endotracheal tubes (with obturator), oral and nasal airways, connectors for masks or endotracheal tubes, sterile anesthetic lubricant (for the endotracheal tube and obturator), syringes (to inflate the tube cuff), tongue blades, topical anesthetic for instillation into the larynx (e.g., LTA kit), ordinary and esophageal stethoscopes, etc.
Monitoring devices for blood pressure and pulse, electrocardiogram, oxygen and carbon dioxide monitors, oxygen alarm, and pulse oximeter
Ordinary intravenous (IV) line, central venous and arterial lines and the trays to insert them, and appropriate gauges.
Ether screen, IV standards, drape clips, padded armboards, etc.
Nasogastric tubes, etc. (as requested)

Special Notes

Induction is facilitated by a quiet atmosphere.

The circulator stands at the head of the table particularly during endotracheal intubation, to assist in patient care measures such as manipulating the trachea (thereby enabling the anesthetist to better visualize the glottis) and injecting premeasured intravenous drugs.

Suction should be ready at all times.

Chapter 6

Conduction Anesthesia

SPINAL, EPIDURAL, CAUDAL

Definition

Central nerve blocks performed by injecting anesthetic solutions intrathecally (into the subarachnoid space), into the epidural space, or into the caudal canal (an extension of the epidural space).

Discussion

These anesthetics are employed for procedures on the lower abdomen and lower extremities. The composition and concentration of the anesthetic solution will determine the duration of the block. The position of the patient immediately following the injection of the anesthetic solution influences the level and distribution of the block.

Preparation of the Patient

Position of the patient is determined by the type of block being administered, procedure being performed, condition of the patient, and preference of the anesthetist. Position may be sitting, lateral, or prone.

Sitting: With back arched and feet supported on a stool (spinal or epidural)

Lateral: With knees, hips, back, and neck flexed (spinal or epidural)

Prone: Flexed at the waist (caudal or hypobaric spinal)

Following the injection of the agent (after an interval determined by anesthetist), the patient is placed in the selected operative position.

For prolonged procedures or for postoperative analgesia, continuous epidural or caudal anesthesia is established by inserting a catheter into the appropriate space at the time of the initial needle placement. Increments of anesthetic solution may then be administered.

Skin Preparation and Draping

Usually performed by the anesthetist. These materials may be included in the prepackaged disposable tray.

Equipment

Stool (for patient's feet, sitting position)
Sitting stool (for anesthetist)

Supplies

Appropriate sterile disposable tray (spinal, epidural, caudal)
Additional agents, needles, catheters, etc. (as requested)

Special Notes

The circulator may be requested to set up an intravenous line.

The circulator is usually requested to assist in maintaining the patient's position during administration of the block.

The circulator (in addition to the anesthetist) should closely observe the patient for signs of respiratory distress caused by the sedation or by the inadvertent administration of a "high" spinal, which would result in depression or paralysis of the respiratory muscles and require immediate intubation and ventillation.

Special care must be taken to protect the patient in order to avoid injuries, that is, burns, neurological damage, pressure sores, or other traumas to the patient who is unable to sense these injuries while receiving an anesthetic.

According to some authorities, in order to avoid postspinal headache, patients may be instructed preoperatively and reminded postoperatively that they should remain at bedrest without raising their heads for 24 to 48 hours.

Adhesive tape secures intravenous line and anesthetic catheter.

Do not dispose of the tray items until the anesthetist has the appropriate information needed for the anesthetic record.

The patient, although often sedated, may be alert enough to hear; therefore, discussion of the diagnosis, other medical information, and idle conversation should be limited accordingly.

The patient's privacy should always be maintained.

REGIONAL, LOCAL, TOPICAL

Definition

Application of an anesthetic agent that may be either injected about a peripheral nerve trunk, adjacent to or directly into the surgical site, or applied directly to the surface to be treated.

Discussion

Regional nerve block (e.g., brachial plexus block, ankle block) is achieved by depositing an agent immediately adjacent to a larger peripheral nerve(s). This anesthetic is used primarily for surgery upon the extremities. Intercostal nerve block or field block is used in limited abdominal surgery (e.g., gastrostomy, inguinal herniorrhaphy).

Local anesthesia refers to the injection of anesthetic agent into or adjacent to the site of surgery so that smaller nerves are directly anesthetized.

In *topical anesthesia* the anesthetic agent is absorbed through the tissue (usually mucous membrane) to anesthetize the area immediately beneath (e.g., ophthalmic, gingival) or to anesthetize a larger nerve trunk that lies close to the surface (e.g., glossopharyn-geal nerve block).

These modalities may be used in combination or con-junction with general anesthesia or heavy sedation. Hyaluronidase (Wydase) may be added to the in-jectable agent to promote more rapid spread and more rapid resolution of the local edema related to the injec-tion. Epinephrine (Adrenalin) added to the anesthetic solution will prolong its effect.

Preparation of the Patient

The patient is positioned to expose the site of the pro-posed injection or application. In local or topical anes-thesia this site is often identical to the site of the surgery, whereas in regional anesthesia the site may be remote from that of surgery.

Skin Preparation

Regional: Performed by the anesthetist or surgeon; when the block is established, the surgical site is pre-pared in the usual fashion.

Local: Skin preparation for the injection and the surgery is usually the same.

Topical: Usually none required.

Supplies

Skin preparation tray (regional or local)
Needles and syringes (regional or local)
Medicine cup (for anesthetic agent)
Sponges
Anesthetic agent(s)

Special Notes

Circulator may be responsible for insertion of an intra-venous line.

Determine type of anesthesia and required supplies prior to bringing patient into the operating room.

Be aware of special needs, for example, use of two tourniquets (or double-cuff tourniquet) or retrograde intravenous block.

The patient, although often sedated, may be alert enough to hear; therefore, discussion of the diagnosis, other medical information, and idle conversation should be limited accordingly.

Observe measures to maintain the patient's privacy.

Part III

SURGICAL PROCEDURES INCLUDING MINIMAL ACCESS PROCEDURES

Operative procedures, as all medical treatments, are performed to provide correction of a problem, while rendering as little harm to the patient as possible. With few exceptions, the paramount need is to expose in order to visualize the operative field while preserving the patient's capacity to heal.

An appropriately placed, carefully performed incision provides the exposure necessary for the execution of a safe and rapid definitive surgical procedure. As the surgery progresses, visualization of the structures is facilitated by the use of traction and countertraction.

A protocol has been developed in the performance of skin (and certain mucosal) incisions. A first scalpel (or "skin" knife) is used and then discarded for a second scalpel (or "deep" knife). Underlying tissues are serially incised and distracted by the use of toothed forceps, retractors, clamps, sponges, and so on, until the surgical site is exposed. In each anatomic site different instruments may be employed, but this general principle is applicable. In specialized procedures, utilizing endoscopes, the operating microscope, electrosurgical equipment, lasers, a plasma scalpel, argon beam coagulator, hydrodissector, intraoperative radiation therapy modalities, ultrasound modalities, and so on, the technique is altered accordingly.

In procedures in which potential contamination is inherent (e.g., intestinal surgery), the wound is protected throughout. When clean closure of the incision is indicated, the operating team regowns and regloves, the field is redraped, and the instruments, electrosurgical pencil, and so on are replaced.

Historically, procedures employing limited incisions have been applied to situations in which the underlying structures are immediately apparent with minimal dissection and manipulation of tissues. Ingenious recently introduced (embellished and reintroduced) techniques of performing lesser and greater procedures via limited access are now commonly utilized in most surgical specialties. Previously, the procedures included thoracoscopic, abdominal, and pelvic laparoscopic surgery, but currently they have been extended to include orthopedic, neurological, otolaryngological, and urological specialties.

The basic tenet of limited access surgery is that the definitive portions of the procedure be accomplished in identical fashion to that of an "open" procedure. If, for whatever reason, inability to safely expose and visualize structures due to uncontrolled hemorrhage, inflammation and sepsis, dense adhesions, obesity, or excessive anesthesia time, or if consequent surgical injury ensues, or the urgency of the situation dictates, or there is equipment failure, the procedure must promptly be converted to the traditional approach. In certain instances a lesser formal incision may be employed with the limited access technique as in "laparoscopic assisted" surgery.

An additional use for limited access surgery is in its diagnostic capabilities with respect to assessment of metastatic disease, infertility, endometriosis, sepsis, the extent of trauma, and so on. Biopsies or fluid samples and cultures can be obtained. Continuation of the limited access procedure or conversion to a standard approach may then be performed accordingly.

TECHNICAL CONSIDERATIONS

Fundamental in limited access surgery is the ability to visualize the operative field. On occasion this may supersede visualization in a comparable open procedure due to the availability of intense illumination, magnification, and capability to see "around" structures. Most often a video camera is incorporated into the specific scope and the image is displayed on two appropriately placed monitors with associated recording and photographic capabilities.

A virtual deluge of instruments for limited access surgery has been introduced with continual modification. Many are precision miniatures of standard instruments with attached pistol grip handles and with the capabilities of locking, rotation, angulation, and electrification. Also available is a great variety of trocars, electrosurgical devices, laser adaptations, hydraulic dissectors, extrudable retractors, and so on.

There has been a trend to substitute reusable instruments for single use items with the obvious exceptions of staplers, cutting-edged instruments, and so on. Indeed, novel technology has been introduced for ultrasonic cleaning and sterilization of these instruments. Special training courses, books and visual aids for physicians and nursing personnel, accreditation, and credentials have accompanied this new technology.

Finally, clinical success, time, and economic limitations rather than innovative scientific advances will establish which limited access procedures will be utilized.

Chapter 7

Neck Surgery

THYROIDECTOMY

Definition

Removal of all or a portion of the thyroid gland.

Discussion

The thyroid is a highly vascular gland composed of two lobes connected by a narrow bridge (isthmus). It is located on the anterior aspect of the trachea adjacent to the second, third, and fourth rings. Thyroid lobectomy is performed for the treatment of some thyroid nodules and carcinomas. Total thyroidectomy is indicated for certain carcinomas and to relieve tracheal or esophageal compression. Infrequently, a portion of the gland may be substernal, necessitating a more extensive procedure.

Procedure

The incision is made above the sternal notch. The platysma muscle is incised and retracted. The strap muscles are separated or divided. Blunt and sharp dissection are employed until the thyroid is exposed. Care is taken to avoid injury to the recurrent and superior laryngeal nerves and the parathyroid glands. The gland is mobilized. All or a portion of the gland is removed. Hemostasis is obtained. The wound may be irrigated, and a drain may be inserted. Incision is closed in layers by interrupted stitches.

Preparation of the Patient

The patient is supine with a rolled sheet or small sand-bag placed between the scapulae (extending the neck). A padded footboard is placed on the table. The table is positioned in reverse Trendelenberg. Arms may be extended on armboards. Apply electrosurgical dispersive pad.

Skin Preparation

Begin at the anterior neck extending upward to just below the infra-auricular border and lower lip, and downward to 2.5 to 5 cm (1 to 2 inches) above the nipples; continue down to the table at the neck, around the shoulders, and at the sides.

Draping

Folded towels, a sterile adhesive plastic drape (optional), and a sheet with a small fenestration.

Equipment

Electrosurgical unit
Suction
Footboard extension (padded) for table

Instrumentation

Thyroid tray
Limited procedure tray
Spring retractor
Right angle clamps with fine points (2)
Lahey clamps (extra available)

Supplies

Basin set
Blades (2) No. 10, (1) No. 15
Needle magnet or counter
Suction tubing
Electrosurgical pencil
Dissectors (e.g., peanut)
Small drain (e.g., 1/4″ Penrose)

Fine suture (e.g., 4-0 silk to mark line of incision) or
marking pen
Bulb syringe

Special Notes

A fine silk suture may be pressed against the neck to
mark the line for incision.

Usually straight Crile or mosquito clamps are used.
Have extra clamps on hand, for the surgeon may prefer
to clamp and cut many times before ligating.

The dressing is secured by a "thyroid collar" (e.g.,
Queen Anne's dressing). After the wound is dressed in
the usual manner, a collar is made with a towel folded
in thirds lengthwise. The towel is wrapped around the
neck, and the ends of the collar are crossed and secured
by adhesive tape.

The scrub person should keep the back table sterile
until the patient is extubated, breathing satisfactorily,
and taken from the room (i.e., prepared for tracheostomy if airway becomes compromised).

In many institutions a tracheostomy tray accompanies the patient to the recovery room and later to the
patient's room until any consideration of airway obstruction secondary to edema or hematoma has passed.

PARATHYROIDECTOMY

Definition

Removal of one or more of the four parathyroid glands
located behind the thyroid gland.

Discussion

Parathyroidectomy is performed to excise adenomas,
carcinomas, and hyperplasia; only normal or atrophic
glands are left intact. Removal of all parathyroid tissue
results in tetany and death.

Procedure

See approach for Thyroidectomy, pp. 48–49. Thyroid
gland is mobilized. Parathyroid glands are identified

and resected as indicated. Some parathyroid tissue (amount is controversial) is left intact. Hemostasis is achieved, the wound may be irrigated, and a drain may be inserted. The incision is closed in layers by interrupted stitches.

Preparation of the Patient, Skin Preparation, Draping, Equipment, Instrumentation, and Supplies

See Thyroidectomy, pp. 48–50.

Special Notes

As for Thyroidectomy, a fine silk suture may be pressed against the neck to mark the line for the incision. A marking pen may be used instead.

Have ready several pathology slips and biopsy containers for the many specimens.

A special "thyroid collar" (Queen Anne's dressing) may be applied after the wound is dressed in the usual manner. A collar is made with a towel folded in thirds lengthwise. The towel is wrapped around the neck, and the ends of the towel are crossed and secured by adhesive tape.

The scrub person should keep the back table sterile until the patient is extubated, breathing satisfactorily, and taken from the room (i.e., prepared for tracheostomy if airway becomes compromised).

THYROGLOSSAL DUCT CYSTECTOMY

Definition

Excision of a cyst and duct in the midline of the neck including a portion of the hyoid bone.

Discussion

The duct is an embryological remnant extending from the foramen caecum at the base of the tongue through the hyoid bone to the thyroid gland. When a ductal sinus or cyst is present, it is usually found inferior to the hyoid bone.

Procedure

An incision is made between the hyoid bone and thyroid cartilage. The platysma muscle is incised and retracted. Strap muscles are separated and divided. Sharp and blunt dissection are employed to mobilize the cyst and duct. A central portion of the hyoid bone is removed to prevent recurrence, and the cephalad portion of the duct is ligated. The specimen is excised. The wound is closed with interrupted stitches. A drain may be employed.

Preparation of the Patient

The patient is supine with a folded sheet (adult), towel (child), or small sandbag placed between the scapulae to extend the neck; the shoulders are lowered (to give better exposure). Arms may be extended on armboards. Additional measures such as padded restraints on extremities may be needed for the pediatric patient. Apply electrosurgical dispersive pad.

Skin Preparation, Draping, and Equipment

See Thyroidectomy, pp. 48–50.

Instrumentation

Limited procedure tray
Minor orthopedic procedures tray
Right angle clamps with fine points (2)

Supplies

Basin set
Blades, adults (2) No. 10, (1) No. 15; children (2) No. 15
Suction tubing
Needle magnet or counter
Electrosurgical pencil
Dissectors (e.g., peanut)
Drain (e.g., 1/4″ Penrose)

Special Notes

Bone cutters, rongeurs, and periosteal elevator from Minor orthopedic procedures tray may be needed to remove a portion of the hyoid bone.

Infrequently, the tract of the duct may be identified by injecting the duct with a solution of methylene blue.

Chapter 8

Breast Procedures

BREAST BIOPSY

Definition

Removal of tissue to determine the nature of a breast lesion.

Discussion

When the lesion is not palpable, prior to the biopsy procedure, the patient is taken to the radiology department where needles are inserted into the breast under imaging techniques to localize the lesion. (In some facilities a stereotactic guided needle biopsy may obviate the need for open surgical biopsy.)

A frozen section can be performed on the specimen immediately, if indicated.

Procedure

The incision is generally made over the lesion. For central lesions, a circumareolar incision may be employed. The lesion is grasped and dissected free. The specimen may be sent for a frozen section. After hemostasis is obtained, a drain may be inserted. Subcuticular tissue is approximated. Skin is closed with fine subcuticular suture or fine interrupted skin stitches. A safety pin or stitch secures the drain.

Preparation of the Patient

Patient is supine with arm on the affected side extended on an armboard; the other arm may be tucked in at the patient's side. Apply electrosurgical dispersive pad.

If local anesthesia is employed, see circulator responsibilites, pp. 34–35.

Skin Preparation

Use a *gentle* circular motion beginning at the lesion extending from neckline to lower ribs, including a wide margin beyond the midline and under the arm down to the table on the affected side. For lesions in the upper outer quadrant, include the axilla.

Draping

Folded towels and sheet with a small fenestration

Equipment

Electrosurgical unit

Instrumentation

Basic/Minor procedures tray

Supplies

Basin set
Blades (2) No. 15
Electrosurgical pencil
Needle magnet or counter
Small drain (e.g., 1/4″ Penrose)
Safety pin

Special Notes

The circulator must confirm with the patient the side of the lesion.

Exercise all precautions in handling excised tissue to avoid misidentification of biopsies when multiple specimens are taken.

The circulator is responsible for the specimen's being sent to the laboratory immediately for a frozen section. Do *not* put the specimen in formalin.

Notify pathologist if the patient is awake.

MASTECTOMY

Definition

Removal of the breast.

Partial Mastectomy (Lumpectomy). Excision of a breast tumor with appropriate tumor-free margins.

Subcutaneous Mastectomy. Removal of all breast tissue; overlying skin and nipple are left intact.

Simple Mastectomy. Removal of entire breast only.

Radical Mastectomy

Modified Radical Mastectomy. Removal of breast and axillary lymph nodes; most frequently performed radical procedure.

Classic Radical Mastectomy. Includes the removal of the entire breast, pectoralis muscles, axillary lymph nodes, fat, fascia, and adjacent tissues. A skin graft may be necessary for skin closure. Less frequently employed, unless there is an invasion of deeper structures.

Extended Radical Mastectomy. En bloc removal of the breast, axillary contents, pectoralis muscles, and internal mammary lymph nodes. Resection of the ribs and sternum may also be included. A skin graft may be required for closure of the wound; rarely performed today.

Discussion

Patients are particularly emotionally affected by any of these procedures. Every effort must be made on the part of the surgical team, particularly the circulating nurse to be understanding and sensitive to the patient's feelings.

Partial mastectomy followed by radiation treatments is now more widely employed.

A *subcutaneous mastectomy* is recommended for patients with small, centrally located, noninvasive lesions including chronic cystic mastitis, gynecomastia, and patients with a strong family history of breast cancer who require prophylactic mastectomy.

A *simple mastectomy* is usually reserved for patients with no lymph node involvement or elderly or poor-risk patients who cannot tolerate a more extensive procedure.

A *radical mastectomy* is performed on patients with malignant lesions in which axillary fat and lymphatic tissues are excised and pectoral muscles may be removed to more widely encompass any potential tumor.

In current practice, when discussed with the patient preoperatively, immediate breast reconstruction may be performed at the time of mastectomy. A prosthesis or a myocutaneous flap or a combination thereof may be employed. When the prosthesis is employed, a muscular pocket is created into which a tissue expander balloon is inserted (to be incrementally inflated postoperatively) to attain appropriate size for insertion of a permanent prosthesis subsequently placed as an outpatient procedure. The pocket created will vary with the patient's breast size and availablity of adjacent musculature. When necessary, a latissimus dorsi myocutaneous (LDM) flap may be used to enhance the symmetry. An alternative to the use of a prosthesis is a transverse rectus abdominus myocutaneous (TRAM) flap, in which case a mesh prosthesis may be necessary to reconstruct the abdominal wall donor site defect as well as additional adjacent tissue mobilization. A greater omentum pedicle graft and free gluteal flap requiring microvascular anastomotic techniques have been used.

Procedure

In *partial mastectomy,* the incision is usually made over the lesion. The skin is elevated and the breast mass is excised. Hemostasis is obtained. The wound may be irrigated. A drain may be inserted. Skin is closed with interrupted stitches. A safety pin or skin stitch secures the drain.

In *subcutaneous mastectomy,* the incision is generally made in the inframammary fold. If the breast is small (or in male patients with gynecomastia), a circumareolar incision may be employed. The skin is elevated, and all subcutaneous and connective tissues are removed with the nipple and the skin left intact. Hemostasis is obtained. The wound may be irrigated. A drain may be inserted. A prosthesis may be inserted at this time. The skin is closed.

In *modified radical mastectomy,* usually a transverse or longitudinal incision is used. Skin flaps are developed and often pectoralis fascia is dissected free from underlying structures. The axillary contents are dissected free from vascular and nervous structures and are removed. Care is taken to avoid injury to the nerve supply to various muscles. After hemostasis is achieved, the skin flaps are approximated over drains or suction catheters (e.g., Hemovac). A skin graft may be required for skin closure.

In *classic radical mastectomy,* additional structures including the pectoralis major and minor muscles and the intervening lymphatic and fatty tissues are excised.

Preparation of the Patient

The patient is supine with arms extended on armboards; a folded sheet is under the shoulder on the affected side. Apply electrosurgical dispersive pad.

Skin Preparation

Using a *gentle* circular motion begin at the lesion extending up to the neckline, and down to the umbilicus with a wide margin beyond the midline. Prepare around the shoulder, under the arm, and down to the table on the affected side. Apply electrosurgical dispersive pad.

Draping

The patient's arm on the affected side is held up in a tube (or impervious) stockinette as a drape sheet is placed under the axilla. The field around the breast is draped with folded towels. The arm is brought through the fenestration of a laparotomy sheet.

Equipment

Electrosurgical unit
Suction

Instrumentation

Major procedures tray
Additional curved Crile clamps and large towel clips
Hemoclip appliers (small, medium, large)
Rake retractors (4 or 6 prong)
Supplies
Basin set
Blades, several No. 10
Electrosurgical pencil
Suction tubing
Needle magnet or counter
Tube (or impervious) stockinette
Hemoclips (small, medium, large)
Electrosurgical pencil holder (optional)
Dermatome (for skin graft) (e.g., Brown, and necessary
    supplies including: mineral oil, saline, tongue blades,
    and petrolatum-impregnated gauze)
Drainage unit (e.g., Hemovac)
Pressure dressing
Marlex mesh, optional
Inflatable breast prothesis (optional)

Special Notes

The circulator must confirm with the patient the side
of the lesion.

If mastectomy is to follow a breast biopsy, the patient
is reprepared, and redraped, the team is regowned and
gloved, and the instruments are changed.

Prepare gently to avoid the potential of dislodging
tumor cells.

The circulator will hold out the prepped arm to receive the double (or impervious) stockinette; the arm is
then held by scrubbed personnel.

Check coagulation and cutting settings on the electrosurgical unit. Often a great deal of the dissection is
performed with the cautery. Keep the electrosurgical

pencil tip clean as necessary. The use of two electro-surgical pencils may be indicated so that a clean tip will always be available. Avoid a burn injury to the patient by protecting the electrosurgical pencil not in use by keeping it in a holder.

Several knife blade changes may be required because of the fibrous nature of the tissues incised; notify the surgeon when a blade is new.

If a skin graft is necessary, one thigh must be prepared and draped along with the main operative site.

Irrigation is usually with water, not saline, to lessen the survival of tumor cells.

Estrogen and progesterone assays may be requested on the specimen.

With breast reconstruction, intravenous fluorescin dye may be employed to determine viability of the flap.

Chapter 9

Abdominal
Extraintestinal Surgery

ABDOMINAL LAPAROTOMY

Definition

An opening made through the abdominal wall into the peritoneal cavity for the purpose of exploration, diagnosis, and treatment.

Procedure

The skin is incised with the "skin" knife. Subcutaneous tissue is incised with the "deep" knife or electrosurgical unit. Blood vessels may be clamped or cauterized. Fascia is incised, and the underlying muscles are retracted or transsected. The surgeon grasps the peritoneum and incises it with the "deep" knife. A scissors (usually a Metzenbaum, infrequently a curved Mayo) and cautery is used to complete the peritoneal incision. The abdomen is explored. Wound edges are retracted accordingly by Deaver and/or Richardson retractors or by a self-retaining retractor (e.g., Balfour). The surgery is performed. The wound and/or peritoneal cavity may be irrigated and the irrigation fluid removed by suction. Drains may be employed, often through stab wound incisions. The peritoneum is usually closed with a continuous suture. Two toothed forceps or several Pean or

Kocher clamps may be used to grasp the peritoneum to assist in its exposure. The abdomen is closed in layers, or less often, in a single layer. The skin is approximated using Adson tissue forceps and suture material or skin staples. For infected cases, skin and subcutaneous tissues may be left open and drained.

Preparation of the Patient

The patient is supine; arms may be extended on armboards. Check with the surgeon regarding insertion of a urinary catheter (e.g., Foley). Apply electrosurgical dispersive pad.

Skin Preparation

Determine site of incision; begin cleansing at this point. Include area from nipples to midthighs and down to the table at the sides. For women, a vaginal preparation may be indicated.

Draping

Four folded towels and a laparotomy sheet

Equipment

Suction
Electrosurgical unit

Instrumentation

Major procedures tray
Self-retaining retractor (e.g., Balfour)
Hemoclip appliers, variety (available)

Supplies

Basin set
Blades (2) No. 10, (1) No. 15
Needle magnet or counter
Suction tubing
Electrosurgical pencil
Hemoclips, variety (available)

Special Notes

Once the abdomen is entered, the only free sponges used are laparotomy pads (lap pads). All x-ray detectable 4″ × 4″ sponges must be mounted on a sponge forceps (frequently referred to as a *spongestick*).

Many surgeons prefer to use lap sponges lightly moistened by warm saline after the peritoneal cavity has been entered.

Carbon dioxide gas (CO_2) is used to establish pneumoperitoneum because it has a record of safety with its property of being absorbed, it is less likely to cause gas embolization, and because it supresses combustion. A CO_2 machine with a controlled rate of flow, pressure, and so on is employed and monitored throughout the procedure.

ABDOMINAL LAPAROSCOPY

Definition

The introduction of a laparoscope through the anterior abdominal wall into the peritoneal cavity or preperitoneal planes for purposes of exploration, diagnosis, and treatment.

Discussion

Common to all abdominal laparoscopic procedures is the need to distend or distract the parietal wall most often by establishing pneumoperitoneum or by the less frequently employed gasless technique. Except for the placement of the laparoscopic ports and the occasional need for ancillary small incisions through which specimens can be retrieved or intestinal anastomosis performed, and so on, the procedures are similar with respect to laparoscopic technique and are distinguished only by the use of instrumentation specific to the procedure.

Because of the rapid evolution of techniques and the wide variety of instrumentation available, only the basics will be covered here as every surgeon has an individual preference for specific technique and instrumentation.

Procedure

Through an appropriate site chosen by its relevance to the proposed procedure and its likelihood of being free of underlying adherent viscera, either an insufflator needle (Verres, etc.) or a trocar is inserted transperitoneally. Another established technique is to employ a minimal incision about the umbilicus penetrating the peritoneum under direct vision. Pneumoperitoneum is established at the site, and additional parts are placed under visual control from within to avoid any visceral trauma. Through these ports of different diameters, instruments are inserted to accomplish the surgery. Currently available trocars feature sharp tips that automatically retract as the peritoneum is pierced and are held in place as they are inserted into the abdominal wall with incorporated screw threads. Stay sutures may be used to further secure these ports. Interchangeable adaptors can alter the internal diameter of the port without having to remove the port. Pneumatic seals (or double seals) prevent leakage of CO_2. Initial insufflation pressure is between 5 and 7 mm Hg and is usually increased to 12 to 13 mm Hg during the definitive procedure. When the surgery is completed, the pneumoperitoneum is released, and the ports are removed and sutured closed. On occasion a port may be removed and its insertion defect enlarged to accommodate the extraction of a large specimen. Following this the wound is closed by standard techniques.

There are infrequent complications related to CO_2 pneumoperitoneum including respiratory compromise and decreased venous return due to elevated intra-abdominal pressure, excessive cooling during lengthy procedures, subcutaneous emphysema, and in patients with respiratory compromise or in ill infants, hypercarbia with ensuing acidosis. In trauma patients with lacerated vessels, gas emboli is a potential risk, and if the diaphragm is injured, pneumothorax can be induced. The effects of CO_2 on the fetus in pregnant patients are not completely understood. A gasless technique employing a mechanical lifting device to establish a working cavity has been developed. This modality avoids any potential physiologic ill effects of carbon dioxide, may cost less, and avoids the need of maintaining pneumatic seals, permitting the use of larger (standard) instruments. A special fan retractor with legs closed is introduced through a minimal incision employing open technique. The retractor is usually placed intraperitoneally or when significant adhesions are anticipated, into the immediate preperitoneal space. The retractor is attached to a mechanical lifting arm previously secured to the table. The fan legs are spread, and the retractor mechanically elevated. A second fan retractor may be employed if necessary, particularly in obese patients or to expose the paracolic gutters. However, exposure may be limited to a single area or quadrant necessitating replacement of the fan retractors. Retraction of adjacent structures requires additional manual effort or gravity effects rather than the gaseous pressure effect of pneumoperitoneum. Particularly in cholecystectomy, inguinal hernia repair, and pelvic surgery, the pneumoperitoneum technique is usually superior. When advantageous, the two techniques can be combined for alternate phases of a procedure.

Recently introduced modalities for use in laparotomy are being adapted for use laparoscopically. Examples include the argon beam coagulator (*which see*) and intraoperative ultrasonographic probes. Laparotomy is also being used to detect radioactive-labeled antibodies to localize tumor deposits either in primary sites or in lymph nodes (e.g., colon anorectal carcinomas), as the instrument is used as a "hand-held" gamma counter.

Preparation of the Patient

The patient is supine and may be placed in the Trendelenburg position. Arms may be extended on armboards. Check with the surgeon regarding the insertion of a urinary catheter (e.g., Foley). Apply electrosurgical dispersive pad.

Skin Preparation

Determine the site of incision; begin cleansing at this point. Include area from nipples to midthighs and down

to the table at the sides. For women, a vaginal preparation may be indicated.

Draping

Four folded towels and a laparoscopy sheet
Camera cable cover

Equipment

Video monitors (2)
Insufflation device (CO_2)
Fiberoptic light source (e.g., Xenon 300 W)
VCR
Mavigraph (optional)
Pressure bag (to facilitate irrigation, optional)
Sequential compression device (optional)
Electrosurgical unit
Suction

Instrumentation

Verres needle
Trocars (5 mm, 10 mm, 12 mm, or Hasson)
Reducers
Dissectors
Graspers
Scissors
Staplers
Clip appliers
Suturing and ligation instruments
Suction—cautery or combination instrument combin-
  ing suction, irrigation, and electrosurgical capabili-
  ties with cord

Supplies

Foam padding for elbows and ankles; blanket may be
  used under knees
Fog reduction agent
Ligation sutures
Foley catheter
Nasogastric tube (optional)
Endoscopic specimen retrieval bag (optional)

Blades (1) No. 10, (1) No. 15 or (1) No. 11
Suction tubing
Clip cartridges

Special Notes

After the patient is in the room, position monitors.

The circulator checks CO_2 level.

Following draping, the scrub person will pass off camera cable, light cord, suction tubing, and electrocautery cord.

The circulator adjusts the insufflator. First adjust to low flow (between 5 and 7 mm Hg), then high flow according to surgeon's directions.

Connect and turn on light source and white balance camera.

The circulator will turn on the VCR (to record) if requested.

Recheck position of monitors so they can be easily viewed.

The circulator connects remaining items: irrigation tubing, suction tubing, and electrosurgical cord.

Keep lens clean as necessary.

The circulator positions the electrosurgical unit.

ABDOMINAL HERNIORRHAPHY

Definition

Repair of a musculofascial defect, through which various organs or tissues may present.

Types

Inguinal (Direct, Indirect) and Femoral. The musculofascial defect is in the groin, the herniated tissues presenting through the posterior inguinal wall medial to the deep inferior epigastric vessels (direct); or through the deep inguinal ring and inguinal canal, emerging at the superficial inguinal ring (indirect); or through the femoral canal (femoral).

Umbilical. Within the umbilicus (or about the umbilicus: paraumbilical) most often seen in children or obese adults.

Epigastric. Defect in the abdominal wall between the xiphoid process and the umbilicus through which fat protrudes.

Incisional (Ventral). A defect within the scar of a surgical incision (abdominal).

Discussion

Hernias are either reducible or irreducible, that is, incarcerated. The contents of an incarcerated hernia may become strangulated, compromising the viability of trapped tissue and necessitating their resection in addition to the herniorrhaphy.

Procedures

Several techniques are employed for each of these hernia types. Usually an incision is made over the site of the defect. Blunt and sharp dissection are employed to expose the hernia sac and surrounding musculofascial defect. With incisional hernias, the peritoneal cavity may be entered. The hernia sac may be allowed to retract, sutured over (imbricated), or excised. The musculofascial defect may be closed employing a wide variety of techniques and suture materials, and occasionally a mesh prosthesis. The subcutaneous tissue and skin are approximated.

Preparation of the Patient

The patient is supine with the arm on the affected side extended on an armboard. Apply electrosurgical dispersive pad. If local anesthesia is employed, see circulator responsibilities, pp. 34–35.

Skin Preparation

Inguinal and Femoral. Begin at the incision extending from umbilicus to midthigh (including a wide margin beyond the midline), and down to the table on the sides; external genitalia are prepped last.

Umbilical. Begin at the incision extending from the nipples to upper thighs, and down to the table at the sides.

Epigastric. Begin at the incision extending from the clavicles to the upper thighs, and down to the table at the sides.

Incisional. Begin at the site of previous incision; prepare widely enough to allow for extension of the incision.

Draping

Folded towels and a fenestrated sheet

Equipment

Electrosurgical unit

Instrumentation

Basic/Minor procedures tray
Self-retaining retractor (e.g., Adson, optional)

Supplies

Basin set
Blades (2) No. 10, (1) No. 15
Needle magnet or counter
Penrose drain (small, for retraction, optional)
Dissectors (e.g., peanut)
Electrosurgical pencil
Skin closure strips (optional)

Special Notes

The small Penrose drain (used to isolate the spermatic cord) is moistened in saline and passed on a Pean clamp.

Synthetic mesh such as Mersilene or Marlex is often used to repair recurrent hernias or large ventral defects.

LAPAROSCOPIC GROIN HERNIORRHAPHY

Definition

Repair of an inguinofemoral musculofascial defect employing laparoscopic technique.

Discussion

Laparoscopic groin herniorrhaphy is among the most controversial laparoscopic procedures being performed. The present techniques of traditional hernia repair are proven techniques, performed without violation of the abdominal cavity, often under local anesthesia. The advantages of a laparoscopic hernia repair are purported to be marked reduction of pain and rapid return to normal activity. The disadvantages are the requirement for general anesthesia and a lack of long-term follow-up data.

Procedure

Following the establishment of a pneumoperitoneum, a 10 to 11 mm laparoscope is inserted through the umbilical port. The patient is placed in the Trendelenburg position, and the abdomen is inspected. A second and third 10 to 11 mm port are created lateral to the rectus sheath at the level of the umbilicus on the side of the defect. Both inguinal rings are examined for hernias. The hernia sac, if present, is retracted out of the inguinal canal, and a segment is excised. Peritoneal flaps are developed by blunt dissection. Care is taken to avoid injury to the spermatic vessels and vas deferens in the male. A piece of mesh (e.g., Marlex, Gortex, or Surgipro) is fashioned to cover the hernial defect and a surrounding rim of the abdominal wall. (Slit[s] may be made in the mesh for the epigastric vessels and the spermatic cord. Some surgeons staple a piece of mesh into the surrounding rim of the abdominal wall as a reinforcement.) The mesh is then inserted via a port and is placed over the hernia defect. Endoscopic staples are employed to staple the mesh to the abdominal wall. Care is again taken to avoid injury to the spermatic vessels, vas deferens, and epigastric and iliac vessels as indicated. The pneumoperitoneum is relaxed. The peritonial flaps are then stapled together to cover the mesh and as an attempt to prevent adhesions to the bowel. Contralateral repair has been advocated by some authorities despite absence of a frank hernia. Some surgeons may repair indirect, direct, and recurrent laparoscopic inguinal hernias by preperitoneal approach.

Hemostasis is verified. The peritoneum is completely deflated, the trocars are removed, and the puncture holes are closed.

Preparation of the Patient

The patient is supine; both arms may be padded and tucked in at the patient's sides. Apply electrosurgical dispersive pad. A Foley catheter is not routinely inserted.

Skin Preparation

Begin at the midline extending from nipples to upper thighs and down to the table at the sides.

Draping

Folded towels and a laparoscopy sheet

Equipment

Electrosurgical unit with foot control
Suction
Fiberoptic light source (e.g., Xenon)
Video monitor(s)
VCR (optional)
Insufflator
Pressure bag (optional)

Instrumentation

Verres needle
Trocars 5 mm, 10 mm, 12 mm
Reducers
Dissectors
Graspers
Scissors
Stapler
Clip appliers
Suction—cautery or combination instrument combining suction, irrigation, and electrosurgical capabilities
Hydraulic dissector (optional)
Telescopes
Camera and cable

Supplies

Foam padding for elbow, blanket for under knees
Fog reduction agent
Blades No. 10 (1), No. 15 (1) or No. 11 (1)
Suction tubing (optional)
Staple cartridges

Special Notes

See Abdominal Laparoscopy, p. 66.

CHOLECYSTECTOMY

Definition

Removal of the gall bladder.

Discussion

This procedure may be performed to treat chronic or acute cholecystitis, with or without cholelithiasis, to remove a malignancy, or to remove polyps. Related procedures include:

Cholecystotomy. The establishment of an opening into the gallbladder to allow drainage of the organ and removal of stones. A tube (e.g., Foley, Pezzer, or Malecot) is then placed in the gallbladder to establish external drainage (cholecystostomy). This is performed when the patient cannot tolerate cholecystectomy.

Choledochoscopy. The insertion of a choledochoscope into the common bile duct in order to directly visualize stones and facilitate their extraction.

Choledochotomy. The opening of the common bile duct to remove stones. It is performed to relieve choledocholithiasis or otherwise drain an obstructed common bile duct. Drainage is usually established by placing a T-tube in the duct (choledochostomy).

Procedure

The incision is right subcostal, right paramedian, or midline. The gallbladder is grasped (generally with a Pean clamp). The cystic duct, cystic artery, and the common bile duct are exposed. The cystic artery is clamped (using two right-angle clamps) and ligated with a suture passed on a long instrument or by He-moclips, as is the cystic duct. The gallbladder is mobilized by incising overlying peritoneum and removed. The underlying liver bed may be reperitonealized. A drain (e.g., Jackson-Pratt) may be employed exiting a stab wound and secured to the skin with a stitch. The wound is closed in layers. The skin is closed by interrupted stitches or skin staples.

Cholangiogram. Performed prior to the ligation of the cystic duct. A catheter is passed through the stump of the cystic duct into the common bile duct. A suture or special cystic duct clamp secures the catheter. Prior to taking x-ray films, all extraneous metal clamps and retractors are removed from the field. The catheter is tested with saline for leakage, and then radiopaque dye is injected. X-rays are taken. The catheter is removed, and the cystic duct is ligated.

Choledochotomy and Choledochoscopy. The common bile duct is exposed and traction sutures are placed through it. A longitudinal incision is made in the duct, and a variety of stone-removing forceps, scoops, and irrigation and balloon catheters may be employed to explore for and extract stones either proximally (hepatic bile ducts) or distally (bile duct). A choledochoscope may also be employed. Further cholangiograms may then be taken. The duct is usually closed over a T-tube drain.

Preparation of the Patient

The patient is supine; both arms may be extended on armboards. Some surgeons position the patient with a roll under the right upper flank, which facilitates interpretation of the cholangiogram, "separating" the biliary tree from the spine. A preliminary x-ray film may be taken to ensure correct placement of the cassette. Apply electrosurgical dispersive pad.

Skin Preparation

Begin at the incision, either right subcostal (most frequently used), right paramedian, or midline; extending from the axilla to just above the pubic symphysis, and down to the table at the sides.

Draping

Folded towels and a laparotomy sheet

Equipment

Roll (for positioning)
Suction
Electrosurgical unit
X-ray cassette

Instrumentation

Major procedures tray
Long Metzenbaum scissors
Hemoclip appliers (various sizes and lengths)
Biliary tract tray (for common duct exploration)

Supplies

Basin set
Blades (1) No. 10, (1) No. 15
Hemoclips (various sizes)
Electrosurgical pencil
Needle magnet or counter
Drain (e.g., Jackson-Pratt)
T-tube (if choledochotomy is done)
Dissectors (e.g., peanut)
Culture tubes (aerobic and anaerobic)

For Cholangiogram
Catheter (surgeon's preference) and radiopaque dye (e.g., Hypaque or Renografin 60)
Small basins (2) for saline and dye
Biliary tract tray
Syringes (2) 30 mL

For Choledochoscopy
Choledochoscope
Normal saline 1000 mL
Flexible tubing (e.g., cystoscopy tubing)
Polyethylene tubing (surgeons preference)
Arterial line pressure bag

Special Notes

Correct positioning of the patient is imperative to assure accurate visualization of the biliary tract.

Test drains for patency.

Drains are anchored with a skin stitch.

Instruments coming into contact with bile are isolated in a basin.

Syringes filled with saline or radiopaque dye must be labeled to avoid confusion and ensure successful x-ray exposures.

A "scout" film is taken before surgery begins.

Observe x-ray precautions, see p. 21.

Protective goggles may be worn for choledochoscopy.

LAPAROSCOPIC CHOLECYSTECTOMY

Definition

Endoscopic excision of the gallbladder.

Discussion

The laparoscopic approach may prove difficult or impossible if the patient is obese or if there are excessive adhesions (related to a previous surgery, recurrent attacks of cholecystitis, and so on), ductal or vascular anomalies exist, unexpected pathology is encountered, acute inflammation distorts normal tissue planes, or there is excessive bleeding or surgical injury. In any of those instances the procedure must be promptly converted to open laparotomy.

Procedure

Pneumoperitoneum is achieved. Usually a 10 to 11 mm trocar is inserted infraumbilically through which a laparoscope with camera is introduced. The laparoscope may be removed and reinserted via a subsequently placed port. The abdomen is explored. A subzyphoid trocar is inserted. The patient's right side is rotated anteriorly 15 to 20°. A third trocar is placed in the right anterior axillary line halfway between the iliac crest and the twelfth rib. A locking grasping forceps is introduced through this port, seizing the fundus of the gall-bladder and distracting it until the hilum can be seen. Local dissection of fat or adhesions may be necessary to achieve visualization of the gallbladder prior to this maneuver. To maintain traction on the gallbladder, the handle of the grasper can be fastened to the drape. A fourth trocar may be inserted 2 to 3 cm below the right costal margin just medial to the shaft of the grasper (holding the gallbladder). By appropriate dissection the hilum of the gallbladder is visualized including the cystic duct and the cystic artery. The cystic artery is divided between clips. A clip is placed on the junction of the cystic duct and gallbladder. A cholangiogram may then be performed.

Cholangiogram. The cystic duct is incised as close to the gallbladder as possible. A cholangiogram catheter is inserted (with or without prior placement of a guide wire) and clipped or held in place with a cholangiogram clamp. Saline may be injected into the catheter to check for leaks. Radiopaque dye (diluted to half strength) is injected after the patient is repositioned as necessary. Standard x-ray films are obtained. (Alternative techniques may be employed.)

Choledochoscopy. The cystic duct is pneumatically dilated through which the common bile duct is cannulated with a choledochoscope or a ureteroscope. A separate camera-monitor system may be utilized. A guide wire is passed via the cystic duct, and the choledochoscope is advanced over the wire. An endoscopic stone basket may be used to retrieve calculi. If the stone is too large to be removed, lithotripsy of the stone may be employed using a mechanical, electrical, or laser energy source (crushing forceps, electrohydraulic lithotripter, or pulse-dye laser). Limitation of choledochoscopy exists due to the size of the instruments currently in use. Postoperatively, extraction of remnants of calculi may be facilitated by endoscopic retrograde cholangiopancreaticography (ERCP) including duodenal papillary sphincterotomy. Some surgeons may perform duct choledochotomy. As indicated, the procedure may require conversion to open laparotomy to correct the common duct pathology. The cystic duct is then ligated and divided. The neck and the fundus of the gallbladder are freed from the liver bed using either monopolar electrocautery or laser dissection. (Before the gallbladder is completely detached, the area may be irrigated to expose sites of bleeding in the liver bed.) A closed suction drain may be passed through the lateral portal in an appropriate position and secured to the skin. When the gallbladder is freed of its attachments, bile and small stones may be aspirated to facilitate its extraction. If very large stones are encountered, the umbilical incision is extended and the gallbladder is removed directly by a large (18 mm) portal. Hemostasis is achieved, and the trocar puncture sites are closed following the release of the pneumoperitoneum.

Preparation of the Patient

The patient is supine as close to the head of the table as possible. Both arms may be padded and tucked in at the sides, unless the patient is obese, in which case, the patient's left arm can be placed on an armboard. A standard table with an x-ray cassette in place or an image intensifier may be used in conjunction with a C-arm. Sequential compression stockings on both legs may be used to avoid pooling of blood in the lower extremities. A nasogastric tube is placed by the anesthetist. Most surgeons request a Foley catheter be inserted. Apply electrosurgical dispersive pad. The table is placed in a Trendelenburg at 5 to 10° to establish pneumoperitoneum and then in reverse Trendelenburg at 10 to 20° to allow the abdominal viscera to gravitate inferiorly, away from the gallbladder. The table may be rotated slightly to the left to increase exposure of the gallbladder and cystic duct.

Skin Preparation

Begin at the midline and extend from axilla to just above the pubic symphysis and down to the table at the sides.

Draping

Folded towels and a laparoscopy sheet

Equipment

Suction
Electrosurgical unit and/or Nd:YAG laser unit (infrequently, optional)
X-ray cassettes
Light source (e.g., Xenon 300 W)
Video monitors (2)
VCR (optional)
Mavigraph (video printer, optional)
CO_2 insufflator
Pressure bag to facilitate irrigation
Sequential compression device

Instrumentation

Major tray (open)
Biliary tract tray (available)
Choledochoscopy tray (available)
Laparoscopy cholecystectomy tray (endoscopic instruments)

 Verres needle
 Hasson trocar (available)
 Trocars (2) 10 or 11-mm (radiolucent cannula sheaths preferred)
 Trocars (2) 5 mm
 Reducer caps
 Dissector clamps (2)
 Grasping clamps (4) (2 traumatic, locking), (2 atraumatic)
 Cholangiography clamp (with nipple for guide wire), several types available
 Maryland clamp (almost right angle)
 Right-angle hook (L shaped) ⎤
 J-hook tip   ⎬ suction electrosurgical dissectors
 Spatula tip   ⎦
 Babcock clamp, 10 mm (atraumatic)
 Babcock clamp, 5 mm
 Allis clamp
 Scissors (3) (hook, straight, micro)
 Metzenbaum double-action shears
 Clip applier

Laparoscopes (2) (0°, and 30° or 40°) and cameras
Extrudable retractors (2) (fan, curved)
Stone basket or 3-prong grasper
Stone-crushing forceps
Suction, irrigation, electrosurgical device

Supplies

Foam padding for elbows, ankles
Pneumatic antiembolitic stockings
Guide wire (e.g., 0.035 mm)
Fog reduction agent
Loop sutures available (e.g., Endoloop)
Cysto tubing (straight, 1000-mL bag normal saline and 3-way stopcock)
Electrosurgical cord
Pressure bag
12 mL syringe, 3-way stopcock, K50 tubing
Catheter, e.g., Taut, No. 5 ureteral catheter open-ended, Karlan
Culture tubes (aerobic, anaerobic)
Video-cassette (optional)
X-ray cassette on table, if image intensifier table not available
Foley catheter
Nasogastric tube (e.g., No. 16)
Ligating clips
Luer lock syringes, 35 mL (2)
Radiopaque dye (e.g., Renographin 60 mixed half strength with normal saline)
Blades (1) No. 10, (1) No. 15, or (1) No. 11
Suction tubing
Endoscopic specimen retrieval bag
Ductal dilating balloon catheter (e.g., 7 Fr)
Skin closure strips

Special Notes

After the patient is in the room, position and connect monitors.

Position electrosurgical unit.

Following draping, the scrub person will pass off camera cable, light cord, Silastic tubing, and suction.

The circulator adjusts insufflator. First low flow (between 5 and 7 mm Hg), then higher flow according to surgeon's instructions.

Connect and turn on light source and white balance camera.

The circulator will turn on the VCR to record, if requested.

The circulator rechecks position of monitors so that they can be easily viewed.

The circulator connects all remaining items: irrigation system, suction tubing, electrosurgical cord.

All non-disposable instruments may be flash-sterilized.

Soak scope and light cord in Steris solution after thorough cleansing.

Use an image intensifier table when possible; if not possible, put cassette in a regular table ahead of time. Have a C-arm available.

Some surgeons may retract the gallbladder with a toothed grasper, which is then fastened to the drape.

Cavitron unit may be requested for stone crushing.

If laser is used, see pp. 619–624 for safety rules.

Some surgeons use 5000 U Heparin in 1 L of 0.9% normal saline for irrigation.

Turn room lights and overhead lights out during procedure; leave one light on overhead for scrub person.

Lights will be turned on again after the gallbladder is out.

Circulator should notify x-ray department regarding cholangiogram.

The scrub person covers the C-arm, if used, and camera holder. A drape covers the x-ray screen.

The circulator should turn off the camera during cholangiogram.

Following the cholangiogram, the circulator reconnects the electrosurgical device and turns on the recorder.

DRAINAGE OF PANCREATIC CYST (PSEUDOCYST)

Definition

Internal drainage of a pseudocyst is performed by anastomosing the cyst wall to an adjacent hollow viscus (stomach, duodenum, jejunum), or less frequently, by external drainage or marsupialization.

Discussion

A pseudocyst of the pancreas is so named because this "cyst" does not have an epithelial lining as does a true cyst. These cysts develop secondary to pancreatic trauma or acute pancreatitis in which pancreatic fluid and/or blood has been encased in adhesions which later form the cyst wall. As the cyst often contains pancreatic enzymes, internal drainage is preferable to external drainage to avoid external fistula and excoriation of the skin.

Procedure

A vertical or transverse incision is made. The cyst is identified and anastomosed to an adjacent viscus. An incision is made into the anterior wall of hollow viscus (e.g., stomach), to gain access to the posterior wall to which the anastomosis is made. Prior to suturing the cyst, the contents are aspirated to facilitate the anastomosis and to avoid spillage of pancreatic fluid into the operative field. If biliary tract disease is responsible for the pancreatitis, a concomitant biliary tract procedure is performed (e.g., cholecystectomy and/or common bile duct exploration). The abdomen is closed in layers. A drain may be used.

Preparation of the Patient

The patient is supine; arms may be extended on armboards. Apply electrosurgical dispersive pad.

Skin Preparation

Begin at the incision (vertical or transverse) extending from nipples to upper thighs, and down to the table at the sides.

Draping

Folded towels and a laparotomy or transverse sheet (depending on incision)

Equipment

Electrosurgical unit
Suction

Instrumentation

Major procedures tray
Biliary tract tray
Hemoclip appliers (variety of sizes and lengths)

Supplies

Basin set
Electrosurgical pencil
Suction tubing
Blades (2) No. 10, (1) No. 15
Needle magnet or counter
Retention type catheter (e.g., Pezzer)
Hemoclips (small, medium, large)
Umbilical tapes
Dissectors (e.g., peanut)

Special Notes

The trocar (on the Biliary tract tray) attached to suction tubing may be used to aspirate the cyst.

PANCREATICODUODENECTOMY (WHIPPLE PROCEDURE)

Definition

Removal of the head of the pancreas, the entire duodenum, the very proximal portion of the jejunum, the distal third of the stomach, and the distal half of the common bile duct, with the re-establishment of continuity of the biliary, pancreatic, and gastrointestinal tracts.

Discussion

This procedure is usually performed for regional malignancy or benign, obstructive, chronic pancreatitis.

Procedure

Approach is through a transverse, midline, or paramedian incision. The operability of the findings is assessed. The distal stomach, extrahepatic biliary tract, the head of the pancreas, and the entire duodenum are mobilized. The distal stomach, the distal common bile duct, and the neck of the pancreas are resected. A total pancreatectomy, splenectomy, cholecystectomy, and vagotomy may be included. If tumor has invaded the base of the mesocolon, portal vein, aorta, vena cava, or superior mesenteric vessels, this procedure is abandoned, and a lesser procedure, usually a bypass (of the biliary tree and/or stomach) will be performed. The proximal end of the jejunum is anastomosed to the distal pancreas. The common bile duct is anastomosed to the jejunum in end-to-side fashion. The distal stomach is anastomosed to the jejunum also in end-to-side fashion. Stapling devices may be utilized in mobilizing and transsecting multiple blood vessels and in the transsection of the stomach and the gastrojejunal anastomosis. Various plastic stents may be placed in the biliary or pancreatic anastomoses. The wound is drained. The abdomen is closed in layers.

Preparation of the Patient

The patient is supine; arms may be extended on armboards. Apply electrosurgical dispersive pad.

Skin Preparation

Begin at incision (transverse, midline, or paramedian) extending from nipples to upper thighs, and down to the table at the sides.

Draping

Folded towels and a laparotomy or transverse sheet (depending upon incision)

Equipment

Electrosurgical unit
Suction

Instrumentation

Major procedures tray
Biliary tract tray
Gastrointestinal procedures tray
Long instruments tray (available)

Harrington retractors
Hemoclip appliers (variety of sizes and lengths)
Automatic stapling device (optional)

Supplies

Basin set
Electrosurgical pencil
Suction tubing
Blades (2) No. 10, (1) No. 15
Hemoclips, variety of sizes
Dissectors (e.g., peanut)
Needle magnet or counter
Staples (optional)
Drains: for retraction (e.g., 1″ Penrose); for drainage
  (e.g., Jackson-Pratt, Hemovac)
Umbilical tapes

Special Notes

Verify with blood bank that number of units of blood ordered are ready and available.
  Weigh sponges.
  Keep accurate record of amount of irrigation used.
  The scrub person may receive specimen in a basin.
  Keep all soiled instruments isolated in a basin.

PANCREATECTOMY

Definition

Removal of the entire pancreas.

Discussion

Partial pancreatectomy usually refers to the removal of the tail portion of the pancreas. The extent of the procedure performed depends upon the site and nature of the lesion. Indications for pancreatectomy include ductal obstruction, pancreatic stones, pancreatic cysts, trauma, benign or malignant tumors, and endocrine tumors. If total pancreatectomy is performed for benign disease or a malignancy restricted to a very distal portion of the pancreas, a small portion at the head of the pancreas may remain and be attached to the duodenum along with the common bile duct.

Procedure

A transverse, midline, or right paramedian incision is made. The abdomen is explored. If total pancreatectomy is to be performed, see Pancreaticoduodenectomy, pp. 81–82. If only the distal portion of the pancreas is removed, the pancreas is mobilized by dissecting it from numerous vascular attachments, transsecting the gland at the appropriate point, and the proximal portion of the pancreas remaining is oversewn. The operative site is usually drained. The wound is closed in layers.

Preparation of the Patient, Skin Preparation, Draping, Equipment, Instrumentation, Supplies, and Special Notes

See Pancreaticoduodenectomy (Whipple Procedure), pp. 82–83.

DRAINAGE OF ABSCESS(ES) IN THE REGION OF THE LIVER

Definition

Evacuation of purulent material within a confined space in or about the liver.

Discussion

The location of the abscess is determined by sonogram, CT scan, or other x-ray study. A radiologist may aspirate and drain the abscess percutaneously. If percutaneous drainage is inadequate, open surgical drainage is peformed. The abscesses are classified as left and right subdiaphragmatic, or subhepatic, and intrahepatic. Multiple abscesses may be present.

Procedure

An incision is made posteriorly along the twelfth rib extraperitoneally, or anteriorly, either extraperitoneally or transperitoneally. The abscess is identified and cultures are taken. The abscess is evacuated and may be irrigated with an antibiotic solution. Drains are placed. The wound is closed in layers.

Preparation of Patient

The patient is supine; arms may be extended on armboards for an upper midline or subcostal approach. For a posterolateral approach, the patient is in the lateral position with the right side uppermost. The left arm is extended on an armboard; the right arm is supported by a Mayo stand padded with a pillow (or a double armboard may be used). The left leg is extended, and the right leg is flexed with a pillow between the legs and padding around the feet and ankles. Position is secured by wide adhesive tape from the shoulders, hips, and legs to the table. Apply electrosurgical dispersive pad.

Skin Preparation

For a *subcostal approach,* begin at the incision extending from axilla to just above the pubic symphysis, and down to the table at the sides.

For a *posterolateral approach,* begin at the incision (eighth interspace) extending from the shoulder to the iliac crest and down to the table anteriorly and posteriorly.

Draping

Folded towels and a laparotomy or transverse sheet (depending on incision)

Equipment

Electrosurgical unit
Suction

Instrumentation

Major procedures tray
Long instruments tray
Biliary tract tray (available)
Harrington retractor

Supplies

Basin set
Electrosurgical pencil
Suction tubing
Blades (2) No. 10, (1) No. 15
Needle magnet or counter
Drainage materials
Culture tubes (aerobic and anaerobic)
Antibiotic irrigation (optional)

Special Notes

Determine position of patient.

All instruments that come in contact with the abscess are isolated in a basin.

"Clean" closure of the abdomen requires regowning, regloving, and redraping and a Basic/Minor procedures tray.

Protect skin under adhesive tape with tincture of benzoin.

HEPATIC RESECTION

Definition

Refers to a small wedge biopsy, local excision of tumors, or a major lobectomy.

Discussion

Indications for hepatic resection include trauma, cysts, or tumors, benign (e.g., hemangioma) and malignant (e.g., primary or secondary, i.e., metastatic). A preoperative CT scan or angiogram delineates the pathology.

Procedure

The incision is determined by the section of the liver to be resected. Feasibility of resection is determined. If a thoracoabdominal incision is employed, the abdominal portion is incised first. The thoracic portion of the incision is made incising the diaphragm. Hepatic artery, portal vein, and major biliary ducts are controlled by vascular forceps or vessel loops. The liver parenchyma is divided, pausing to ligate major vascular and biliary channels. Careful technique is necessary when approaching the posterior surface where the hepatic veins enter the inferior vena cava. If bleeding is excessive, the vena cava may be controlled by the insertion of balloon catheters intracavally. After hemostasis is obtained and the bile ducts are ligated, the exposed parenchyma may be covered by greater omentum or absorbable hemostatic agents. The area is drained. The abdomen is closed in layers.

Preparation of Patient

For partial left lobe excision a subcostal approach is employed; the patient is supine with arms extended on armboards. For major resection the approach is thoracoabdominal; the patient is in a modified (45°) lateral position with right side uppermost. The left arm is extended on an armboard; the right arm is supported by a Mayo stand padded with a pillow (or a double armboard may be used). The left leg is extended, and the right leg is flexed with a pillow between the legs and padding around the feet and ankles. The position is secured by wide adhesive tape from the shoulders, hips, and legs to the table. Apply electrosurgical dispersive pad.

Skin Preparation

For a subcostal approach begin at the incision extending from axilla to just above the pubic symphysis, and down to the table at the sides. For a posterolateral approach begin at the incision (eighth interspace) extending from the shoulder to the iliac crest, and down to the table anteriorly and posteriorly.

Draping

Folded towels and a transverse or laparotomy sheet

Equipment

Electrosurgical unit
Suctions (2)

Hypothermia mattress (available)
Manometer (for measuring portal pressure)
Cell saver (optional)

Instrumentation

Major procedures tray
Long instruments tray
Gastrointestinal procedures tray
Biliary tract tray (available)
Thoracotomy tray (for thoracoabdominal approach)
Hemoclip appliers (various sizes and lengths)

Supplies

Basin set
Blades (3) No. 10
Electrosurgical pencil
Suction tubing
Hemoclips (various sizes)
Dissectors (e.g., peanut)
Needle magnet or counter
Hemostatic agents (e.g., Helistat, Hemostat, Thrombo-
   stat, Avitene, cryoprecipitate)
Vessel loops (optional)

For Thoracoabdominal Approach, Add
   Chest tubes (e.g., Argyle)
   Intrapleural sealed drainage unit (e.g., Pleurevac)
   Y-connector
   Bulb syringe

Special Notes

Inquire if a hypothermia mattress is necessary.
   Confirm with blood bank that the number of units or-
dered are ready and available.
   Special liver sutures are available.
   Cavitron or plasma scalpel or argon beam coagulator
may be employed.
   Weigh sponges.
   Keep accurate record of the amount of irrigation used.
   Protect skin under adhesive tape with tincture of
benzoin.

SPLENECTOMY

Definition

Removal of the spleen.

Discussion

Most common indication for splenectomy is accidental injury. Other indications include hematologic disorders, tumors, cysts, or splenomegaly, and in staging of Hodgkin's disease. Splenectomy may also be indicated as the result of trauma during surgery, as in gastrectomy or mobilization of the splenic flexure of the colon; an attempt is made to preserve the traumatized spleen with suture techniques and hemostatic agents. Splenectomy is avoided whenever possible to avoid the necessity for indefinite protection against pneumococcal pneumonia. Accessory spleens may be present in perisplenic tissues; rarely they are found in more removed sites.

Procedure

A midline or left subcostal incision is made. The spleen is identified and the splenic hilum is isolated, taking care not to injure the tail of the pancreas. The splenic vessels (may be multiple) are divided and ligated. The enlarged spleen may be adherent to surrounding structures including the parietal peritoneum and diaphragm. The spleen is removed. The wound may be irrigated. Hemostasis is achieved, and the wound is closed in layers. If optimal hemostasis cannot be achieved or there is a question of pancreatic injury, a closed suction unit may be employed.

Preparation of the Patient

The patient is supine; arms may be extended on armboards for an abdominal approach. Rarely, a thoracoabdominal approach is indicated for massive splenomegaly.

Skin Preparation

Begin at the incision extending from the axilla to just above the pubic symphysis, and down to the table at the sides.

Draping

Folded towels and a laparotomy or transverse sheet (depending on incision)

Equipment

Electrosurgical unit
Suction
Cell saver (optional)

Instrumentation

Major procedures tray
Gastrointestinal procedures tray
Long instruments tray (available)
Harrington retractor
Hemoclip appliers (various sizes and lengths)
Automatic stapling device (optional)

Supplies

Basin set
Electrosurgical pencil
Suction tubing
Blades (2) No. 10, (1) No. 15
Hemoclips (various sizes)
Dissectors (e.g., peanut)
Hemostatic agents (e.g., Thrombostat, Avitene, Heli-stat)
Needle magnet or counter
Drains; for retraction (e.g., 1″ Penrose); for drainage (e.g., Jackson-Pratt or Hemovac)
Umbilical tapes
Staples (optional)

Special Notes

Verify with the blood bank that the number of units of blood ordered are ready and available.

Weigh sponges.

Keep an accurate record of the amount of irrigation used.

The scrub person may receive specimen in a basin.

LAPAROSCOPIC SPLENECTOMY

Definition

Endoscopic removal of the spleen.

Discussion

Laparoscopic splenectomy has been performed in patients with idiopathic thrombocytopenic purpura (ITP) or as part of a staging procedure (as for Hodgkin's disease). The splenic tissue should be entirely removed (including possible accessory spleens) to avoid the occurrence of postoperative splenosis. When the procedure is part of a staging laparoscopy, it is performed with bi-lobar superficial and deep hepatic biopsies peri/para-aortic and pelvic lymph node sampling is taken. Large or adherent spleens are often difficult to remove laparoscopically, necessitating an open procedure.

Procedure

Pneumoperitoneum is created, and a 10- to 11-mm trocar is inserted in the midline 2 to 3 cm above the umbilicus. The additional trocars are then inserted. The abdomen is explored, with emphasis placed on identifying any accessory spleen, which is critical in the treatment of patients with ITP.

A window into the lesser sac is created adjacent to the greater curvature of the stomach. The vessels are clipped and cut to create an appropriate-sized window. The 30° telescope is introduced into the lesser sac. The splenic artery is meticulously dissected and clipped but not yet transsected. The splenic vein is also clipped. The telescope is withdrawn from the lesser sac, and dissection of the spleen is initiated. Retraction is required on both sides of the spleen. Through the most lateral port on the right, an endoscopic Babcock is used to grasp the greater curvature of the stomach (opposite the hilum of the spleen), retracting it medially. An endoscopic extrudable fan retractor is inserted via the most lateral port on the left side to retract the spleen upward and laterally. Any additional vascular supply to the spleen (which can be variable) is identified, clipped, and divided. Electrosurgery should be avoided in controlling these large vessels. Care is taken to avoid injury to the tail of the pancreas. The peripheral attachments or perisplenic adhesions are then severed, the previously controlled hilar vessels are transsected, the spleen removed through an ancillary incision, or in ITP, when the anatomy of the specimen is not a factor, the spleen may be morcellated within a specimen bag and removed via a port. If visualization is inadequate or bleeding excessive, the procedure must be promptly converted to an open approach. After hemostasis is assured, the pneumoperitoneum is released and the wounds closed in the usual manner.

Preparation of the Patient

The patient is supine, and the arms are tucked in at the patient's sides unless the patient is obese and then the right arm may be placed on an armboard. Sequential compression stockings may be put on both legs to avoid pooling of blood in the extremities. A nasogastric tube is usually placed by the anesthetist. Apply electrosurgical dispersive pad. Initially the patient is placed in Trendelenburg 5 to 10° to allow the viscera to gravitate inferiorly. The table may be rotated to the right to increase exposure.

Skin Preparation

Begin at the midline extending from the axilla to the pubic symphysis and down to the table at the sides.

Draping

Folded towels and a laparoscopy sheet
Camera cable cover (with ties, plastic)

Equipment

Padding for elbows and ankles
Suction
Electrosurgical unit
Light source (e.g., Xenon 300 W)
Video monitors (2)
VCR (optional)

Mavigraph (optional)
CO_2 insufflator
Silastic and suction tubing with 3-way stopcock
Sequential compression device

Instrumentation

Major tray (opened)
Verres needle
Hasson trocar
Trocars (2) 10 to 11 mm
Trocars (2) 5 mm
Reducer caps
Extrudable fan-shaped retractor, endoscopic
Unipolar electrosurgical dissector, endoscopic (1)
Telescope(s)
Light cord
Camera
Graspers, endoscopic
Scissors, endoscopic
Clip applier, endoscopic
Endoscopic stapling device

Supplies

Fog reduction agent
Silastic tubing (straight, 1000-mL bag normal saline,
    3-way stopcock)
Pressure bag
Electrosurgical cord
Foam padding for elbows and ankles
Pneumatic antiemboletic stockings
Clip cartridges (ligating)
Staple cartridge
Video-cassette (optional)
Foley catheter
Nasogastric tube (e.g., 16 Fr)
Suction tubing
Skin closure strips

Special Notes

After the patient is in the room, position and correct the
monitors.

Position the electrosurgical unit.

Following draping, the scrub person passes off the camera cable, light cord, and Silastic tubing.

The circulator adjusts insufflator; first low flow (between 5 and 7 mm Hg), then higher flow according to surgeon's directions.

Connect and turn on the light source and white balance camera.

The circulator turns on the VCR, if requested.

The circulator rechecks the position of the monitors to see that they can be easily viewed.

The circulator corrects all remaining items: irrigation system, suction tubing, and electrosurgical cord.

All instruments (nondisposable) may be flash-sterilized.

Soak scope(s) and cord(s) in Steris solution after thorough cleansing.

Turn room and overhead lights out during the procedure; leave one light on for the scrub person. Lights will be turned on again when the procedure is completed.

Verify with the blood bank that the blood ordered is available.

Chapter 10

Gastrointestinal Surgery

ESOPHAGOSCOPY

Definition

Endoscopic visualization of the esophagus.

Discussion

Esophagoscopy is performed to diagnose malignancies, esophagitis (noting reflux), hiatal hernia, strictures, and varices; to remove tissues or secretions for study; for direct therapeutic manipulations such as removal of a foreign body, injection or coagulation of varices, or insertion of a plastic prosthesis to relieve strictures. Flexible fiberoptic esophagoscopy is most often performed in the gastrointestinal (GI) laboratory. Most often diagnostic procedures are performed employing a flexible fiberoptic scope in the gastrointestinal laboratory rather than in the operating room.

Procedure

The surgeon applies topical anesthesia (usually a spray). The head of the table is lowered. The patient's head is held by an assistant, and it is raised or lowered as the endoscopist directs until the esophagoscope is passed (the neck will be extended).

The entire esophagus including the esophagogastric junction and proximal stomach may be examined. Manipulations for diagnosis and treatment are performed. The scope is removed.

Preparation of the Patient

The patient is supine with shoulders even with or a little over the break at the head of the table to permit lowering of the head. Anesthesia is usually topical with sedation and/or analgesia administered intravenously by the anesthetist. See Bronchoscopy, pp. 246–249, for topical anesthesia tray.

Draping

Patient may be covered with a drape sheet. A drape sheet covers the back table.

Skin Preparation

None.

Equipment

Fiberoptic light source
Suction

Instrumentation

Fiberoptic esophagoscope, suction, biopsy forceps, sponge carriers, grasping forceps, dilators, and bougies
Fiberoptic light cord

Supplies

Small basin (with saline and syringe)
Lubricating jelly
Bronchoscopy sponges (on carrier)
Aspirating tubes (e.g., Leuken's)
Specimen containers
Needle, e.g., 25 gauge (to remove biopsy)
Suction tubing
Topical anesthetics (as for Bronchoscopy, pp. 246–249)

Special Notes

Check with surgeon regarding topical anesthesia.

Gloves are worn.

Protective goggles should be worn.

Pass forceps in the closed position, and guide them into the scope as requested.

Remove specimens from forceps with a needle to avoid damaging cells.

Hold aspirating tubes upright, and pinch off suction tubing as necessary to prevent aspiration of specimen.

Careful labeling and handling of specimens is essential. (Have several labels and requisitions ready.)

GASTROSCOPY

Definition

Endoscopic visualization of the stomach and proximal duodenum.

Discussion

Gastroscopy is performed for diagnosis, aspiration of gastric contents, removal of a foreign body, or tissue biopsy. Flexible fiberoptic gastroscopy is usually performed in the gastrointestinal (GI) laboratory or at the patient's bedside. For percutaneous gastrostomy, which is aided by the passage of a fiberoptic gastroscope, see Gastrostomy, pp. 114–115.

Preparation of the Patient, Skin Preparation, and Draping

See Esophagoscopy, p. 96.

Equipment

Electrosurgical unit
Fiberoptic light source
Suction

Instrumentation

Rigid fiberoptic gastroscope, suction-electrocoagulator and cord, biopsy forceps, grasping forceps, cautery
Fiberoptic light cord

Supplies

Small basin (with saline and syringe)
Lubricating jelly
Needle, e.g., 25 gauge (for specimen removal)
Specimen containers
Aspirating tubes
Suction tubing
Topical anesthetics (as for Bronchoscopy, see pp. 246–249)

Special Notes

See Esophagoscopy, p. 97.

COLONOSCOPY

Definition

Endoscopic visualization of the large intestine from rectum to cecum (and occasionally the very terminal ileum).

Discussion

Total colonoscopy is usually performed in the gastrointestinal (GI) laboratory or the radiology department. Exceptions to this include colonoscopy performed during open laparotomy or certain pediatric examinations when general anesthesia is required. Colonoscopy limited to the distal colon may be performed in the operating room by inserting only a portion of the colonoscope or by employing a flexible fiberoptic sigmoidoscope. See Sigmoidoscopy, below, for Procedure, Preparation of the Patient, Skin Preparation, Draping, Equipment, Instrumentation, and Supplies.

SIGMOIDOSCOPY

Definition

Endoscopic visualization of the anal canal, rectum, and sigmoid colon.

Discussion

This procedure is performed for diagnosis, excision of polyps, biopsy of lesions, and so on. Sigmoidoscopy is performed in the operating room under sedation or anesthesia when the patient is unable to tolerate the procedure because of pain and tenderness, or for biopsy, polypectomy, and so on, when these procedures are too risky outside the operating room environment.

Procedure

Rigid Sigmoidoscopy. The anus is digitally lubricated and examined. Anoscopy may be performed. The sigmoidoscope is inserted and advanced under direct visualization until obstructed by an unyielding angulation of the lumen or to the full length of the scope. Definitive inspection of the mucous membrane is done as the scope is withdrawn. Air may be insufflated to distend the lumen for better visualization. A variety of instruments may be used via the scope, for example, biopsy forceps, suction-electrocoagulator, snare, or clip applicator. Scopes are usually 18 to 19 mm in diameter; larger diameters to 30 mm may be employed when anesthesia is given.

Flexible Sigmoidoscopy. Digital examination and anoscopy are performed. The tip of the scope is inserted, and under direct visualization the scope is advanced by various torquing and advancement motions to the length of the scope (30 or 65 cm) or until resistance, patient discomfort, or inability to see the lumen ahead is reached. Definitive examination is done on withdrawal. Various accessory instruments (e.g., electrosurgical biopsy forceps, snare, cautery, cytology brush, or irrigating tube) may be employed.

Preparation of the Patient

Positions for rigid sigmoidoscopy include jackknife, modified lateral/Sims', or lithotomy. The modified lateral/Sims' position is generally preferred for flexible sigmoidoscopy, although the jackknife position may be employed. Apply electrosurgical dispersive pad.

Jackknife. The table is flexed, and the patient is prone with arms extended on armboards angled toward the head of the table with the hands pronated. A pillow is placed in front of the legs, and a roll is placed at the ankles. Buttocks are distracted by 3-inch or 4-inch adhesive tapes anchored to the underside of the table (pull tapes toward patient's head before anchoring them for maximal exposure) when surgery (e.g., hemorrhoidectomy) is performed. When general anesthesia is employed, chest rolls are required.

Lithotomy. The patient's legs are placed in stirrups, and the buttocks are elevated by a folded towel. Buttocks may be distracted by 3-inch or 4-inch adhesive tapes anchored to the stirrups.

Modified Lateral/Sims'. The patient lies on the left side with left arm extended on an armboard and the right arm flexed over it on a pillow (or double armboard may be used). The back is angled so that the anal canal area extends just over the table's edge. The left leg is straight and the right leg is flexed, or both legs may be flexed with a pillow between the knees; additional padding is required at feet and ankles. Buttocks are distracted by a 3-inch or 4-inch adhesive tape on the right buttock (uppermost) anchored to the underside of the table.

Skin Preparation

None

Draping

Patient may be covered with a drape sheet. A drape sheet covers the back table.

Equipment

Stirrups or pillow and rolls for positioning
Double armboard, optional

Rigid
  Fiberoptic light source
  Suction
  Electrosurgical unit

Flexible

Fiberoptic light source with a combined air insufflation and irrigation capacities

Suction (connects directly to the channel of the scope)

Electrosurgical unit

Instrumentation

Rigid

Sigmoidoscopy tray, suction-electrocoagulator and cord, biopsy forceps, snare, clip applicators, grasping forceps

Flexible

Flexible sigmoidoscope, electrosurgical biopsy forceps, suction, endoscopy snare, polyp grasper, irrigating tube, cytology brush

Supplies

Gloves
Lubricant
Suction tubing
Long cotton swabs

Special Notes

Protect skin under adhesive tape with tincture of benzoin.

Adequate padding is required for female breasts and male genitalia.

Gloves are worn.

Protective goggles should be worn.

Lubricate scope.

Clean scope immediately following use.

Rigid. Assist surgeon as necessary guiding suction, forceps, and so on, into scope, and removing biopsies as necessary.

Flexible. Be prepared to help stabilize scope. Assist surgeon by passing biopsy forceps, endoscopic snare, polyp grasper, and so on, as necessary.

The surgeon may direct the scrub person to open and close the endoscopy snare and biopsy forceps.

ESOPHAGEAL HIATAL HERNIORRHAPHY

Definition

Repair of the esophageal diaphragmatic aperture to prevent herniation of the stomach into the thorax.

Discussion

Esophageal hiatal hernia is often detected in patients who are asymptomatic. Indications for surgical repair include clinical symptoms such as gastroesophageal reflux, chest pain, and so on, with radiographic, endoscopic, and intestinal physiologic and manometric findings. On occasion, the apparent herniation of the stomach into the thoracic cavity is due to a foreshortened esophagus. Numerous procedures have been devised to correct this condition by transabdominal, transthoracic, or laparoscopic approach. The recurrence rate is relatively high. No single procedure has been determined to be best.

Procedure

A transabdominal approach will be described. The upper abdomen is exposed through a midline, paramedian, or high transverse incision. The esophagocardiac region is exposed by either retraction or mobilization of the left lobe of the liver. The herniated stomach is reduced, and the posterior mediastinal space is entered exposing the distal esophagus. The crural fibers of the esophageal hiatus of the diaphragm are exposed and, with the stomach distracted inferiorly, approximated (usually with nonabsorbable suture) inferior and posterior to the distal esophagus. The distal esophagus may be sutured to reflected portions of the peritoneum, phrenicoesophageal ligament, and to the gastric cardia maintaining an acute esphagogastric angle. Care must be taken to avoid making the repair too tight and to injuring the vagus nerves. The anesthetist may be asked to pass a large-diameter esophageal bougie to determine that the hiatus is not unduly compromised.

Preparation of the Patient, Skin
Preparation, Draping, Equipment,
Instrumentation, and Supplies

See Vagotomy and Pyloroplasty, pp. 106–108.

LAPAROSCOPIC FUNDOPLICATION (NISSEN PROCEDURE)

Definition

Endoscopic wrapping of the gastric fundus about the cardia to correct gastroesophageal reflux and/or hiatal hernia.

Discussion

This procedure is used to treat gastroesophageal reflux disease and certain presentations of an esophageal hiatal hernia by physically reestablishing the gastroesophageal angle and a barrier to intrathoracic gastric displacement.

Procedure

Pneumoperitoneum is established, and ports are placed as for Laparoscopic Vagotomy, pp. 109–110. The left lobe of the liver is retracted, and incising of the triangular ligament is done as necessary. The esophageal hiatus is visualized. The gastric cardia is distracted with reduction of the hiatal hernia, if present, and the phrenoesphageal ligament is incised. The left gastric artery and vegal nerve branches are displaced. A window is dissected past the distal esophagus through which a drain or soft catheter (e.g., 12 or 14 Fr) is placed to provide traction on the esophagus. The stomach may be mobilized by dividing the short gastric vessels on the greater curvature. If the esophageal hiatus is enlarged, several sutures may be placed to minimize the crural defect. A 50 to 60 Fr esophageal dilator is passed transorally. The gastric fundus is seized by an atraumatic grasping forceps passed posterior to the esophagus. An adjacent portion of the fundus is seized anterior to the esophagus and apposed to the posteriorly seized segment and sutured or stapled incorporating the esophagocardiac wall, completing the fundoplication. The drain or catheter and esophageal dilators are removed. After the surgical field is inspected for hemostasis and irrigated as necessary, pneumoperitoneum is released, and the ports are closed in the usual manner.

Preparation of the Patient

The patient is supine; arms are padded and may be tucked in at the patient's sides unless the patient is obese, in which case the right arm may be placed on an armboard. Sequential compression stockings may be put on both legs to avoid pooling of blood in the extremeties. A nasogastric tube is usually placed by the anesthetist. Apply electrosurgical dispersive pad. The table is placed in Trendelenburg 5 to 10° to establish pneumoperitoneum and then in reverse Trendelenburg 10 to 20° to allow the viscera to gravitate inferiorly. The table may be rotated slightly to the right to increase exposure.

Skin Preparation

Begin at the midline extending from the axilla to the pubic symphysis and down to the table at the sides.

Draping

Folded towels and laparoscopy sheet
Camera cable cover (with ties, plastic)

Equipment

Padding for elbows and ankles
Suction
Electrosurgical unit
Light source (e.g., Xenon 300 W)
Video monitors (2)
VCR (optional)
Mavigraph (optional)
CO_2 insufflator
Pressure bag to facilitate irrigation

Silastic and suction tubing with 3-way stopcock
Sequential compression device

Instrumentation

Major tray (open)
Verres needle
Hasson trocar
Trocars 10 to 11 mm (2)
Trocars 5 mm (2 or 3)
Reducer caps
Dissector clamps, endoscopic, with unipolar cautery (2)
Dissector hook, endoscopic
Grasping clamps (4) (2 traumatic, locking; 2 atrau-
    matic), endoscopic
Irrigation, suction, electrosurgical device, endoscopic
    J-hook tip, endoscopic, or right-angle electrosurgical
    dissector with suction, irrigation
Babcock clamp 10 mm (atraumatic), endoscopic
Babcock clamp 5 mm (atraumatic), endoscopic
Allis clamp
Scissors (3) (hook, straight, and micro), endoscopic
Clip applier, endoscopic
Laparascope(s) and camera(s)
Stapling device (e.g., endo GIA), endoscopic
Extrudable fan retractor, endoscopic

Supplies

Fog reduction agent
Silastic tubing (straight, 1000-mL bag normal saline,
    3-way stopcock)
Pressure bag
Electrosurgical cord
Foam padding for elbows and ankles
Pneumatic antiembolitic stockings
Clip cartridges (ligating)
Staple cartridge
Video-cassette (optional)
Foley catheter
Nasogastric tube (e.g., 16 Fr)
Suction tubing
Skin closure strips

Special Notes

After the patient is in the room, position and connect monitors.

Position electrosurgical unit.

Following draping, the scrub person passes off the camera cable, light cord, Silastic tubing.

The circulator adjusts insufflator; first low flow (between 5 and 7 mm Hg), then higher flow according to surgeon's instructions.

Connect and turn on the light source and white balance camera.

The circulator turns on VCR, if requested.

The circulator rechecks the position of the monitors to see that they can be easily viewed.

The circulator connects all remaining items: irrigation system, suction tubing, electrosurgical cord.

All instruments (nondisposable) may be flash-sterilized.

Soak scope(s) and cord(s) in Steris solution after thorough cleansing.

Turn the room lights and overhead lights out during the procedure; leave one light on for the scrub person. Lights will be turned on again when the procedure is completed.

VAGOTOMY AND PYLOROPLASTY

Definition

Vagotomy. The transection of the vagus nerves (or peripheral divisions) performed at the level of the distal esophagus, or at the gastric cardia, to reduce gastric secretion in patients with peptic ulcers.

Pyloroplasty. The enlargement of the gastric outlet, which will enhance emptying of the stomach.

Discussion

Vagotomy may be truncal or selective. In truncal vagotomy the main trunks of the vagus nerve are interrupted, including branches to the stomach and other abdominal viscera. Selective vagotomy (of which there are several modifications) is performed about the gastric cardia, so that primarily gastric vagal nerves are interrupted. Pyloroplasty is performed in conjunction with vagotomy to enhance gastric emptying, which is otherwise delayed when vagus nerves have been transsected.

Procedure

The upper abdomen is exposed through a midline, paramedian, or high transverse incision. Physical findings are assessed, and either truncal or selective vagotomy is performed. Hemoclips are applied to the severed nerve trunks. Small sections of vagus nerve are sent to pathology to confirm that neural tissue was actually divided. Pyloroplasty is then performed. The most commonly performed procedure is Heinieke-Mikulicz, in which the pyloroduodenal junction is incised longitudinally and closed transversely. In patients with severe bleeding, a gastrotomy or duodenotomy may be necessary to identify and control the bleeding site.

Preparation of the Patient

The patient is supine; arms may be extended on armboards. Apply electrosurgical dispersive pad.

Skin Preparation

Begin at the midline extending from axilla to the pubic symphysis, and down to the table at the sides.

Draping

Folded towels and a laparotomy or transverse sheet

Equipment

Electrosurgical unit
Suction

Instrumentation

Major procedures tray
Long instruments tray
Gastrointestinal procedures tray

Blunt nerve hook (e.g., Smithwick)
Hemoclip appliers (various sizes and lengths, especially long)

Supplies

Basin set
Blades (3) No. 10, (1) No. 15
Needle magnet or counter
Suction tubing
Electrosurgical pencil
Penrose drains (2) long, 1″ (for traction on esophagus)
Hemoclips (assorted sizes)

Special Notes

Left and right vagus nerve specimens must be kept separate and labeled accurately.

LAPAROSCOPIC VAGOTOMY

Definition

The endoscopic transection of the vagus nerves (or peripheral divisions) at the level of the distal esophagus
or gastric cardia.

Discussion

There are numerous procedures and their modifications to diminish gastric acid secretion as related to
peptic ulcer disease. Many of these modifications can be
performed laparoscopically. Most often interruption of
the vagus nerves or branches thereof must be accomplished. Selective vagotomy versus truncal (complete)
vagotomy permits gastric emptying without the need
for an accompanying drainage procedure (pyloroplasty,
gastricjejunostomy, partial gastrectomy, and so on) unless advanced peptic ulcer disease with fibrosis or
stricture are present, in which case the latter may be
necessary. In some instances within several hours of
perforation of a peptic ulcer, vagotomy may be combined with the application of an omental patch to the
site of the perforation.

Procedure

Pneumoperitoneum is established in the umbilical or supraumbilical position. Additional ports are established inferior to the left and right costal margins midaxillary line, subzyphoid and midleft upper quadrant. After the abdomen is explored and the feasibility of the laparoscopic procedure is determined, through a right subcostal port an extrudable fanshaped retractor is inserted to displace the left lobe of the liver (dividing the triangular ligament if necessary). A 30° scope is preferred by most surgeons. A large-bore nasogastric tube or esophageal dilator may be passed by the anesthetist to facilitate traction on the stomach. As indicated, an endoscope may be passed to dilate the pyloric channel.

The lesser sac is entered, and the tissues along the lesser curvature to the esophageal hiatus are dissected. The left gastric vein may be divided between sutures or clips. The left margin of the right crus of the diaphragm and the stomach are retracted to the left. The paraesophageal tissues are dissected to expose the esophagus, which is retracted to the left. The posterior vagus nerve is identified, divided, and ligated with clips. A section is sent for histologic confirmation. The anterior vagus nerve is now exposed. Most often a selective vagotomy is elected (versus truncal). Branches to the other viscera (including the nerve of Laterget) are preserved. Gastric branches are identified (employing dissection of the gastric serosa as necessary), clipped, and divided. Hemostasis is assured, irrigation employed accordingly. Pneumoperitoneum is released, and ports are closed.

An alternative procedure is the Post Truncal Vagotomy with Anterior Serotomy (Taylor's Procedure). The procedure is identical to that described above to the point of the division of the posterior vegal trunk. As branches of the anterior vagus nerve are often imbedded within the seromuscular layer of the stomach, preventing division of the individual branches, a seromyotomy 1.5 cm from the lesser curvature from the cardia to a point proximal to the pylorus (5–7 cm) is made. Care is taken to avoid penetration of the mucosa. The seromyotomy is then repaired with staples or a running suture. Methylene blue dye may be instilled into the stomach via nasogastric tube to verify integrity of the gastric repair. A fibrin sealant (e.g., Tisucol) may be applied to the tissue line. A variant of the procedure is to distract a seromuscular strip (in lieu of seromyotomy), excising it using a multifire linear stapler, thus interrupting the intramural vagal branches.

After the vagotomy is complete, a congo red test may be performed. In addition to histologic confirmation that the nervous tissue was removed, testing for gastric acidity may be done intraoperatively. Pentagastrin (to stimulate gastric acid production) 6 μg/kg is given subcutaneously. Twenty minutes prior to the testing, the stomach is lavaged through the laparascope with sodium bicarbonate solution to remove residual acid. Congo red dye is instilled into the stomach to coat the gastric mucosa. If vagotomy is complete, the red dye remains unchanged. If even partial innervation remains, the affected area will turn black as seen via the scope and additional nerve transection may be done.

Hemostasis is assured. The pneumoperitoneum is released. Ports are closed in the usual manner.

Preparation of the Patient

The patient is supine; arms may be padded and tucked in at the patient's sides unless the patient is obese, and then the right arm may be placed on an armboard. Sequential compression stockings may be put on both legs to avoid pooling of blood in the lower extremeties. A nasogastric tube is placed by the anesthetist. A Foley catheter may be inserted. Apply electrosurgical dispersive pad. The table is placed in a Trendelenburg 5 to 10° to establish pneumoperitoneum and then in reverse Trendelenburg 10 to 20° to allow the abdominal viscera to gravitate inferiorly. The table may be rotated slightly to the right to increase exposure of the stomach.

Skin Preparation

Begin at the midline extending from axilla to the pubic symphysis and down to the table at the sides.

Draping

Folded towels and a laparoscopy sheet
Camera cable cover (with ties, plastic)

Equipment

Suction
Electrosurgical unit
Light source (e.g., Xenon 300 W)
Video monitors (2)
VCR (optional)
Mavigraph (optional)
CO_2 insufflator
Pressure bag to facilitate irrigation
Silastic and suction tubing
Sequential compression device

Instrumentation

Major tray (open)
Verres needle
Hasson trocar
Trocars 10 to 11 mm (2)
Trocars 5 mm (2 or 3)
Reducer caps
Dissector clamps, endoscopic (2)
Dissector hook, endoscopic
Grasping clamps (4) (2 traumatic, locking; atraumatic),
    endoscopic
Irrigation, suction, electrosurgical device, endoscopic
J-hook tip, endoscopic
Babcock clamp 10 mm (atraumatic), endoscopic
Babcock clamp 5 mm (atraumatic), endoscopic
Allis clamp, endoscopic
Scissors (3) (hook, straight, micro), endoscopic
Clip applier, endoscopic
Laparoscope(s) and camera(s)
Stapling device (e.g., endo GIA) endoscopic, available
Extrudable fan retractor, endoscopic

Supplies

Fog reduction agent
Silastic tubing (straight, 1000-mL bag normal saline,
    3-way stopcock)

Electrosurgical cord
Pressure bag
Foam padding for elbows and ankles
Pneumatic antiembolitic stockings
Clip cartridge (ligating)
Staple cartridge
Video-cassette (optional)
Foley catheter
Nasogastric tube (e.g., No. 16)
Luer lock syringes (2)
Methylene blue dye
Congo red dye
Suction tubing
Suture material (optional)
Fibrin sealant (e.g., Tisuol)
Skin closure strips

Special Notes

After the patient is in the room, position and connect monitors.

Position the electrosurgical unit.

Following draping, the scrub person passes off the camera cable, light cord, and Silastic tubing.

The circulator adjusts the insufflator, first low flow (between 5 and 7 mm Hg), then higher flow according to the surgeon's instructions.

Connect and turn on the light source and white balance camera.

The circulator turns on the VCR to record, if requested.

The circulator rechecks the position of monitors so they can be easily viewed.

The circulator connects all remaining items: irrigation system, suction tubing, electrosurgical cord.

All instruments (nondisposable) may be flash-sterilized.

Soak scope(s) and light cord(s) in Steris solution after thorough cleansing.

Turn the room lights and overhead lights out during procedure; leave one light on overhead for the scrub person. Lights will be turned on again when the procedure is completed.

CLOSURE OF A PERFORATED PEPTIC ULCER

Definition

Surgical closure of a perforated gastric or duodenal ulcer.

Discussion

A complication of peptic ulcer disease in spontaneous perforation with escape of gastroduodenal secretions is peritonitis. The presentation may be mild with spontaneous closure of the perforation treated by nonsurgical means to extensive life-threatening peritonitis. Less often a gastric malignancy may present in similar fashion. Numerous surgical procedures are described for this condition. When preexisting peptic ulcer disease has been present and peritoneal irritation is limited, a vagotomy (see pp. 106–108) may be performed.

Procedure

An upper abdominal incision (midline, right paramedian) is made. The site of perforation identified. Fluid and debris are aspirated. If not already partially adherent to the perforation, a portion of adjacent greater omentum (or gastrocolic ligament, etc.) is sutured or stapled to the stomach or duodenum surrounding the perforation. If malignancy is suspected, appropriate biopsies may be taken. Concomitant vagotomy may then be performed (see Vagotomy, pp. 106–108). After hemostasis is assured and drains (if any) are placed, the wound is closed in the usual manner.

Preparation of the Patient, Skin Preparation, Draping, Equipment, Instruments, Supplies, and Special Notes

See Vagotomy and Pyloroplasty pp. 106–108.

LAPAROSCOPIC CLOSURE OF A PERFORATED ULCER (WITH VAGOTOMY)

Definition

Closure of perforated stomach or duodenal ulcer and excision of vagus nerve and its branches performed laparoscopically.

Discussion

Limitations to this approach include advanced peritonitis, dense adhesions, and so on.

Procedure

Pneumoperitoneum and ports are established as for Laparoscopic Vagotomy (see, p. 108). The pathology is assessed, and fluid is aspirated and sent for culture. The peritoneal cavity may be irrigated. The site of the perforation is closed with endoscopic sutures if feasible. An omental patch is then stapled or sutured over the site of the perforation. The lesser employed alternative technique is to pass an endoscope transorally through which a grasping forceps is placed from within the stomach or duodenum into the peritoneal cavity seizing (with laparoscopic guidance) a portion of omentum, which is then retracted onto the perforation. The patch is secured with endoscopic suture or staples, and the endoscope withdrawn. Vagotomy may then be performed; as described in Laparoscopic Vagotomy, pp. 108–110. A closed suction drain may be placed. After release of pneumoperitoneum, the ports are closed in the usual manner.

Preparation of the Patient, Skin
Preparation, Draping, Equipment,
Instruments, Supplies and Special Notes

See Laparoscopic Vagotomy, pp. 110–112.

GASTROSTOMY

Definition

Establishment of an artificial opening into the stomach exiting onto the skin of the abdominal wall.

Discussion

A gastrostomy, either temporary or permanent, is used to drain the stomach or allow for liquid feedings for patients with esophageal stricture or tumor. A catheter (e.g., Foley) maintains the patency of the gastrostomy tract. Recently, *percutaneous gastrostomy,* a nonoperative method, has been employed. A flexible fiberoptic gastroscope is passed into the stomach, which is distended with air. The lighted tip of the scope is impacted on the gastric wall. A second operator passes a catheter through a percutaneous stab wound, aiming at the transilluminated gastroscope tip. Gastrostomy is often performed as an adjunct to a more extensive procedure. In a debilitated patient, gastrostomy may be performed under local anesthesia.

Procedure

A gastrostomy (feeding) as an isolated procedure is performed through a limited transverse left upper abdominal incision. The peritoneal cavity is entered, the gastric wall is identified, and concentric purse-string sutures are placed. A small incision is made into the stomach (within the innermost purse-string suture) through which a catheter is passed. The purse-string sutures are secured. The catheter can exit through the incision or preferably a separate stab wound. The gastric wall is sutured at a few points to the peritoneal surface of the stab wound. The abdomen is closed in layers.

Preparation of the Patient

The patient is supine; arms may be extended on armboards. Apply electrosurgical dispersive pad.

Skin Preparation

Begin at the incision (usually transverse left upper abdominal) extending from nipples to upper thighs, and down to the table at the sides.

Draping

Folded towels and a transverse sheet

Equipment

Suction
Electrosurgical unit

Instrumentation

Major procedures tray
Hemoclip appliers

Supplies

Basin set
Blades (2) No. 10, (1) No. 15
Needle magnet or counter
Gastrostomy catheter (e.g., Foley, Pezzer)
Electrosurgical pencil
Suction tubing
Hemoclips (assorted)
Catheter plug

Special Notes

Have suction ready as soon as the incision into the stomach is made.

GASTRECTOMY

Definition

Removal of the stomach and reestablishment of the continuity of the gastrointestinal tract.

Discussion

Subtotal (partial) gastrectomy refers to the excision of a portion of the stomach performed primarily for peptic ulcer disease or tumor of the distal stomach. A vagotomy (see pp. 106–107) may be included. Gastrointestinal continuity is reestablished by anastomosing of the gastric remnant to the proximal duodenum (Bilroth I) or to the proximal jejunum (Billroth II, or a modification of it). When treating malignancies, the greater omentum, lymph nodes, and adjacent organs (e.g., spleen) are removed.

    Total gastrectomy is often performed because of malignancy or uncontrollable bleeding. Continuity of the gastrointestinal tract is established by anastomosing distal esophagus to the proximal jejunum, usually with the creation of a pouch or reservoir. (The duodenum or an isolated segment of colon can also replace the resected stomach.) The lymph nodes, adjacent organs, and greater omentum are removed when treating malignancies.

Procedure

The incision may be upper midline or bilateral subcostal. For total gastrectomy a thoracoabdominal incision may be necessary. The pathology is identified, and its operability assessed. The stomach is mobilized by clamping and dividing the vascular attachments. The greater omentum and sometimes the spleen are resected in continuity with the stomach en bloc when malignancy is present. According to the extent of the resection and the type of anastomosis to be fashioned, the duodenum or jejunum is mobilized and anastomosed to the gastric remnant (or distal esophagus) anterior or posterior to the transverse colon. A retrocolic anastomosis requires an incision to be made in a relatively avascular portion of the transverse mesocolon. Anastomosis is facilitated by the use of automatic stapling devices, or a wide variety of sutures and suturing techniques may be employed. A side-to-side jejunal pouch may be required when total gastrectomy is performed. A drain (e.g., Jackson-Pratt or Hemovac) is inserted. If the pleural space has been entered, an intrapleural sealed drainage unit (e.g., Pleurevac) is necessary. The wound is closed in layers. Drains are anchored.

Preparation of the Patient

For an upper midline or bilateral subcostal approach, the patient is supine. For a thoracoabdominal approach, the patient is in a modified (45°) lateral/Sims' position with the left side uppermost. The right arm is on an armboard; left arm is supported by a Mayo stand padded with a pillow (or a double armboard may be used). The right leg is extended, and the left leg is flexed with a pillow between the legs and padding around the feet and ankles. A pillow folded longitudinally may be necessary to support the back. The position is secured by wide adhesive tape from the shoulders, hips, and legs to the table. Apply electrosurgical dispersive pad.

Skin Preparation

For an upper midline or bilateral subcostal approach, begin at incision extending from the axilla to just above the pubic symphysis, and down to the table at the sides. For a thoracoabdominal approach, begin at the incision extending from the shoulder to the iliac crest, and down to the table anteriorly and posteriorly.

Draping

Folded towels and a transverse or laparotomy sheet

Equipment

Suction
Electrosurgical unit
Pillows, pads for positioning (for thoracoabdominal approach)

Instrumentation

Major procedures tray
Long instruments tray
Gastrointestinal procedures tray
Hemoclip appliers (various sizes and lengths)
Long blunt nerve hooks (2, e.g., Smithwick)
Automatic stapling devices (optional)
Large self-retaining retractor (e.g., Balfour)

Supplies

Blades (2) No. 10, (1) No. 15
Basin set
Needle magnet or counter
Suction tubing
Electrosurgical pencil
Hemoclips (variety)
Staples (optional)

For Thoracoabdominal Approach, Add
  Chest tubes (e.g., Argyle)
  Intrapleural sealed drainage unit (e.g., Pleurevac)
  Y-connector
  Bulb syringe

Special Notes

Check that blood has been ordered and is available.
Weigh sponges.

Keep an accurate record of irrigation fluid used.

Have rubber-shod clamps ready (prevents tissue damage to bowel).

Keep all soiled instruments isolated in a basin.

Have long, free ties ready.

Frozen section may be requested.

Surgeon may request a "clean" closure of the abdomen; this requires regowning, regloving, redraping, and a Basic/Minor procedures tray.

SMALL-BOWEL RESECTION

Definition

Excision of a segment of the small intestine to remove an obstruction, a gangrenous portion of the bowel, a perforation, or source of a hemorhhage, and so on. The remaining small bowel is anastomosed to a segment of more distal small bowel or colon.

Discussion

Small-bowel resection is infrequently performed as an isolated procedure as for inflammatory bowel disease, rare primary tumors, and mesenteric infarctions. More often, the small bowel is resected in the course of other procedures because of adhesive obstructive bowel disease, tumors of adjacent organs, and inflammatory processes as diverticulitis or tubo-ovarian abscess.

Procedure

As an Isolated Procedure. An incision is made so that the entire small bowel is accessible, especially if the patient has had previous surgery and there are adhesions. The mesentery is divided, ligating vascular structures; the affected segment is excised, and continuity of the bowel is restored by suturing the ends of the remaining small bowel together. An automatic stapling device may be employed, or one- or two-layered anastomoses may be performed. The abdomen is closed in layers.

As Part of Another Procedure. Similar steps are taken leaving the resected segment attached to the adherent organ also to be resected (e.g., colon, ovary).

Preparation of the Patient

The patient is supine; arms may be extended on armboards. Apply electrosurgical dispersive pad.

Skin Preparation

Begin at the incision (usually right paramedian) from nipples to upper thighs, and down to the table at the sides.

Draping

Folded towels and a laparotomy sheet

Equipment

Suction
Electrosurgical unit

Instrumentation

Major procedures tray
Long instruments tray
Gastrointestinal procedures tray
Hemoclip appliers (variety)
Self-retaining retractor (e.g., Balfour)
Automatic stapling devices (optional)

Supplies

Basin set
Blades (2) No. 10, (1) No. 15
Hemoclips (assorted sizes)
Electrosurgical pencil
Needle magnet or counter
Staples (optional)

CUTANEOUS ILEOSTOMY

Definition

Formation of temporary or permanent opening of the ileum, which is brought out onto the abdomen as a stoma.

Discussion

Cutaneous ileostomy is performed to divert the fecal stream in resection of the colon and rectum (permanent end ileostomy); to protect a distal anastomosis, for example, ileo-anal (temporary loop ileostomy); or to relieve inflammatory bowel disease of the colon with or without distal resection. A continent ileostomy (Koch pouch) consists of a stoma in continuity with a pouch of folded and sutured ileum that serves as a reservoir. The patient catheterizes the stoma to empty the pouch.

Procedure

The abdomen is entered, usually through a right paramedian or midline incision. A disc of skin and subcutaneous fat is excised at the ileostomy site; the anterior rectus sheath is incised and a small fragment removed. The incision is deepened into the peritoneum. The ileum is cleared of its mesentery for several centimeters and divided, and the proximal end is passed through the stoma site onto the abdominal wall. The distal end of the ileum, unless resected, is sutured or stapled closed. The proximal end is everted on itself and sutured circumferentially. The mesentery of the terminal ileum is sutured to the parietal peritoneum to prevent internal hernia. Alternatively, a loop ileostomy may be performed. The abdomen is closed. An ileostomy appliance is placed over the stoma.

Preparation of the Patient

The patient is supine; arms may be extended on armboards. Apply electrosurgical dispersive pad.

Skin Preparation

Begin at midline extending from above nipples to the upper thighs, and down to the table on the sides.

Draping

Folded towels and a laparotomy sheet

Equipment

Suction
Electrosurgical unit

Instrumentation

Major procedures tray
Long instruments tray
Gastrointestinal procedures tray
Hemoclip appliers (various sizes and lengths)
Automatic stapling device (optional)

Supplies

Basin set
Blades (3) No. 10, (1) No. 15
Needle magnet or counter
Electrosurgical pencil
Suction tubing
Hemoclips (various sizes)
Marking pen (optional)
Staples (optional)
Ileostomy appliance (e.g., Karaya Seal)

APPENDECTOMY

Definition

Excision of the appendix, usually performed to remove the acutely inflamed organ.

Discussion

An incidental appendectomy may be performed in conjunction with other abdominal surgery.

Procedure

An incision is made in the right lower abdomen either transversely oblique (McBurney) or vertically for primary appendectomy. The appendix is identified and its vascular supply ligated. The appendix is ligated, that is, the stump is tied off with absorbable suture. The appendix is removed, and the stump may be inverted in the cecum, cauterized with chemicals or electrocoagulation, or simply left alone after ligation. Another technique is to devascularize the appendix and invert the entire appendix into the cecum. The wound is closed in layers except when an abscess has occurred with acute appendicitis, in which case the skin and subcutaneous tissues are often left open. A drain may be placed into the abscess cavity exiting through the incision or a stab wound. Antibiotic irrigation may be used.

Preparation of the Patient

The patient is supine; arms may be extended on arm-boards. Apply electrosurgical dispersive pad.

Skin Preparation

Begin in lower right quadrant (McBurney incision is most frequently used) extending from nipples to upper thighs, and down to the table at the sides.

Draping

Folded towels and a laparotomy sheet

Equipment

Electrosurgical unit

Instrumentation

Basic/Minor procedures tray

Supplies

Basin set
Blades (3) No. 10
Needle magnet or counter
Electrosurgical pencil
Culture tube (aerobic and anaerobic)
Drain (e.g., Penrose, 14", optional)
Antiobiotic irrigation (optional)

Special Notes

Instruments used for amputation of the appendix are to be isolated in a basin.

LAPAROSCOPIC APPENDECTOMY

Definition

Endoscopic excision of the appendix.

Discussion

Indications for laparoscopic appendectomy are the same as for the traditional procedure. Controversy exists, however, as to the propriety of performing laparoscopic appendectomy in that the standard open procedure can often, by a small incision, be accomplished in less time with minimal postoperative morbidity and less operating room anesthesia cost. When the preoperative diagnosis is in doubt, the laparoscopic approach is very useful especially in the female patient to exclude gynecologic and other entities, some of which can then be treated laparoscopically (e.g., ovarian torsion or cyst). Some authorities suggest that laparoscopic visualization is superior to the traditional small incision approach in instances of obesity and to expose a retrocecal appendix. However, when an abscess or significant adhesions are encountered and the definitive operative area cannot be defined expeditiously or if a mucocele or neoplasm is found, conversion to an open procedure is necessary. Incidental appendectomy may be performed in conjunction with other laparoscopic procedures.

Procedure

Pneumoperitoneum is established. Abdominal exploration is performed through a 10/11 mm or 12 mm port. If appendicitis is confirmed, additional ports in the suprapubic area (5 mm) and right subcostal at the anterior axillary line (12 mm) are established. Additional right or left lower quadrant ports may be required. The cecum is retracted superiorly via a right subcostal port employing an atraumatic instrument (e.g., endoscopic Babcock). After appropriate dissection the appendiceal tip is distracted by grasping forceps (or by endoscopic loop ligature if edematous). The mesoappendix is exposed and a "window" made in an avascular site. Using an endoscopic gastrointestinal stapler or between serial clips, the mesoappendix (including the appendiceal artery) is divided. An endoscopic loop ligature of chromic catgut may be secured about the appendiceal base, and with an endoscopic gastrointestinal stapler

placed just distal to the same, the appendix is amputated. Alternatively, additional suture loop can be employed, and the appendix divided by endo laser fiber or
electrocautery or scissors. The appendiceal stump may
be cauterized. During the procedure the port functions
can be alternated. The specimen is withdrawn into the
trocar sleeve (of the selected port). If the appendix is severely inflamed or edematous, an endoscopic specimen
pouch can be employed. Hemostasis is assured. Local
irrigation and suction may be done and a drain placed
as indicated. Pneumoperitoneum is released and the
wounds closed in the usual manner.

Preparation of Patient

The patient is supine; both arms may be padded and
tucked in at the patient's sides. Apply electrosurgical
dispersive pad. Foley catheter is not routinely placed.

Skin Preparation

Begin at the midline extending from the nipples to the
upper thighs and down to the table at the sides.

Draping

Folded towels and a laparoscopy sheet
Camera cable cover

Equipment

Video monitor
Insufflation device (CO_2)
Fiberoptic light source (e.g., Xenon 300 W)
VCR
Electrosurgical unit

Instrumentation

Minor tray
Verres needles
Trocars (5 mm, 10 mm, 12 mm, or Hasson)
Reducers
Dissectors
Scissors

Stapler

Single clip appliers and Multifire gastrointestinal appliers

Endoscopic suturing and ligation instruments

Telescope

Camera and cable

Suction, cautery with cord

Supplies

Foam padding for elbows and ankles; blanket under knees

Blades (1) No. 10, (1) No. 15, (1) No. 11

Suction tubing

Single clip cartridge

Endoscopic chromic loop ligatures (optional)

Multifire gastrointestinal staple cartridge

Skin closure strips

CO_2 tubing

Culture tubes

COLOSTOMY

Definition

Formation of a permanent or temporary opening into the colon brought out onto the abdominal wall as a stoma.

Discussion

A colostomy is intended to be either permanent or temporary. A *temporary colostomy* is performed to divert the fecal stream from the distal colon, which may be obstructed by tumor or inflammation or which may require being "put at rest" because of an anastomosis or a pouch procedure. A temporary colostomy may be created in the transverse colon or the sigmoid colon. The proximal and distal portions of the colon remain connected (loop colostomy) or separated (double barrel colostomy). In a Hartmann procedure a sigmoid colostomy is formed, and the distal end of the colon is either brought out as a mucous fistula or closed and returned intraperitoneally.

A *permanent colostomy* is performed to treat malignancies of the colon; other indications include irrevocable rectal stricture, irrevocable anal incontinence, and inflammatory bowel disease. A permanent colostomy can be fashioned similar to a temporary colostomy but most often is an end colostomy.

Procedure

The incision depends on the segment of the colon to be used, unless performed in conjunction with another procedure. The segment of colon is mobilized. The colon can be brought out through the main incision or through an adjacent site from which a disc of skin and subcutaneous tissue has been excised. The underlying rectus fascia, muscle, and peritoneal layers are incised to accommodate the colon. The appropriate segment of the colon is excised between clamps (atraumatic clamps may be used on the retained portions of bowel), or an automatic stapling device may be employed. An "end" segment or loop of colon is brought through the stoma site and (usually) sutured to the peristomal skin. In a loop colostomy a rod or bridge may be placed under the colon to avoid retraction. The wounds are closed, and a colostomy pouch is applied over the stoma.

Preparation of the Patient

The patient is supine; arms may be extended on armboards. Apply electrosurgical dispersive pad.

Skin Preparation

Begin at the incision (check with surgeon) extending from nipples to upper thighs, and down to the table at the sides.

Draping

Folded towels and a laparotomy or transverse sheet (depending on incision)

Equipment

Electrosurgical unit
Suction

Instrumentation

Major procedures tray
Long instruments tray
Gastrointestinal procedures tray
Self-retaining retractor (e.g., Balfour), optional

Supplies

Basin set
Blades (2) No. 10
Suction tubing
Electrosurgical pencil
Penrose drain, 1″ (retraction on colon)
Glass rod and tubing with colostomy pouch (e.g., Karaya Seal or plastic bridge) and loop colostomy set (e.g., Hollister)

Special Notes

Instruments used on the bowel are isolated in a basin. Specimen may be received in a basin.

"Clean" closure of the abdomen requires regowning, regloving, and redraping and the use of a Basic/Minor procedures tray.

CLOSURE OF COLOSTOMY

Definition

Reestablishment of colonic continuity and the repair of the abdominal wall.

Discussion

This procedure can be simple or involved, particularly the anastomosis between a sigmoid end colostomy and the proximal rectal remnant.

Procedure

For an *end colostomy* an incision circumscribes the stoma, which is dissected free of abdominal wall structures. An appropriate incision is made to enable intra-abdominal dissection, permitting anastomosis at the site of the distal colon. The distal segment is mobilized and anastomosed to the proximal end; an end-to-end automatic stapling device can facilitate the procedure. The wound is closed; subcutaneous tissue and the skin of the stoma site can be left open to avoid infection.

For a *loop* or *double barrel colostomy,* an elliptical incision is made about the stoma(s). The colonic loop is dissected free of scar tissue and skin, and the anastomosis is performed. The proximal and distal segments may need to be resected in order to perform anastomosis on a well-vascularized bowel of satisfactory diameter. The abdomen is closed, often leaving the subcutaneous tissue and skin packed open to prevent wound infection.

Preparation of the Patient

The patient is supine; arms may be extended on armboards. Apply electrosurgical dispersive pad.

Skin Preparation

Cover colostomy stoma with a sponge soaked in preparation solution. Begin just beyond the perimeter of the stoma extending from nipples to midthighs, and down to the table at the sides. Cleanse the area immediately around the stoma and the stoma itself last. Discard each sponge after cleansing the stoma.

Draping

Folded towels and a laparotomy or transverse sheet

Equipment

Electrosurgical unit
Suction

Instrumentation

Major procedures tray
Long instruments tray
Gastrointestintal procedures tray
Automatic stapling device (optional)
Self-retaining retractor (e.g., Balfour) (optional)

Supplies

Basin set
Blades (3) No. 10, (1) No. 15
Needle magnet or counter
Suction tubing
Electrosurgical pencil
Staples (optional)
Packing (e.g., Adaptic dressing, 4″ × 4″ sponges) (optional)

Special Notes

Instruments used on the bowel are isolated in a basin.

"Clean" closure of the abdomen requires regowning, regloving, and redraping and the use of a Basic/Minor procedures tray.

RIGHT HEMICOLECTOMY

Definition

Resection of the right half of the colon (a portion of the transverse colon, the ascending colon, the cecum) and a segment of the terminal ileum and their mesenteries. An anastomosis is performed between the ileum and the transverse colon (ileocolostomy).

Discussion

Indications for right hemicolectomy are tumors, bleeding, inflammation, or trauma; obstruction is less often encountered than in the left half of the colon.

Procedure

A right paramedian, midline, or oblique right midabdominal incision is made. The distal small bowel and the midtransverse colon are identified, and their vascular attachments ligated and divided. The appropriate segment of colon is excised between clamps (atraumatic clamps may be used on the portions of the retained bowel), or an automatic stapling device may be employed. The terminal ileum and midtransverse colon are anastomosed by various suture techniques or staples. Care is taken to avoid injury to structures including the right ureter, duodenum, inferior vena cava, and common bile duct. The incision is closed in layers.

Preparation of the Patient

The patient is supine; arms may be extended on armboards. Check with the surgeon regarding insertion of a Foley catheter before beginning to prepare the patient. Apply electrosurgical dispersive pad.

Skin Preparation

Begin at the incision (right paramedian, midline, or oblique right midabdominal) extending from nipples to upper thighs, and down to the table at the sides.

Draping

Folded towels and a laparotomy sheet

Equipment

Electrosurgical unit
Suction

Instrumentation

Major procedures tray
Long instruments tray
Gastrointestinal procedures tray
Hemoclip appliers (various sizes and lengths)
Automatic stapling devices (optional)
Harrington retractor
Self-retaining retractor (e.g., Balfour)

Supplies

Basin set
Blades (3) No. 10, (1) No. 15
Electrosurgical pencil
Suction tubing
Needle magnet or counter
Hemoclips (various sizes)
Staples (optional)

Special Notes

The scrub person may receive specimen in a basin.
Instruments used on the colon are isolated in a basin.
"Clean" closure of the abdomen requires regowning, regloving, and redraping and a Basic/Minor procedures tray.

TRANSVERSE COLECTOMY

Definition

Resection of a segment of the transverse colon with an end-to-end anastomosis to reestablish continuity of the colon.

Discussion

Transverse colectomy is usually performed as treatment for a malignancy or a stricture caused by inflammatory bowel disease.

Procedure

A vertical or transverse incision may be used. The transverse colon and hepatic and splenic flexures are mobilized by dividing vascular mesenteric attachments and supporting connective tissues. The appropriate segment of colon is excised between clamps (atraumatic clamps may be used on the portions of the retained bowel), or an automatic stapling device may be employed. An anastomosis is fashioned between the proximal and distal colon, and the mesenteric defect closed; sufficient mobility must be achieved to enable the anastomosis to be tension free. Injury to the stomach, pancreas, spleen, and superior mesenteric vessels is avoided. The wound is closed in layers.

Preparation of the Patient

The patient is supine; arms may be extended on armboards. Check with surgeon regarding insertion of a Foley catheter before beginning preparation. Apply electrosurgical dispersive pad.

Skin Preparation

Begin at the incision (midline or transverse) extending from nipples to upper thighs, and down to the table at the sides.

Draping

Folded towels and a transverse or laparotomy sheet (depending on incision)

Equipment

Electrosurgical unit
Suction

Instrumentation

Major procedures tray
Gastrointestinal procedures tray
Automatic stapling device (optional)
Hemoclip appliers (various sizes)
Harrington retractor
Self-retaining retractor (e.g., Balfour)

Supplies

Basin set
Blades (3) No. 10
Suction tubing
Electrosurgical pencil
Hemoclips (various sizes)
Needle magnet or counter
Staples (optional)

Special Notes

Instruments used on the colon are isolated in a basin.
Specimen can be received in a basin.
Ends of the bowel may be covered with lap pads or surgical gloves and tied with umbilical tape to prevent contamination of the abdomen.
"Clean" closure of the abdomen requires regowning, regloving, and redraping and a Basic/Minor procedures tray.

ANTERIOR RESECTION OF THE SIGMOID COLON AND RECTUM

Definition

Involves the excision of the sigmoid colon and when applicable the rectosigmoid and the proximal two-thirds of the rectum with the anastomosis of the distal descending or proximal sigmoid colon to the remaining segment of the rectosigmoid or rectum.

Discussion

This procedure is performed for benign (e.g., diverticulitis) or malignant conditions.

Procedure

A vertical or transverse incision can be used. The lower descending, sigmoid, and rectosigmoid colon (and proximal rectum) are mobilized by dividing mesenteric vascular attachments. In procedures for malignancy, greater portions of the mesentery are excised to include additional lymph-node-bearing tissue. The ureters are identified and protected. The appropriate segment of colon is excised, and the bowel is anastomosed with sutures or staples. Tension is avoided on the anastomosis by mobilizing more proximal colon as necessary. The abdomen is closed in layers.

Preparation of the Patient

The patient is supine; arms may be extended on armboards. Check with surgeon regarding insertion of a Foley catheter before beginning preparation. Apply electrosurgical dispersive pad.

Skin Preparation

Begin at the incision (vertical or transverse) extending from nipples to upper thighs, and down to the table at the sides.

Draping, Equipment, Instrumentation, and Supplies

See Right Hemicolectomy, p. 131.

ABDOMINOPERINEAL RESECTION OF THE RECTUM

Definition

Excision of the rectum, usually including a portion of the sigmoid colon, through an abdominal (anterior) and a perineal approach.

Discussion

This procedure is performed most often for the treatment of rectal malignancy but also for inflammatory bowel disease, irreversible sphincter injuries, and so on. Abdominoperineal resection of the rectum may be combined with resection of the proximal colon as well.

Procedure

A vertical or transverse abdominal incision is made. The extent and level of the pathology is determined. The portion of the colon to be removed is mobilized by dividing the mesenteric vascular attachments to the bowel, carrying the dissection to the rectum. The ureters and other adjacent organs are identified and otherwise avoided unless they are to be removed. The colon is transsected proximally. The distal portion (the transsected end of which is protected from spillage by use of lap pads, clamps, and/or a rubber glove secured by umbilical tapes) is dissected into the depths of the pelvis transsecting the lateral rectal stalks (middle hemorrhoidal vessels) to the level of the coccyx. Perirectal connective and adipose tissue are removed with malignancies. In benign disease the dissection stays close to the bowel wall. A stoma site is fashioned by excising a disc of skin and tunneling into the peritoneum through the rectus muscle. The end of the proximal portion of the colon (or ileum) is passed through the tunnel without tension and assuring good vascularity is sutured to the peristomal skin. The abdomen may then be closed, or if simultaneous perineal dissection is performed, the "abdominal" surgeon remains to assist from above. As the perineal portion is completed, the surgeon above closes the abdomen. The "perineal" surgeon closes the anus with a heavy-gauge pursestring suture. An elliptical saggital incision is made into the perianal and perirectal tissues and deepened, incising the levator muscles; the pelvis is entered, and the previously dissected distal colon and proximal rectum are passed into the perineal wound. The rectum is excised avoiding the urethra and prostate or vagina. Hemostasis is achieved. The perineal wound is closed in layers over one or more drains. A colostomy pouch is placed over the stoma.

Preparation of the Patient

The patient is usually in a modified lithotomy/Sims' position with the sacrum elevated on folded towels or a sandbag, or the procedure is begun with the patient supine and later moved to a lithotomy or modified lateral/Sims' position. Check with the surgeon regarding insertion of Foley catheter before beginning the preparation. Apply electrosurgical dispersive pad.

Skin Preparation

Modified Lithotomy. Begin at the incision (midline, left paramedian, or transverse) extending from the nipples to lower thighs; and down to the table at the sides. Prepare genitalia (add a vaginal preparation for females), extending to the table at the perineal area; prepare anus last, and discard each sponge.

Supine. Begin at the pubic symphysis extending downward over the labia. Cleanse each inner thigh working toward the perineum. Prepare vagina, then perineum, and anus last (discarding each sponge).

Modified Lateral/Sims'. Begin at suprapubic area extending from the iliac crest to midthighs, and down to the table anteriorly and posteriorly. Prepare genitalia and anus last.

Draping

Modified Lithotomy. Drape sheet (under buttocks), leggings, folded towels (abdomen), and a laparotomy or transverse sheet (a hole will be cut for perineal exposure).

Supine. Folded towels and a laparotomy or transverse sheet.

Modified Lateral/Sims'. Folded towels and a laparotomy or transverse sheet.

Lithotomy. Same as modified lithotomy

Equipment

Electrosurgical unit
Suction
Stirrups (depending on position)

Instrumentation

Major procedures tray
Long instruments tray
Gastrointestinal procedures tray
Basic/Minor procedures tray for perineal approach (when both abdominal and perineal approach are performed)
Hemoclip appliers (various sizes and lengths)
Large retractors (e.g., Harrington, Israel, Balfour)

Supplies

Basin set
Blades (4) No. 10, (1) No. 15
Needle magnet or counter (2 for simultaneous approach, 3 for "clean" setup)
Electrosurgical pencils (2 for simultaneous approach, 3 for "clean" setup)
Pouch for electrosurgical pencils
Suction tubing
Hemoclips (assorted sizes)
Extra glove and umbilical tape (for proximal end of a specimen before it is passed through the perineal wound)
Vessel loop or umbilical tape (retraction)
Marking pen (stoma site), optional
Colostomy pouch (e.g., Karaya Seal)
Drainage supplies (e.g., Penrose, Hemovac, Foley catheter)

Special Notes

For modified lithotomy position, the abdominal and perineal approaches are performed by two teams simultaneously (a second scrub nurse is necessary). For a two-stage procedure the patient is prepared and draped for the second stage after the abdomen is closed.

Isolate all instruments used on the colon in a basin.

The scrub person may receive specimen in a basin.

Since there are two separate surgical fields, additional care must be exercised to avoid confusion when counting sponges, needles and sharps, and instruments.

"Clean" closure of the abdomen requires regowning, regloving, and redraping and a Basic/Minor procedures tray.

Using a pouch prevents inadvertent activation of a second electrosurgical pencil not in use.

LAPAROSCOPIC-ASSISTED COLON RESECTION

Definition

Excision of a segment of the large intestine incorporating endoscopic technique and a minilaparotomy incision or large-bore laparoscopic port.

Discussion

Most commonly performed procedures on the colon can be technically accomplished by laproscopic or laparoscopic-assisted approach. It is not yet known as to whether a "proper" cancer resection can be performed laparoscopically. The laparoscopic approach may not be appropriate in cases of severe obesity, extensive adhesions, severe inflammation, or colonic perforation with peritonitis or in malignancy when the primary tumor is large or assosiated with adjacent organ involvement or when wide dissection is necessary. If upon assessment of the pathology the laparoscopic approach is likely to compromise the proposed procedure or in the case of hemmorhage or if excessive anesthesia time accumulates, the laparoscopic procedure must be promptly converted to an open procedure.

Procedures may be completed entirely by laparoscopic approach or may be combined with a minilaparotomy incision or use of a large port. Similarly, creation or elimination of a stoma and procedures in which instruments may be inserted transanally are combined with the laparoscopic approach. The selection of trocar sites will vary with the patient's habitus, the pathology, previous surgery, and preference of the surgeon and may need to be repositioned during the course of the procedure.

If after placement of the camera the involved colonic segment is deemed to be mobile or in a redundant loop and a limited procedure is indicated, the segment may be delivered extracorporeally via a minilaparotomy procedure accomplished without further laparoscopic maneuvers. When a small lesion has been identified colonoscopically and requires segmental excision, ethylene blue dye can be injected into the adjacent bowel wall to facilitate identification on laparoscopic exploration. Similarly, if laparoscopic visualization cannot identify a smaller lesion or its regional location is not established with respect to deciding procedure of choice, intraoperative colonoscopy can be performed to verify the level of pathology.

The more commonly performed laparoscopic (or laparoscopic-assisted) colonic procedures will be described, again noting yet unresolved controversies to the propriety of this approach for malignancy and certain other conditions. Various modifications or combinations of these basic procedures, for example, total abdominal colectomy with ileorectal anastomosis or end ileostomy with proctocolectomy, will not be described.

Procedure

Right Hemicolectomy. Pneumoperitoneum is established through the umbilicus. Three additional 10- to 11 mm ports are placed: suprapubic, right subcostal at the midclavicular line, and right subziphoid. The table is adjusted with the right side elevated to allow gravity to assist in the exposure of the immediate operative area, and later placed in reverse Trendelenburg. After assessment of the pathology, the cecum and proximal ascending colon are placed on traction as the lateral attachments are dissected. Care is taken to avoid injury to the ureter and duodenum as the dissection is continued about the terminal ileum, hepatic flexure, and proximal transverse colon. Division of the mesenteric vessel is then accomplished. Employing appropriate stapling devices, the segment of colon is resected and the specimen removed via a large port or minilaparotomy incision in the right upper quadrant. The anastomosis can then be performed intracorporeally or extracorporeally by delivering the bowel through the minilaparatomy incision. The mesenteric defect is repaired, and after hemostasis is assured, the pneumoperitoneum is released. The trocar sites and minilaparatomy sites are closed.

Left Hemicolectomy or Sigmoid Resection. This procedure is similar to a right hemicolectomy. Pneumoperitoneum is established, and the ports are placed on the left side (umbilical, left upper quadrant midclavicular line, left para umbilical, left midclavicular line, and left suprapubic). The table is adjusted with the left side up and later placed in reverse Trendelenburg. The left colon is mobilized (avoiding injury to the spermatic or ovarian vessels, ureter, stomach, and spleen). After dissection has been completed, resection and anastomosis are performed as in right hemicolectomy. If the distal sigmoid colon is included in the resection, see Low Anterior Resection (to follow).

Low Anterior Resection. The patient is positioned in modified lithotomy possibly providing access to the anterior abdomen and perineum. Pneumoperitoneum is established. Patient is placed in reverse Trendelenburg. Ports are similar to that of left hemicolectomy. The sigmoid colon and rectum are mobilized, taking care to avoid injury to gonadal vessels, ureters, and internal female genitalia. The mesenteric structures are divided and the specimen resected and delivered through a large-bore port, minilaparatomy incision, or transanally via the distal rectal remnant. Anastomosis is performed employing an intraluminal end-to-end stapler inserted transanally. The anastomosis is begun by extracting the proximal end of the resected bowel via a large-bore post or minilaparatomy incision. The staple line placed at the time of division of the colon is excised and the separated anvil of the stapler secured by hand-sewn pursestring suture or automatic pursestring suture device. The stapler is inserted transanally, and its trocar is extended perforating the stapled end of the rectal segment. Employing a modified anvil grasper to stabilize the proximal segment, end-to-end anastomosis is completed in the standard fashion. The tissue rings are inspected and the anastomosis tested employing a sigmoidoscope or bulb syringe. After hemostasis is assured, the pneumoperitoneum is released and the access ports closed.

Hartmann's Procedure and Reversal of Hartmann's Procedure. The conduction of the Hartmann's procedure is identical to low anterior resection as described above with the exception that the distal rectal segment is closed or on occasion is brought out onto the abdominal wall as a mucous fistula. The proximal segment is brought out as an end colostomy. To reverse this procedure, that is, to restore continuity, the colostomy (proximal colon segment) is anastomosed to the rectal remnant. The pelvis is inspected and the closed rectal remnant identified. If visualization is inadequate, adherent viscera and adhesions must be dissected to expose the proximal portion of the rectal segment. To facilitate identification of the rectal segment, a blunt instrument, large-bore catheter, or sigmoidoscope is inserted transanally to "tent" the apex of the segment. When this dissection is complete, the previously established colostomy stoma is dissected free from the abdominal wall with laparoscopic assistance if necessary. Any questionably viable colon is excised. The anvil of the intraluminal stapler is placed within this proximal segment secured by a pursestring suture. This segment with the anvil is replaced intraperitoneally. The assistant surgeon then passes the trocar of the intraluminal stapler through the apex of the closed rectal segment. Care is taken to assure that no extraneous tissues or structures overlie the site of the anastomosis. The anastomosis is completed as in a low anterior resection above.

Laparoscopically Assisted Abdominal Perineal Resection of the Rectum. The surgery is initially identical to low anterior resection except that the distal dissection is performed as low as feasible; the specimen is left in situ as the proximal end is transsected. The proximal segment is then brought out as an end colostomy at a previously selected stoma site in the left lower quadrant.

Preparation of the Patient

For right and left hemicolectomy the patient is supine with the table in Trendelenburg.

With laparoscopic low anterior resection, the patient is in modified lithotomy with the table in Trendelenburg.

The patient is supine for the Hartmann's procedure. To reverse the Hartmann's procedure (closure of colostomy), the patient is placed in lithotomy using Allen-Llyod-Davies stirrups. Insert a Foley catheter. Apply electrosurgical pad.

Skin Preparation

For the right and left hemicolectomy and Hartmann's procedure, begin at the umbilicus extending from nipples to upper thighs and down to the table at the sides. For the low anterior resection, begin at the umbilicus extending from nipples to the pubic symphysis, and down to the table at the sides. Follow this with a vaginal preparation (women) and include the genitalia. Cleanse each inner thigh. Prepare the perineum and anus last, discarding each sponge after wiping the anus.

Draping

For right and left hemicolectomy and Hartmann's procedures. Folded towels and a laparoscopy sheet.

For low anterior resection. Drape sheet under buttocks, and a special laparoscopy sheet with attached leggings.

Instruments

Major procedures tray (open)
Long instruments tray
Gastrointestinal procedures tray
Laparoscope with camera and cord, endoscopic
Verres needle
Endoscopic blunt tip trocar
Endoscopic 10 to 11 mm or 10 to 12 mm sharp trocar (4)
Endoscopic Babcock clamps, 10 mm (2)
Endoscopic curved scissors, 5 mm
Endoscopic right-angle dissector, 10 mm
Endoscopic Kelly clamp, 10 mm
Endoscopic multiple clip applier
Endoscopic right angle and hook suction–electrosurgical dissectors
Endoscopic hook scissors
Endoscopic extrudable fan retractor
Endoscopic grasping clamps (2)
Endoscopic dissecting clamps (2)
Endoscopic probe with suction, irrigation
Endoscopic ligate and divide stapler
Endoscopic linear cutter (intracorporeal)
Endoscopic linear cutter (extracorporeal)
Endoscopic intraluminal end-to-end stapler
Endoscopic modified anvil grasper
Endoscopic needle driver

Supplies

Padding foam for pressure points
Sandbag under sacrum (only for Abdominal Perineal)
Suction tubing
Endoscopic suture loops
Fog reduction agent
Foley catheter
Nasogastric tube (e.g., No. 16)
Blades (2) No. 10, (1) No. 15, (1) No. 11
Endoscopic specimen retrieval bag
Pneumatic antiemboletic stockings

Equipment

Suction tubing
Sequential pressure device

Light source (e.g., Xenon 300 W)
Video monitors (2)
VCR
Mavigraph (video printer, optional)
CO_2 insufflator
Methylene blue dye
Skin closure strips (optional)
Silastic tubing

Special Notes

After the patient is in the room, position and connect the monitors.

Position electrosurgical unit.

Following draping, the scrub person passes off the camera cable, light cord, and Silastic tubing.

The circulator adjusts the insufflator: first low flow (between 5 and 7 mm Hg), then higher flow according to the surgeon's instructions.

Connect and turn on the light source and white balance camera.

The circulator rechecks the position of monitors.

The circulator then connects all remaining items: suction tubing, electrosurgical cord, and so on.

All instruments (nondisposable) may be flash-sterilized.

Soak scope(s) and light cord(s) in Steris solution after thorough cleansing.

The circulator turns the lights on and off as requested. One light will remain on for the scrub person.

TRANSANAL ENDOSCOPIC MICROSURGERY

Definition

Application of endoscopic surgical techniques via transanally placed rectoscope.

Discussion

For rectal and rectosigmoid lesions to the level of 20 cm proximal to the anus, which otherwise would be excised by an open (transperitoneal or transsacral) approach, or for a lesion not technically feasible to be adequately treated by the usual transanal exposure, special instrumentation has been devised permitting the use of endoscopic surgical instruments in a well-visualized gas-distended operative field. Up to four instruments may be manipulated in parallel fashion simultaneously by the operator and assistant. A unit is utilized that continuously monitors intrarectal pressure and insufflates with carbon dioxide to maintain an appropriate pressure to keep the rectum distended, thus permitting visualization and responding to the introduction of instruments and need for suctioning blood or fumes as well. Visualization is by means of binocular stereoscopic optics to which a side arm or teaching attachment or video monitor can be adapted. An irrigating device to cleanse the lens is also a part of the system. A Morton arm retractor stabilizes the scope after it is positioned transanally. Most often this technique is employed for sessile lesions too large to be safely and/or adequately excised or electrofulgerated via a standard sigmoidoscope. Benign and limited malignancies may be so treated. Preoperative evaluation may, in addition to biopsy, include transrectal ultrasonography to determine the depth of mural invasion and lymph nodal involvement, which would influence the operative approach. The position of the lesion will also influence the positioning of the patient for ease of access (i.e., prone, lithotomy, or lateral). Transanal endoscopic rectopexy in which the posterior rectal wall is incised and the rectum fixed to the presacral ligaments has been described. In most instances when violation of a full-thickness segment of rectal wall is anticipated, preoperative preparation and postoperative care is similar to that for a formal colon surgery. If during the course of the procedure the peritoneum is entered, immediate repair is performed.

Procedure

This procedure would be performed on a patient with a transanal sessile tumor of the midrectum. After induction of anesthesia, the patient is positioned to best visualize the lesion with respect to the operative field (e.g., prone for an anterior lesion). The special rectoscope is inserted and secured. Carbon dioxide pressure of 150 mbar is maintained. Employing various grasping and electrosurgical cutting instruments, the lesion is circumscribed and excised. Depending on the size and depth of the defect thus created, after hemostasis is obtained, suture repair is then undertaken. Clips are used to secure the suture ends rather than standard knots. If the procedure cannot easily be accomplished, a standard surgical procedure may have to be performed.

Preparation of the Patient

The patient is in prone, lithotomy, or lateral positioning, depending upon the orientation of the lesion. A Foley catheter is inserted. Apply electrosurgical dispersive pad.

Skin Preparation

Preparation is minimal. Cleanse the area from the level of the umbilicus to the level of midthighs. Discard each sponge after wiping the anus.

Draping

Drapes used for transuretheral resection with integrated pouches and openings

Equipment

Stirrups with padding for lithotomy
Padding for elbows and ankles
Pillow for between the legs in lateral position
Martin arm (self-securing adjustable retractor mount)
Endoscopic combination unit (monitors intrarectal pressure, provides gas insufflation to maintain desired pressure with connections for optic rinsing and suction)
Electrosurgical unit
Monitor (1)
VCR (optional)
Special roller pump suction device (e.g., Wolf) (functions without causing total decompression)

Instrumentation

Special operating rectoscope with binocular optics with rigid (for video adaptation) and flexible sideport viewing
Endoscopic grasping instruments
Endoscopic suction-electrosurgical, irrigator
Endoscopic hook and microscissors
Endoscopic needle driver
Endoscopic clip applicators
Endoscopic teaching arm (flexible or rigid) may be attached to direct viewing of video monitoring
Endoscopic camera

Special Notes

The endoscopic combination unit is positioned on the surgeon's left side. It is controlled by the surgeon using the double footswitch.

The optic irrigator, controlled by a single footswitch, is used by the assistant.

The light source, monitor, and camera control system are positioned on the surgeon's right side.

The U-shaped double ball joint (Martin arm) is attached to the table with the V-groove clamp approximately 20 cm below the anus.

The surgeon sits on an adjustable chair.

The scrub person sits on the right behind the surgeon, and passes instruments from the right.

HEMORRHOIDECTOMY

Definition

Excision of the veins of the anus and associated overlying skin and anoderm (externally) and mucous membrane (internally).

Discussion

Hemorrhoidectomy refers to the removal of the hemorrhoidal tissues including the enlarged veins within. Hemorrhoids may be treated with concomitant anal conditions such as fissure (anal ulcer) and fistula.

Anesthesia may be regional, local, or general (or a combination). Following the induction of anesthesia, proctosigmoidoscopy is performed.

Procedure

The proximal portions of the hemorrhoidal complex are suture-ligated, and the hemorrhoid is excised by scalpel, cautery, or laser. Less often cryosurgery is employed (usually reserved for limited outpatient procedures). If the anus is stenotic, the distal internal sphincter may be incised. A mucous membrane flap and/or skin flaps may be employed to cover denuded areas. Care is taken not to excise too much skin, anoderm, or mucous membrane and to avoid injury to the sphincter mechanism.

Preparation of the Patient

See Sigmoidoscopy, pp. 99–100.

Skin Preparation

Preparation is minimal. Begin inside tape margins, discarding each sponge after wiping the anus.

Draping

Jackknife. Folded towels and a laparotomy sheet
Lithotomy. Drape sheet under buttocks, leggings, folded towels, drape sheet over abdomen
Modified Lateral/Sims. Folded towels and a laparotomy sheet

Equipment

Stirrups or pillow and roll for positioning
Electrosurgical unit

Instrumentation

Rectal procedures tray
Rectal retractors, including Sims, Hill-Ferguson, and
   Sawyer
Curettes

Supplies

Blades (1) No. 10, (1) No. 15
Needle magnet or counter
Small basin
Hemostatic agent (e.g., Surgicel, Gelfoam)
Suction tubing
Electrosurgical pencil
Lubricant
Pressure dressing (e.g., petrolatum-impregnated
    gauze, 4″ × 4″ sponges)

Special Notes

Protect skin under adhesive tape with tincture of benzoin.

Be prepared for sigmoidoscopy prior to procedure.

Lubricate retractors.

Carbon dioxide laser may be used. See Appendix, pp.
619–624, for safety precautions.

If the primary pathology is anal fissure or fistula, the
basic setup is essentially the same as when hemorrhoids are the primary pathology.

PILONIDAL CYSTECTOMY AND SINUSECTOMY

Definition

Refers to the removal of a cystic mass containing hair,
skin, tissue debris, and so on, most often located in the
sacroccocygeal area.

Discussion

Pilonidal cysts are most frequently found in the sacro-
coccygeal region, but they can occur about the perineum,
hands, and so on. When acutely or chronically infected,
surgical treatment is indicated. These cysts may be very
extensive with multiple and deep side tracts. Pilonidal
cyst disease is not related to the gastrointestinal tract,
but it is included here for convenience.

Procedure

An incision is made about the cyst or into the cyst directly. Necrotic tissue, hair, tissue debris, and so on are

curetted and/or excised. The cyst wall is sometimes excised. The wound can be packed open, partially closed, or completely closed by means of tissue flaps.

Preparation of the Patient

The patient is in a jackknife position (the table is flexed) with arms extended on armboards angled toward the head of the table and the hands pronated, a pillow in front of the legs, and a roll at the ankles. Buttocks are distracted by 3- or 4-inch adhesive tapes anchored to the underside of the table (pull tapes toward patient's head before anchoring for maximal exposure).

Skin Preparation

Begin at the sacrum extending from the iliac crests to the upper thighs. Cleanse anus last, discarding each sponge afterward.

Draping

Folded towels and a laparotomy sheet

Equipment

Pillow and roll for positioning
Electrosurgical unit
Suction

Instrumentation

Rectal procedures tray
Extra probes (available)
Curettes

Supplies

Small basin
Blades (1) No. 10, (2) No. 15
Suction tubing
Electrosurgical pencil
Needle magnet or counter
Methylene blue with needle and syringe (optional)
Pressure dressing

Special Notes

Protect skin under adhesive tape with tincture of benzoin.

THIERSCH PROCEDURE

Definition

Placement of a circumanal device to restrict complete rectal prolapse (procidentia).

Discussion

Prosthetic materials include various sutures, fascia, Mersilene tape, folded Marlex mesh, vascular prostheses, and so on. The Thiersch procedure often ultimately fails when the prosthetic material extrudes with ensuing local infection. The procedure may be repeated after the infection subsides.

Procedure

Two incisions, 1 cm each, are made diametrically opposite around the anus. A large curved hemostat is passed deep in the perianal tissues external to the sphincter (avoiding the vagina), encircling the sphincter, and exiting the opposite incision. The prosthetic material is passed through the tunnel created by the clamp. This maneuver is repeated for the other hemi-circumference (prosthesis completely encircles the anal canal). The prosthetic ends are sutured (or stapled) after an appropriate degree of constriction is determined. The sutured segment is replaced deep in the wound. Wounds may be irrigated with an antibiotic solution. The wounds are closed.

Preparation of the Patient

The procedure may be performed under regional, local, or general anesthesia. The patient may be in the jack-knife, lithotomy, or modified lateral position (see Sigmoidoscopy, pp. 99–100). A sigmoidoscopy may be performed prior to the procedure.

Skin Preparation

Preparation is minimal. Begin inside tape margins, discarding each sponge after wiping the anus.

Draping

Jackknife. Folded towels and a laparotomy sheet
Lithotomy. Drape sheet under buttocks, leggings, towels, drape sheet over abdomen
Modified Lateral. Folded towels and a laparotomy sheet

Equipment

Electrosurgical unit
Suction
Pillow and roll or stirrups (for positioning)

Instrumentation

Rectal procedures tray
Rectal retractors, including Sims, Hill-Ferguson, and
   Sawyer
Ligature carrier (optional)

Supplies

Blades (1) No. 10, (2) No. 15
Needle magnet or counter
Small basin
Suction tubing
Electrosurgical pencil
Lubricant
Prosthesis
Antibiotic irrigation and bulb syringe (optional)

Special Notes

Protect skin under tape with tincture of benzoin.
   Be prepared for sigmoidoscopy prior to the procedure.
   Lubricate retractors.
   Check with the surgeon regarding prosthesis material.

RIPSTEIN PROCEDURE (PRESACRAL RECTOPEXY)

Definition

An anterior (abdominal) approach to correct complete rectal prolapse (procidentia) by mobilizing the rectum within the abdomen (and pelvis) and fixing it to the presacral fascia and periosteum by an encircling band of material such as a Teflon, Marlex, or Mersilene mesh.

Discussion

If the sigmoid colon is extremely redundant, a portion of it may be resected. Accordingly, low anterior resection (see p. 134) with extensive mobilization of the distal rectum may be performed without requiring placement of a prosthetic mesh altogether and is currently considered by some to be the procedure of choice for complete rectal prolapse.

Procedure

A vertical or transverse incision is used. The rectum is dissected from its supporting tissue attachments. A mesh of Marlex (or Mersilene, Teflon, etc.) is sutured (or stapled) to the presacral periosteum, taking care to avoid the local venous plexus. The mesh is placed about the bowel to anchor it to the sacrum without restricting the rectum too tightly. A resection proximally may be performed. The abdomen is closed in layers.

Preparation of the Patient

The patient is supine; arms may be extended on armboards. Check with the surgeon regarding insertion of a Foley catheter. Apply electrosurgical dispersive pad.

Skin Preparation

Begin at the incision (vertical or transverse) extending from nipples to upper thighs, and down to the table at the sides.

Draping

Folded towels and a laparotomy or transverse sheet

Equipment

Electrosurgical unit
Suction

Instrumentation

Major procedures tray
Long instruments tray
Gastrointestinal procedures tray (available)
Harrington retractor
Self-retaining retractor (e.g., Balfour)
Hemoclip appliers (assorted sizes and lengths)
Stapler (fascia)

Supplies

Basin set
Electrosurgical pencil
Blades (3) No. 10
Suction tubing
Needle magnet or counter
Hemoclips (variety)
Mesh or banding materials
Staples (optional)

Special Notes

Check with the surgeon regarding prosthetic material
to be used.

PERINEAL RESECTION OF THE RECTUM FOR COMPLETE RECTAL PROLAPSE (PROCIDENTIA)

Definition

Excision of the prolapsed segment of the rectum.

Discussion

Complete excision of the prolapsed rectal segment may
be accomplished by a perineal approach. This is particularly applicable in medically compromised patients in

whom an abdominal procedure entails a significantly longer term result than the encirclement procedure (see Thiersch, p. 151).

Procedure

The lithotomy position is preferred as the prolapse is accentuated. The prone position can be employed. The patient has been prepared as for formal colon resection; a Foley catheter is placed. A circumferential incision is made proximal to the dentate line through the full thickness of the rectum. The prolapse is distracted and amputated at an appropriate level, taking care to obtain hemostasis of the messenteric vessels. A peritoneal defect, if created, is repaired. As indicated, a levatorplasty is preferred. The rectal continuity is then restored by primary anastomosis.

Preparation of the Patient, Skin Preparation, Draping, Equipment, and Instrumentation

See Hemorrhoid Surgery, p. 148.

Special Notes

In addition to the hemorrhoid instruments, a pediatric Deaver and malleable retractors may be required.

Chapter 11

Gynecologic and Obstetric Surgery

DILATATION OF THE CERVIX AND CURETTAGE OF THE UTERUS (D & C)

Definition

The gradual enlargement of the cervical canal and removal (by scraping) of endocervical or endometrial tissue for histolologic study.

Discussion

The procedure is usually performed to diagnose cervical or uterine malignancy, control dysfunctional uterine bleeding, complete incomplete abortion, aid in evaluating infertility, and relieve dysmenorrhea. Fractional curettage differentiates between endocervical and endometrial lesions.

Procedure

A weighted speculum is placed in the vaginal vault. The cervix is grasped with a tenaculum. A sound is passed through the cervical canal into the uterine cavity to determine its depth and angulation. The cervix is dilated with graduated dilators. The uterine cavity may be explored with stone forceps. The uterine cavity is then curetted. Curettings are removed with stone forceps and collected on Telfa placed in the posterior fornix. A small serrated curette is used to scrape the uterine walls again; or, when a D & C is performed to remove placental tissue, a large, blunt curette and ovum forceps are used.

If a fractional D & C is performed, endocervical curettings are obtained *before* the uterus is sounded to avoid bringing endometrial cells into cervical os.

Preparation of the Patient

Following the administration of regional or general anesthesia, the patient is positioned in lithotomy. Arms may be extended on armboards.

Skin Preparation

Begin at the pubic symphysis and extend downward over the labia. Cleanse each inner thigh. Vaginal vault and cervix are cleansed using spongesticks (three). The perineum and anus are cleansed with the remaining sponges. Discard each sponge after wiping the anus. The patient's bladder is usually drained with a straight catheter.

Draping

Drape sheet under the buttocks, leggings, and drape sheet over the abdomen

Equipment

Stirrups

Instrumentation

Dilatation and curettage (D & C) tray

Supplies

Telfa (for specimen)
Perineal pad
T-binder or sanitary napkin belt

Special Notes

Stirrups are well padded to avoid nerve damage.

Lift both legs at the same time when putting the patient in stirrups to prevent postoperative lumbosacral strain.

Raise and lower legs slowly to prevent disturbances caused by rapid alterations in venous return.

Instruments are set up on back table for the surgeon; usually a scrub person is not required.

CONIZATION OF THE UTERINE CERVIX

Definition

The excision of tissue about the cervical os.

Discussion

This procedure is performed to diagnose and/or treat conditions such as cervicitis, epithelial dysplasia, and carcinoma in situ. *Cold conization* refers to scalpel and scissors dissection. *Hot cone* refers to tissue removal by use of electrocautery.

Procedure

A weighted speculum is placed in the vaginal vault. The outer portion of the cervix is grasped with a tenaculum. Dilatation and Curettage (see pp. 156–157) is performed. The cervix may be stained with Schiller's or Lugol's solution. Sutures are placed at 3 o'clock and 9 o'clock positions. The cervix may be injected circumferentially with a phenylephrine (Neo-Synephrine) solution. The uterine canal is carefully sounded. An incision is made circumferentially around the cervical os using a knife or cautery. Alternatively, a cervical cyst may be electrodesicated with a needle electrode. Bleeding may be controlled with sutures and/or ball electrode desiccation or a hemostatic agent.

Preparation of the Patient

Following the administration of regional or general anesthesia, the patient is positioned in a lithotomy.

Arms may be extended on armboards. Apply electro-surgical dispersive pad.

Skin Preparation

Preparation may be omitted (check with the surgeon); see Dilatation and Curettage, p. 157, for vaginal preparation.

Draping

Drape sheet under the buttocks, leggings, and drape sheet over the abdomen

Equipment

Stirrups
Electrosurgical unit

Instrumentation

Dilatation and curettage (D & C) tray
Cervical cone tray

Supplies

Telfa (for specimen)
Electrosurgical pencil (with blade, needle, and/or ball tip)
Blade No. 11
Small basin(s)
Schiller's or Lugol's solution (optional)
Long cotton-tipped applicators (optional)
Neo-Synephrine 1:20,000 (reduces bleeding) with needle and syringe (optional)
Hemostatic agent (e.g., Surgicel, Thrombostat), optional
Perineal pad
T-binder or sanitary napkin belt

Special Notes

See Dilatation and Curettage, p. 158.

THERAPEUTIC ABORTION BY SUCTION CURETTAGE

Definition

The vacuum aspiration of uterine contents usually performed to terminate early pregnancy.

Discussion

Procedure is also performed for missed and incomplete abortions.

Procedure

This procedure is similar to dilatation and curettage until the cervix is dilated. An appropriate suction curette is inserted through the dilated cervix into the uterine cavity. The controlled suction apparatus is activated. The curette is rotated 360° with a back-and-forth motion while traction is maintained on the cervix. The endometrial cavity is curetted with a sharp curette, and a brief suction curettage is repeated.

Preparation of the Patient, Skin Preparation, and Draping

See Dilatation and Curettage, p. 157.

Equipment

Stirrups
Controlled suction apparatus (e.g., Berkely Vacurette
   Machine)

Instrumentation

Dilatation and curettage (D & C) tray
Disposable vacuum curettes (assorted sizes, curved
   and straight)
Aspiration tubing

Supplies

Lubricant
Perineal pad
T-binder or sanitary napkin belt

Special Notes

See Dilatation and Curettage, p. 158.

Evacuation is done using all available vacuum (in Berkely unit, better than 73 cm of mercury is recommended).

The surgeon connects a suction tip to the aspiration tubing. The circulator or scrub person attaches tubing to controlled suction unit and activates it on the surgeon's request.

A gauze tissue bag is used inside the collection bottle to collect specimen. Send gauze tissue bag and contents to pathology laboratory.

MARSUPIALIZATION OF BARTHOLIN'S DUCT CYST

Definition

The incision and drainage of a vulvovaginal cyst and the suturing of the cyst wall to the edges of the incision.

Discussion

The cyst wall is composed primarily of the duct of the gland; by not excising the cyst, the secretory function of the gland may be preserved.

Procedure

A vertical incision is made in the vaginal mucosa over the center of the cyst (outside the hymenal ring). The cyst is incised and drained. The lining of the cyst is everted and sutured to the vaginal mucosa with interrupted stitches. If cystectomy is necessary, the cyst is mobilized using sharp and blunt dissection. The intact cyst is excised. The mucosa is approximated; a drain may be inserted.

Preparation of the Patient

Following the administration of local, regional, or general anesthesia, the patient is positioned in a lithotomy. Arms may be extended on armboards. Apply electrosurgical dispersive pad.

Skin Preparation

See Dilatation and Curettage, p. 157. The patient's bladder may be catheterized with a straight catheter; check with the surgeon.

Draping

The patient is draped with a sheet under the buttocks, leggings, and a fenestrated sheet. The surgeon and the assistant may be seated. A drape sheet is fastened beneath the fenestration; the sheet lies across the surgeon's lap and an instrument lap tray is placed on the surgeon's lap. Some surgeons prefer to stand, eliminating the need for the extra drape sheet and lap tray.

Equipment

Stirrups
Electrosurgical unit

Instrumentation

Cervical cone tray

Supplies

Culture tubes (2) (aerobic and anaerobic cultures) and swabs
Smear slides (2)
Disposable syringe and long 15 or 18 gauge needle (optional)
Lap tray (optional)
Electrosurgical pencil
Drain (e.g., Penrose ¼″, optional)
Perineal pads
T-binder or sanitary napkin belt

Special Notes

Stirrups are well padded to avoid nerve damage.

Lift both legs at the same time when putting the patient in stirrups to prevent postoperative lumbosacral strain.

Raise and lower legs slowly to prevent circulatory disturbances due to rapid alterations in venous return.

CULDOSCOPY

Definition

Culdoscopy is the introduction of an endoscope through the posterior vaginal wall, which provides visualization of the pelvic structures.

Discussion

Once frequently employed as a diagnostic tool, culdoscopy has largely been replaced by laparoscopy in which the positioning of the patient is easier and better visualization of the pelvis is achieved. See Laparoscopy, pp. 167–170, for Procedure, Preparation of the patient, Instrumentation, and Supplies.

VAGINAL HYSTERECTOMY

Definition

Removal of the uterus through a vaginal approach.

Discussion

Indications for this procedure include diseases of the uterus restricted to benign conditions in which the uterus is not greatly enlarged, and conditions in which poor pelvic muscular support is present, necessitating anterior and posterior colporrhaphy.

Procedure

A weighted vaginal speculum is placed in the vaginal vault. The cervix is grasped with a tenaculum. Dilatation and curettage may be performed. A phenylephrine (Neo-Synephrine) solution may be injected into the vaginal incision sites. An incision is made anterior to the cervix in the vaginal wall. The bladder is reflected from the cervix using sharp, then blunt dissection, exposing the peritoneum of the anterior cul-de-sac, which is then incised, posteriorly. The uterosacral ligaments are ligated and divided. The uterus is placed on traction. The cardinal ligaments and uterine arteries are ligated and divided, and the uterus is delivered. If the ovaries are to be preserved, the ovarian vessels are preserved, and the remaining structures in the broad ligament are ligated and divided. After the specimen is removed, the incisions into the cul-de-sac and vaginal apex are repaired. The uterosacral and round ligament stumps may be sutured to the angles of the vaginal vault closure. An anterior and/or posterior colporrhaphy may be performed (see pp. 166–167). The vagina may be packed.

Preparation of the Patient

Following the administration of regional or general anesthesia, the patient is positioned in lithotomy. Arms may be extended on armboards. Apply electrosurgical dispersive pad.

Skin Preparation

Begin at the pubic symphysis and extend downward over the labia. Cleanse each inner thigh. The vaginal vault and cervix are then cleansed using spongesticks (three). The perineum and anus are cleansed with the remaining sponges. Discard each sponge after wiping the anus. The bladder may be drained with a straight catheter.

Draping

The patient is draped with a sheet under the buttocks, leggings, and a fenestrated sheet. Usually the surgeon and the assistant are seated. A drape sheet is fastened beneath the fenestration; the sheet lies across the surgeon's lap, and an instrument lap tray is placed on the surgeon's lap. Some surgeons prefer to stand, eliminating the need for the extra drape sheet and lap tray.

Equipment

Electrosurgical unit
Suction
Stirrups

Instrumentation

Vaginal hysterectomy tray

Supplies

Blades (2) No. 10
Needle magnet or counter
Basin set
Lap tray (optional)
Neo-Synephrine 1:20,000, with local syringe and needle (optional)
Suction tubing
Electrosurgical pencil
Foley catheter drainage unit
Gauze packing (e.g., 1", optional)
Vaginal cream
Perineal pad
T-binder or sanitary napkin belt

Special Notes

In addition to the operative permit, a sterilization permit may be required.

Stirrups are well padded to avoid nerve damage.

Lift both legs at the same time when putting the patient in stirrups to prevent postoperative lumbosacral strain.

Raise and lower legs slowly to prevent circulatory disturbances due to rapid alterations in venous return.

Instruments for the lap tray often include a weighted speculum, a tenaculum, retractors, curved Mayo scissors, and hysterectomy clamps (e.g., Heaney, curved Kocher).

ANTERIOR AND/OR POSTERIOR COLPORRHAPHY

Definition

Repair and reinforcement of musculofascial support of the bladder and the urethra (anteriorly) and distal rectum (posteriorly), preventing protrusion of the structures through the vaginal wall.

Discussion

Cystocele (or cystourethrocele) presents with symptoms of nuisance protrusion anteriorly into the vagina with urinary retention and/or stress incontinence. *Rectocele* presents posteriorly and may be associated with difficulties in defecation. These conditions may present simultaneously or independently to varying degrees. An associated *enterocele* (herniation through the recto-uterine pouch) may also occur. This latter entity can also present with uterine prolapse or in patients in whom hysterectomy has been performed. Multiparity is the most common cause for these entities. Repair may be peformed to correct any of these conditions alone, in combination, or to complement a vaginal hysterectomy.

Procedure

The cervix (if present) is grasped with a tenaculum. For *anterior colporrhaphy* the anterior vaginal mucosa is incised in the midline. The incision is deepened into the musculofascial wall reflecting the bladder anteriorly, mobilizing the urethra, and exposing the urethrovesical junction. Plication sutures are placed in the musculofascial tissues to restore the urethrovesical angle and support of the bladder. Care is taken not to overtighten the repair. Excess of the previously stretched vaginal mucosa is excised, and the mucosal incision is approximated.

For *posterior colporrhaphy* an incision is made at the mucocutaneous junction reflecting the attenuated vaginal mucosa proximally to expose the rectocele. Perirectal fascia is separated from the mucosa and plicated.

The levator muscles are approximated at the midline to an appropriate degree of tension. The excess vaginal mucosa is excised, and the mucosal incision is closed. A vaginal pack may be placed.

Preparation of the Patient

Following the administration of regional or general anesthesia, the patient is positioned in a lithotomy. The arms may be extended on armboards. Apply electrosurgical dispersive pad.

Skin Preparation

Begin at the pubic symphysis and extend downward over the labia. Cleanse each inner thigh. The vaginal vault and cervix are then cleansed using spongesticks (three). The perineum and anus are cleansed with the remaining sponges. Discard each sponge after wiping the anus. Patient is catheterized with an indwelling or straight catheter.

Draping, Equipment, Instrumentation, and Supplies

See Vaginal Hysterectomy, pp. 163–165.

Special Notes

Stirrups are well padded to avoid nerve damage.

Lift both legs at the same time to prevent postoperative lumbosacral strain.

Raise and lower legs slowly to prevent circulatory disturbances due to rapid alterations in venous return.

Instruments for the lap tray often include a weighted speculum, a tenaculum, retractors, curved Mayo scissors, and Allis clamps.

PELVIC LAPAROSCOPY/PELVISCOPY

Definition

The introduction of an endoscope through the anterior abdominal wall following the establishment of a pneumoperitoneum.

Discussion

Pelvic laparoscopy permits visualization of the pelvic structures without open laparotomy. It is useful in the diagnosis of causes of infertility, ectopic pregnancy, pelvic masses (benign and malignant), endometrial implants, etiology of the acute abdomen, pelvic pain, and so on. An expanding number of therapeutic modalities includes various fertility procedures (ovarian drilling, laser-assisted neosalpingostomy and fimbroplasty, salpingo-ovariolysis, in vitro fertilization, and so on); other salpingo-ovarian procedures (complete and partial excision, drainage and excision of cysts, correction of torsion, endo-ovarian procedures as for sterilization, treatment of ectopic pregnancy, and so on, endometrial cysts, drainage of tubo-ovarian abcess); uterine nerve ablation for intractable dysmenorrhea, myomectomy, copolsuspension, pelvic lymphadenectomy, hysterectomy (and laparoscopic-assisted vaginal hysterectomy); procedures for endometriosis; and so on. Appendectomy and other general surgical procedures may be combined with the gynecologic surgery as applicable. Laparoscopic hysterectomy (pp. 176–180) will be described in detail, the techniques of which can be modified accordingly to other of the more commonly performed gynecologic laparoscopic procedures.

Procedure

The vagina is retracted, and the anterior lip of the cervix is grasped with a tenaculum. A self-retaining cannula is inserted in the cervix. Pneumoperitoneum is established as for abdominal laparoscopy (pp. 62–64). The pelvis is explored, and the definitive procedure is performed. At the completion of the procedure, the gas is permitted to escape through the sleeve. Incisions are closed with a subcuticular stitch or skin closure strips.

Alternatively, a trocar with an automatically retracting cutting tip is inserted in the inferior umbilicus and directly advanced intraperitoneally. The surgeon or the assistant surgeon may apply manual traction to the abdominal wall to minimize visceral injury during the puncture.

Preparation of the Patient

Following the administration of local, regional, or general anesthesia, the patient is placed in a modified lithotomy (45°) position. Arms may be extended on armboards. The table is positioned in Trendelenburg; for extreme Trendelenburg, shoulder braces are required. Apply electosurgical dispersive pad.

Skin Preparation

Begin at the umbilicus extending from nipples to pubic symphysis, and down to the table at the sides. Follow this by a vaginal preparation beginning at pubic symphysis and extending down over the labia. Cleanse each inner thigh. Prepare vaginal vault and cervix using spongesticks (three). Perineum and anus are prepared last, discarding each sponge after wiping the anus. Catheterize patient with a straight catheter.

Draping

Drape sheet under the buttocks, and a special laparoscopy sheet

Equipment

Insufflation device
Fiberoptic light source
Electrosurgical unit
Suction
Shoulder braces (optional)

Instrumentation

Laparoscopy instrumentation as for Abdominal Laparoscopy, p. 65.
Uterine retractor, tenaculum, and uterine manipulator
For *chromotubation* (infertility detection): Intrauterine cannula (e.g., Cohen)

Supplies

Suction tubing (for uterine manipulator)
Blade No. 15 or No. 11
Skin closure strips (optional)
For *infertility* add: Plastic tubing, syringe containing
  dye (e.g., methylene blue)

Special Notes

Lift both legs at the same time when putting the patient in stirrups to prevent postoperative lumbosacral strain.

Raise and lower legs slowly to prevent circulatory disturbances due to rapid alterations in venous return.

Laparoscope lens warmer may be used. Antifogging solution may be applied to lens before use and wiped off to prevent fogging (e.g., Elvis, Fred).

Regarding insufflation device: Check the amount of gas in tanks before starting, tighten all connections, and prefill unit with carbon dioxide.

TOTAL ABDOMINAL HYSTERECTOMY

Definition

Removal of the entire uterus through an abdominal incision.

Discussion

Some indications for total abdominal hysterectomy are endometriosis, adnexal disease, postmenopausal bleeding, dysfunctional uterine bleeding, and benign and malignant tumors.

Procedure

A Pfannenstiel, vertical, midline, or paramedian incision is employed. The peritoneal cavity is entered, and a self-retaining retractor is placed. The patient is placed in Trendelenburg position, and the intestines are protected with warm moist (saline) laparotomy pads. The round ligaments of the uterus are ligated, divided, sutured, and tagged with a hemostat. After identifying the ureters, the broad ligaments are incised, and the bladder is reflected from the anterior aspect of the cervix. The infundibulopelvic ligaments are ligated and divided. If the ovaries are to be preserved, the ovarian ligament is ligated and divided adjacent to the uterus (avoiding the ureters). The uterosacral ligaments are ligated and divided. The cardinal ligaments are likewise divided. The vagina is incised circumferentially and the uterine specimen removed. A free sponge (soaked in preparation solution) may be placed in the vagina prior to closure. After hemostasis is secured, the vaginal cuff is closed; a drain may be used. The stumps of the uterosacral and round ligaments are sutured to the angles of the vaginal closure. The pelvic peritoneum is approximated, and the wound is closed. The free sponge is removed.

Preparation of the Patient

The patient is supine; arms may be extended on armboards. Apply electrosurgical dispersive pad.

Skin Preparation

A vaginal and an abdominal preparation (separate trays) are required. Put the patient's legs in a froglike position and prepare as for Dilatation and Curettage, p. 157. Insert a Foley catheter and connect to continuous drainage. Return the patient's legs to their original position, and replace the safety belt. For abdominal preparation begin at the incision (usually Pfannenstiel) extending from nipples to midthighs, and down to the table at the sides.

Draping

Folded towels and a transverse or laparotomy sheet

Equipment

Suction
Electrosurgical unit

Instrumentation

Major procedures tray
Abdominal hysterectomy tray
Self-retaining retractor (e.g., Balfour or O'Connor-O'Sullivan)

Supplies

Blades (3) No. 10
Basin set
Needle magnet or counter
Suction tubing
Electrosurgical pencil
Foley catheter drainage unit
Perineal pad

Special Notes

Sterilization permit may be required in addition to the routine surgical permit.

Have spongesticks available throughout procedure.

Instruments that come in contact with the cervix or vagina are isolated in a basin.

Specimen may be received in a basin.

Counts are taken three times (at closure of vaginal cuff, peritoneum, and skin).

If a "free sponge" has been placed in the vagina prior to closure, it is included in the sponge count and *must* be removed from the vagina at the termination of the procedure before the patient leaves the room.

SALPINGO-OOPHORECTOMY

Definition

The removal of a fallopian tube and corresponding ovary.

Discussion

Salpingo-oopherectomy is performed for a variety of nonmalignant diseases that include acute and chronic infections, cysts, tumors, and hemorrhage (tubal pregnancy). Malignancy of a tube or ovary will usually necessitate hysterectomy with excision of the opposite adnexae.

Procedure

A low midline, paramedian, or Pfannenstiel incision is employed. The peritoneal cavity is entered, and a self-retaining retractor is placed. The patient is placed in Trendelenburg position. The intestines are protected by laparotomy pads. If adhesions are present, the affected tube and ovary are isolated from surrounding organs. The infundibulopelvic ligament is ligated and divided as is the broad ligament attachment of the tube and ovary. The tube and ovary are excised. The site of adnexal excision may be reperitonealized. The wound is closed in layers. For details of laparoscopic approach, see laparoscopic hysterectomy, pp. 176–180.

Preparation of the Patient

The patient is supine; arms may be extended on armboards. Apply electrosurgical dispersive pad.

Skin Preparation, Draping, and Equipment

See Total Abdominal Hysterectomy, p. 171.

Instrumentation

Major procedures tray
Self-retaining retractor (e.g., Balfour or O'Connor-O'Sullivan)
Somer's clamp

Supplies

Blades (2) No. 10, (1) No. 15
Basin set
Needle magnet or counter
Suction tubing
Electrosurgical pencil

Special Notes

For bilateral salpingo-oophorectomy, a sterilization permit in addition to the routine surgical permit may be required.

Have spongesticks available throughout the procedure.

TUBAL STERILIZATION

Definition

The interruption of the fallopian tubes resulting in sterilization.

Discussion

Puerperal sterilization is best performed 24 to 36 hours after vaginal delivery, although it is performed at other times, that is, during cesarean section or as an elective surgery. Approaches include minilaparotomy, laparoscopy, and posterior colpotomy. For details of laparoscopic approach, see Laparoscopic Hysterectomy, pp. 176–178.

Procedure

Minilaparotomy. A small incision is made suprapubically. An opening is made into the peritoneal cavity. Each tube is grasped with a Babcock forceps, and the tubal procedure performed (excision of, cauterization of, or application of a clip on a section of tube). The peritoneum is approximated. The wound is closed in layers.

Posterior Colpotomy. A weighted speculum is placed in the vagina. The cervix is retracted anteriorly with a tenaculum. A transverse incision is made into the vaginal mucosa posterior to the cervix and extended through the peritoneum to enter the cul-de-sac. Each tube is grasped with a Babcock forceps and the tubal procedure performed. The colpotomy site is closed with through-and-through sutures including vaginal mucosa and peritoneum.

Preparation of the Patient

Minilaparotomy. Patient is supine; arms may be extended on armboards.

Posterior Colpotomy. Patient is in lithotomy; arms may be extended on armboards.

Patient may be catheterized with a straight catheter; check with the surgeon. Apply electrosurgical dispersive pad.

Skin Preparation

Minilaparotomy. Begin at the incision (check with surgeon) extending from nipples to midthighs.

Posterior Colpotomy. Begin at pubic symphysis and extend downward over the labia. Cleanse each inner thigh. Use spongesticks (three) to cleanse vaginal vault and cervix. The perineum and anus are cleansed with remaining sponges; discard each sponge after cleansing the anus.

Draping

Minilaparotomy. Folded towels and laparotomy sheet

Posterior Colpotomy. Drape sheet under buttocks, leggings, and drape sheet over the abdomen

Equipment

Minilaparotomy. Electrosurgical unit

Posterior Colpotomy. Suction, electrosurgical unit

Instrumentation

MINILAPAROTOMY
Basic/Minor procedures tray
Hemoclip appliers (small, medium)

POSTERIOR COLPOTOMY
Cervical cone tray
Babcock forceps (long)
Weighted speculum
Hemoclip appliers, long (small, medium)

Supplies

MINILAPAROTOMY
Blades (2) No. 15
Basin set
Needle magnet or counter
Electrosurgical pencil
Hemoclips (small, medium)

POSTERIOR COLPOTOMY
Blade No. 10
Suction tubing
Needle magnet or counter
Basin set
Electrosurgical pencil
Hemoclips (medium)

Special Notes

Put specimens in separate containers labeled right and left tube segment.

LAPAROSCOPIC HYSTERECTOMY AND LAPAROSCOPIC-ASSISTED VAGINAL HYSTERECTOMY WITH OR WITHOUT SALPINGO-OOPHORECTOMY

Definition

Excision of the uterus (with or without excision of the uterine tubes and ovaries) by laparoscopic approach with varying components of transvaginal manipulation and/or operative maneuvers.

Discussion

To minimize postoperative morbidity with the avoidance of a laparotomy incision and to directly identify pelvic structures to minimize intraoperative trauma, the laparoscopic approach is employed. Whereas vaginal hysterectomy (see pp. 163–164) likewise avoids an abdominal incision in situations in which the uterus is unduly enlarged (e.g., fibromyomata), uterine descensus is minimal, prior cesarean section, pelvic adhesions secondary to surgery or inflammatory disease, endometriosis, intestinal pathology, and so on. The vaginal approach may be either unsafe or technically infeasible. In these circumstances mobilization of pelvic structures under direct visualization laparoscopically with the delivery of a specimen vaginally or through a large-bore part would be a satisfactory alternative to formal laparotomy. In addition, certain phases of the procedure such as making the colporrhaphy incision, securing uterine vessels, and closure of the vaginal cuff can be done vaginally (LAVH). Finally, anterior and posterior colporrhaphy (see p. 166) may be performed in conjunction with hysterectomy. Supracervical hysterectomy, in which the epithelium of the endocervical canal is ablated but the cervix and its supporting ligaments retained, has been reintroduced. The employment of laparoscopic hysterectomy in cases of malignancy is currently controversial.

Procedure

Following the establishment of pneumoperitoneum (see pp. 62–64) with a 10 to 11 mm trocar, additional 12 mm trocars are inserted at the lateral borders of the rectus muscles, inferior to the level of the umbilicus and suprapubically (optional). The abdomen is explored. An optional intrauterine cannula for facilitation of uterine manipulation (e.g., Kronner Manipujector or Valtchev uterine mobilizer) may be placed transvaginally. If intra-abdominal adhesions are present, enterolysis is performed so that the uterus and adnexal structures can be freely moved (directly or by means of the uterine manipulator). The various supporting ligaments are transsected (see Abdominal Hysterectomy, pp. 170–171). The ligaments are divided employing a linear endoscopic multiple clip applier. The tubes and ovaries may be preserved or excised accordingly. The uterovesical fold is placed under tension directly or by employing the intrauterine manipulator, and a peritoneal bladder flap is developed using an electrosurgical endoscopic scissors. A hydrodissector may be used for this maneuver as well. The uterosacral and cardinal ligaments are transsected, the ureters having been identified. The uterine vessels are tied and cut close to the uterine wall. Pressure is placed on the vagina superiorly, and a posterior colpotomy incision is made electrosurgically. Moist packing is inserted vaginally to minimize the loss of pneumoperitoneum. Colpotomy is completed anteriorly and laterally, and the uterine specimen is delivered vaginally or transabdominally through a large-bore port (e.g., 30 mm). The colpotomy incision is closed transvaginally or by endoscopic suture technique, suspending the corners to the uterosacral ligament remnants when applicable. Pneumoperitoneum is restored and the bladder flap reapproximated laparoscopically with staples (e.g., endoscopic hernia stapler). If the uterine specimen is too large to be passed intact through the colpotomy incision, the uterus can be morcellated within a specimen bag and then withdrawn vaginally or through a large-bore port. Alternatively, as in vaginal hysterectomy, the colpotomy incision, division of uterosacral and cardinal ligaments and ligation of the uterine vessels, extraction of the specimen (as noted), and closure of the vaginal cuff may be performed transvaginally. If supracervical hysterectomy is performed, after the uterine corpus is amputated, the epithelium of the endocervical canal is ablated (e.g., reaming technique employing a serrated edge macromorcellator).

Procedures as myomectomy and the various procedures involving the tubes and ovaries are performed according to the general format described above with additional instrumentation and microinstrumentation as necessary. The definitive portions of these procedures is performed as in the corresponding open procedures and will not be further addressed. After the pelvis is irrigated and suctioned, the pneumoperitoneum is released, and the trocar sites are repaired. Anterior and posterior colporrhaphy may be performed (see pp. 166–167).

Preparation of the Patient

Following the administration of general anesthesia, the patient is placed in a modified lithotomy position using Allen stirrups, if possible. The arms are padded and may be tucked in at the patient's sides. The table is placed in Trendelenburg. Apply electrosurgical dispersive pad.

Skin Preparation

Begin at the umbilicus extending from the nipples to the pubic symphysis extending down over the labia, discarding each sponge after wiping the labia. Cleanse each inner thigh. Prepare the vaginal vault and cervix using spongesticks (three). The perineum and anus are prepared last, discarding each sponge after wiping the anus. Catheterize patient with a straight catheter.

Draping

Drape sheet under the buttocks and a special laparoscopy sheet.

Equipment

Stirrups (e.g., Allen)
Video monitors (1 or 2)
VCR (optional)
Mavigraph (video printer) (optional)
CO_2 insufflator
Light source (e.g., Xenon 300 W)
Electrosurgical unit
Suction
Pressure bag

Supplies

Foam padding for elbows and ankles
Silastic tubing
Antifog agent
Knife blades (1) No. 10, and/or (1) No. 15
Endoscopic sutures (loop), available
Suction tubing
Foley catheter (e.g., No. 16)
Camera cable cover (plastic with ties)
Endoscopic multifire hernia stapler (optional)

Endoscopic clip applier with medium and large clips
Endoscopic specimen retrieval bag (optional)

Instruments

Major tray (open)
Vaginal hysterectomy tray (open)
D & C tray (open)
Uterine manipulator
10 to 11 mm trocar
12 mm trocars (2)
5 mm trocar
Convertors
Endoscopic shears with unipolar cautery
Endoscopic microscissors
Endoscopic right-angle scissors
Endoscopic grasper (2)
Suction-irrigation device
Forward 0° telescope
Camera
Macromorcellator (available)

Special Notes

In addition to the operative permit, a sterilization permit may be required.

Pad ankles well to avoid nerve damage.

Lift both legs at the same time when putting the patient in stirrups to avoid postoperative lumbosacral strain.

HYSTEROSCOPY

Definition

The visual examination of the uterine cavity by means of a hysteroscope.

Discussion

Hysteroscopy is performed for diagnostic and therapeutic purposes as well as in conjunction with hysterosalpingography, laparoscopy, or formal laparotomy. Indications include evaluation of bleeding (after nondiagnostic dilatation and curettage), directed biopsy, evaluation of the endocervix versus the endometrium, and infertility evaluation (noting adhesions, congenital abnormalities, infection, etc.).Excision or ablation of polyps and other lesions (including submucosal fibromyomata), division of a congenital uterine septum, lysis of adhesions, retrieval of a retracted intrauterine device, and so on can be performed. Complications include perforation of the uterus, bleeding, embolization or dissection of the distensive media, and laser injury to adjacent structures. Concomitant laparoscopy can be useful to observe and correct these problems. Contraindications include severe bleeding, acute infection, cervical stenosis, and malignancy.

Visualization of the endometrial surfaces depends upon the ability to distend the uterus with a variety of media. Carbon dioxide is commonly employed; dextran–70 32% in D10W (Hyskon) has good visual properties, is nonconductive, and does not mix with blood or aqueous fluids, but it is sticky, viscous, and complicates instrument cleaning. Glycine 1.5%, Sorbitol 3%, normal saline, and Ringer's solution also are used. A rigid fiberoptic-lighted scope with a range of viewing angles (e.g., 10° to 45°) and diameters of 6 to 8 mm are used. Scopes with multiple channels permit fluid circulation and use of as many as three endoscopic instruments, and scopes similar to the urologic resectoscope are employed for therapeutic purposes. When diagnosis only and/or limited biopsy is indicated, a flexible fiberoptic scope similar to the choledochoscope can be employed. A video system can be adapted as well.

The pressure and flow rate of the media distending the uterus must be monitored to prevent uterine injury, osmotic related fluid changes, and embolization through intrauterine absorbtion or extravasation into the peritoneum. When using CO_2, the pressures must not exceed 200 mm Hg or a flow rate greater than 80 to 100 mL/min. This requires equipment specific for hysteroscopy, not that used for higher flow rate laparoscopic procedures. As smoke, foam, and bleeding are produced during various operative procedures (e.g., electroablation of endometrium), a liquid medium is preferably controlled, for example, by a Hamou Hysteromat.

An increasing array of therapeutic instruments including probes, aspirators, biopsy forceps, graspers, microscissors, electrosurgical tips, loops, and laser fibers (Argon, KTP 532, Nd:YAG) may be used through the scope under direct observation. See the Appendix for laser precautions, pp. 619–624.

Procedure

Under general anesthesia (paracervical blocks with sedation and other modalities are less often employed), the bladder is emptied and the cervix grasped and dilated according to the diameter of the scope to be used. Excessive dilatation will lead to loss of distending medium. The distending medium is deployed, and under direct visualization this situation is assessed and diagnostic and therapeutic measures performed.

Preparation of the Patient (Apply electrosurgical dispersive pad), Skin Preparation, and Draping

See Dilatation and Curettage (D & C), p. 157.

Equipment

Adequate padding for arms and legs
Stirrups (Allen may be preferred)
Nd:YAG laser unit
Electrosurgical unit

Instrumentation

D & C tray
Hysteroscope and sheath
Cup forceps (assorted)
Alligator forcep
Light cord
Cannulas, for example, aspirating
Scissors
Connectors

Laser fiber (600 mm Nd:YAG)
Caps and nipples, if required

Supplies

30 mL syringe
Silastic tubing
Hyskon or Ringer's lactate and/or saline
Flexible needle
Perineal pad
Foley catheter or special intrauterine balloon catheter,
    available

Special Notes

Stirrups are well padded to prevent nerve damage.

Lift both legs at the same time when putting the patient in stirrups to prevent postoperative lumbosacral strain.

Raise and lower legs slowly to prevent disturbances caused by rapid alterations in venous return.

Hyskon is always used with the resectoscope.

Monitor the amount of medium or media being used.

Inspect instruments after use for breakage with possible retention of a foreign body in the uterine cavity.

Have catheter (Foley or intrauterine) available for intrauterine tamponade if bleeding. (It may be left in postoperatively, to be deflated gradually.)

Prophylactic antibiotics may be requested.

Be aware that sudden loss of intrauterine pressure may indicate perforation.

Instruments, especially optics, must be cleaned immediately post use, particularly if Hyskon is used. A proteolytic enzyme wash is available for cleansing.

TUBOPLASTY OF THE FALLOPIAN TUBES

Definition

The reestablishment of patency to the fallopian tubes.

Discussion

Tuboplasty is usually performed when the patient seeks a reversal of a sterilization procedure. Success depends upon the amount of tubal destruction.

Procedure

Usually a Pfannenstiel incision is employed. The peritoneal cavity is entered, and a self-retaining retractor is placed. Tubal patency may be demonstrated by the injection of methylene blue through a cervical cannula. Tuboplasty is performed according to the site obstruction, for example, cornual resection with reimplantation, tubal resection with anastomosis, or fimbrioplasty. The operating microscope is often used. A laser beam may be directed through the microscope to open adhesions of the fimbria and to lyse lesions within the tubes; for laser precautions, see Appendix pp. 619–624. The abdomen is closed in layers. The cervical cannula is removed.

Preparation of the Patient

Following the induction of anesthesia, a catheter or cannula is inserted in the cervix for subsequent instillation of dye. If this step is to be included, the patient must initially be placed in a lithotomy position. After the catheter (connected to extension tubing and a syringe filled with dye) is secured, the patient is returned to the supine position. The safety belt is replaced. Care is taken not to dislodge the catheter. Apply electrosurgical dispersive pad.

Skin Preparation

If the catheter will be inserted into the cervix, a vaginal preparation is required in addition to the abdominal preparation; see Dilatation and Curettage, p. 157. For abdominal preparation, begin at the incision (usually Pfannenstiel) extending from nipples to midthighs, and down to the table at the sides.

Draping

Folded towels, transverse or laparotomy sheet, and microscope cover

Equipment

Stirrups
Suction
Electrosurgical unit
Microscope

Instruments

Dilatation and curettage (D & C) tray
Major procedures tray (includes probe)
Microinstruments (e.g., smooth and toothed forceps, tying forceps, Castroviejo needle holder, scissors)
Beaver knife handle
Mosquito hemostats (6 curved, 2 straight)
Frazier suction tips (assorted)

Supplies

Basin set
Blades (2) No. 10, (1) No. 15, (1) No. 11
Beaver blade
Needle magnet
Electrosurgical pencil (blade and needle tips)
Suction tubing
Pediatric Foley or special cannula, extension tubing, syringe eyedropper
Dye (e.g., methylene blue)
Perineal pad

Special Notes

Stirrups are well padded to avoid nerve damage.

Lift both legs at the same time when putting the patient in stirrups to prevent postoperative lumbosacral strain.

See Appendix, pp. 619–624 for laser precautions.

Raise and lower legs slowly to prevent disturbances due to rapid alterations in venous return.

While the patient is in the lithotomy position, an extension tubing is connected to the catheter or cannula. A syringe filled with dye solution is attached to the catheter. During the abdominal phase of the procedure, the circulator may be requested to inject the dye.

PELVIC EXENTERATION

Definition

The en bloc removal of the rectum, distal sigmoid colon, the urinary bladder and the distal ureters, internal genitalia, pelvic lymph nodes, pelvic peritoneum, a portion of the levator muscles, and the creation of an ileal or colonic loop urinary diversion; the hypogastric vessels are no longer removed.

Discussion

The primary indication for this procedure is radioresistant or recurrent cervical carcinoma. Total pelvic exenteration implies the excision of the internal genitalia, rectum, and bladder, necessitating a permanent colostomy and a urinary diversion. If malignancy has spread beyond the pelvis or there are significant medical risks, this procedure is abandoned. The rectum may be spared, and anterior exenteration is performed. Posterior exenteration is ususally not performed for gynecologic malignancy, but it may be done for rectal malignancy. The morbidity and mortality for this procedure is significant.

Procedure

A generous midline incision is employed. The abdomen is explored. Frozen section may be done. The order of the procedure varies with the operator. The urinary diversion (see Ileal Conduit, pp. 228–229) may be done first or later in the procedure. Pelvic lymphadenectomy is done, removing the fatty tissues about the iliac vessels extending into the obturator fossa. The ligamentous attachment of the uterus and adnexae are separated from the pelvic wall, and the rectum is mobilized from its posterior and lateral attachments (see Ab-

dominoperineal Resection, pp. 135–138). The bladder
and urethra are mobilized and excised (see Cystectomy,
pp. 212–2130). From the perineal approach (often by a
second team), the anus and distal rectum are excised
(see Abdominoperineal Resection, pp. 135–138). The
distal vagina may be preserved or reconstructed later
on. The specimen is removed en bloc. A colostomy is created and the pelvic floor closed. The abdomen is closed
in layers. Appropriate stomal pouches are applied.

Preparation of the Patient

A nasogastric tube, urinary catheter, and rectal tube
may be inserted before surgery. Antiembolic stockings
may be requested. Central venous pressure monitoring
is established. Following the administration of general
anesthesia, the patient is placed in a modified lithotomy position with the legs tilted forward. Folded towels may be used to elevate the buttocks. The legs and
feet are padded with towels or foam pads to avoid injury at pressure points. The table may be in Trendelenburg. Apply electrosurgical dispersive pad.

Skin Preparation

Begin at the midline extending from nipples to knees,
and down to the table at the sides. Prepare perineum
and genitalia next; a vaginal preparation is required
for women. Cleanse the anus last, discarding each
sponge after use.

Draping

The patient is draped with a sheet under the buttocks
and leggings. The abdomen is draped with folded towels and individual drape sheets or a laparotomy sheet.
If a laparotomy sheet is used, it will be cut to expose the
patient's perineum (for an eliptical incision below the
anus).

Equipment

Electrosurgical unit
Suctions (2)

Stirrups
Scales (to weigh sponges)

Instrumentation

Major procedures tray
Long instruments tray
Vascular procedures tray
Kidney tray
Gastrointestinal procedures tray
Abdominal hysterectomy tray (female)
Abdominal prostatectomy tray (male)
Self-retaining retractors (e.g., Balfour, O'Connor-
    O'Sullivan)
Hemoclip appliers (all sizes and lengths)

Supplies

Blades (4) No. 10, (1) No. 15, (1) No. 11, (1) No. 12
Basin set
Needle magnet or counter
Suction tubing
Electrosurgical pencils (2)
Pouches (2) for electrosurgical pencils
Dissectors (e.g., peanut)
Penrose drains, umbilical tapes, and vascular loops (for
    retraction)
Hemoclips, all sizes
Graduate
Asepto syringe
Robinson catheters, various sizes (available)
Pouches for colostomy and urostomy (e.g., Karaya Seal)
T-binder

Special Notes

Confirm with laboratory that blood is available as ordered.
    Weigh sponges.
    Keep an accurate record of amount of irrigation used.
    Be prepared for many frozen sections.
    Keep all soiled instruments isolated in a basin.

Clean closure of the abdomen requires regowning, regloving, and redraping and the use of a Basic/Minor procedures tray.

Check specimen for instruments and sponges.

SHIRODKAR PROCEDURE

Definition

The placement of an encircling tape ligature at the level of the internal os to maintain the integrity of the cervical canal.

Discussion

This procedure is performed to correct the incompetent cervix during mid or latter pregnancy to prevent spontaneous abortion. Incompetency is related to previous laceration or congenital weakness. The procedure is best performed before the cervix actually dilates.

Procedure

A transverse incision is made in the vaginal mucosa at its junction with the anterior aspect of the cervix. The bladder is reflected away. A similar incision is made posteriorly. A tape ligature is passed on a ligature carrier to encircle the cervix with both ends exiting in the anterior incision. The tape is tightened and sutured. The posterior portion of the tape loop may be sutured to the vaginal mucosa. The mucosal wounds are closed. Thus, a tape ligature encircles the cervix (cerclage). An alternate procedure, McDonald, may be employed, in which a suture of Mersilene (No. 4) is placed in a pursestring fashion around the four quadrants of the cervix and tied to effect competency.

Preparation of the Patient

Following the administration of regional or general anesthesia, the patient is placed in a lithotomy position. Arms may be extended on armboards. Apply electrosurgical dispersive pad.

Skin Preparation

Extreme care must be taken to do the vaginal preparation *very gently*. Begin at the pubic symphysis and extend down over the labia. Cleanse each inner thigh. Gently cleanse vaginal vault and cervix with spongesticks (three). The perineum and anus are cleansed with the remaining sponges. Discard each sponge after wiping the anus.

Draping

Drape sheet under the buttocks, leggings, and a drape sheet over the abdomen

Equipment

Stirrups
Electrosurgical unit (optional)

Instrumentation

Dilatation and curettage (D & C) tray
Cervical cone tray
Short Heaney retractors
Ligature carrier

Supplies

Tape ligature (e.g., 5mm Mersilene tape)
Perineal pad
T-binder

Special Notes

See Dilatation and Curettage, p. 157–158.

CESAREAN SECTION

Definition

Delivery of the fetus through incisions in the abdominal wall and the uterus.

Discussion

There are numerous indications for this means of delivery, including mechanical (cephalopelvic) disproportion, fetal distress, malrotation, and placenta previa. Previous cesarean section is no longer regarded as an absolute indication for this procedure.

Procedure

A low transverse or vertical incision consistent with the estimated size of the fetus is made. The rectus muscles are separated and the peritoneum incised. The bladder is reflected from the lower uterine segment and the uterus incised. The amniotic sac is entered and fluid aspirated. The fetal head is delivered using manual pressure or by obstetric forceps and counterpressure on the fundus. The newborn's airway is aspirated gently, and the delivery is completed. Oxytocin is usually administered intravenously. The umbilical cord is clamped and cut. The baby is transferred to the neonatal team. Hemostasis is secured and the placenta delivered. Tubal ligation may be performed. The uterine incision is closed in a single or a double layer. The previously incised peritoneum at the lower uterine segment is sutured to its anatomic position. The wound is closed in layers.

Preparation of the Patient

The patient is supine; arms may be extended on armboards. Insert a Foley catheter and connect it to continuous drainage.

Skin Preparation

Begin at the incision (infraumbilical vertical or low transverse) extending from nipples to midthighs, and down to the table at the sides. Do not prepare the vagina.

Draping

The patient is draped with folded towels and a laparotomy (or transverse) sheet. An additional sheet is needed to cover a second back table for the infant.

Equipment

Suction
Electrosurgical unit
Heat lamps and bassinet with a warmer
Identification bands (3)
Ink pad (for footprint, single use) (optional)

Instrumentation

Cesarean section tray
Delivery forceps
Cord clamp

Supplies

Basin set
Electrosurgical pencil
Suction tubing
Blades (2) No. 10
Bulb syringe (to aspirate infant's nose and mouth)
Test tubes (2, for cord blood)
Drain (e.g., Penrose), optional

Special Notes

Have Oxytocin, usually 20 units, ready for the anesthetist to administer intravenously. This will help the uterus to contract, minimize blood loss, and aid in expulsion of the placenta.

Once the uterus is opened, immediate suctioning is necessary.

Following delivery of the infant, the cord is clamped and cut, and the infant is given to the pediatrician.

Records pertaining to the birth are completed according to hospital policy.

Two newborn identification bands are put on the infant, and one newborn identification band is put on the mother (in addition to her own armband), before either mother or infant leaves the delivery room.

Cord blood is sent to the laboratory in two test tubes.

As soon as the head is delivered, the scrub person hands the bulb syringe to the surgeon to aspirate amniotic fluid from the infant's nose and mouth. The bulb syringe is passed off the table with the infant.

For prophylaxis of gonococcal or Chlamydial ophthalmia neonatorum, erythromycin 0.5% ointment, tetracycline 1% ointment, or silver nitrate 1% solution (single use tubes or ampules) is instilled into each conjunctival sac.

Counts are taken prior to the closure of the uterus, the peritoneum, and the skin.

Chapter 12

Genitourinary Surgery

HYPOSPADIAS REPAIR

Definition

Refers to the correction of a condition in which the distal urethra terminates at some point on the ventral surface of the penis proximal to its normal position.

Discussion

This condition is a relatively common congenital anomaly. Hypospadius can be noted distally (glandular), mid-penile, penoscrotal, and perineal. The ventral aspect of the penis is often shortened, causing a downward curvature (chordee). When very distal, the deformity is minimal and may not require correction; proximal locations necessitate surgery to avoid difficulty in urination and coitus. Continence is usually not affected because the urinary sphincters are not involved. Circumcision should not be performed on infants with hypospadias to preserve skin useful in correcting the deformity. Correction may be delayed until full penile growth occurs.

Procedure

The chordee is repaired by lysing the fibrous tissue on the ventral aspect of the penis. The absent portion of the urethra is reconstructed out of the foreskin. In circumcised patients, other tissues, for example, a segment of vein, ureter, or skin from a non-hair-bearing area such as the inner aspect of the arm may be used. An incision is made on the ventral aspect of the penis. The reconstructed urethra, splinted from within by a catheter, is placed in a tunnel over which the remaining foreskin is grafted. Numerous procedures can be used according to the severity of the defect; some require a second stage to restore urethral continuity.

Preparation of the Patient

The patient is supine with the legs apart; arms may be extended on armboards. The safety strap is replaced above the patient's knees. Children are maintained in a froglike position; care must be taken to adequately secure the child (see Pediatric General Information, pp. 518–520) while preventing trauma to skin and pressure points. Apply electrosurgical dispersive pad (pediatric size for children).

Skin Preparation

Begin cleansing the ventral surface of the penis extending from the umbilicus to lower thighs, and down to the table at the sides. Cleanse rectum last (discarding sponges afterward).

Draping

Cuffed towel under the scrotum, folded towels around pubic area, and a laparotomy sheet (adults) or a pediatric laparotomy sheet (children)

Equipment

Electrosurgical unit

Instrumentation

ADULTS
Basic/Minor procedures tray
Urethral sounds

INFANTS AND CHILDREN
Pediatric minor procedures tray
Lacrimal duct probes

Supplies

Blades (2) No. 15
Needle magnet or counter
Basin set
Catheter (e.g., Foley)
Electrosurgical pencil

EPISPADIAS REPAIR

Definition

Correction of a congenital absence of the dorsal wall of
the urethra proximal to the glans; uretha opens on the
dorsal aspect of the penis.

Discussion

This deformity most often occurs at the abdominope-
nile junction and can be associated with deformities of
the bladder and urinary sphincter. Circumcision
should not be performed on infants with epispadias to
preserve skin useful in correcting the deformity. Repair
is necessary to effect continence and ability to copulate.

Procedure

If a lesser deformity exists distally, the tissues are mobilized, sutured over the defect, and the meatus opened
at the tip of the glans. For more proximal defects the
urethra is corrected in similar fashion to that employed
for hypospadias (see pp. 194–195). A suprapubic incision is made to expose the prostatic urethra. Redundant tissue of the prostatic urethra is excised. Catgut
sutures approximate the prostatic urethra and vesical
neck over a probe or catheter, re-creating the continence mechanism. A suprapubic cystostomy is placed
to provide temporary urinary diversion. The wound is
closed.

Preparation of the Patient, Skin
Preparation, Draping, Equipment,
and Instrumentation

See Hypospadias Repair, pp. 194–195.

Supplies

Blades (2) No. 15
Needle magnet or counter
Basin set
Electrosurgical pencil
Catheters: urethral (e.g., Foley) suprapubic cystostomy
   (e.g., Pezzer, Malecot)

CIRCUMCISION

Definition

The excision of the foreskin.

Discussion

Circumcision may be performed as a prophylactic
health measure, to correct phimosis (constriction of the
foreskin), to treat recurrent balanitis (inflammation of
the glans penis), or as a religious rite.

Procedure

If phimosis is present, a dorsal slit is made. Adhesions
are lysed. A circumferential incision is made at the re-
flection of the foreskin excising it. Hemostasis is achieved
and the wound approximated using absorbable suture.

Preparation of the Patient, Skin
Preparation, Draping, and Equipment

See Hypospadias Repair, pp. 194–195.

Instrumentation

ADULTS
Limited procedure tray
Probe and grooved director

INFANTS AND CHILDREN

Pediatric minor procedures tray
Circumcision clamp (e.g., Gomco, Plastibell)

Supplies

Blades (2) No. 15
Electrosurgical pencil
Needle magnet or counter
Basin set
Catheter, for example, Foley (adult)

Special Notes

Consider the special needs of the Jewish patient for ritual circumcision.

PENILE IMPLANT

Definition

Insertion of a prosthesis in the penis for the treatment of impotence.

Discussion

Although the procedure permits the patient to engage in sexual intercourse, it does not treat the underlying cause. Many varieties of prostheses are available including semirigid, flexible, and dynamic (inflatable prosthesis with reservoir).

Procedure

A Foley catheter is usually inserted. If a single-rod prosthesis is used, a dorsal incision is made proximal to the glans, and a tunnel is made between the corpora cavernosa. Hemostasis is achieved. Using a double rod prosthesis requires incisions made into the corpora cavernosa; the tunnel is dilated with a clamp and Hegar dilators. The prosthesis is inserted. When using a dynamic (inflatable) prosthesis, the tunica albuginea incision is made toward the base of the penis or in the low suprapubic region. The corpora cavernosa are dilated, and the prosthesis cylinders are placed. The reservoir is placed in the prevesical space, and the pump is placed in the scrotum via subcutaneous tunnels also made through the initial incision. The wounds are closed.

Preparation of the Patient

The patient is supine with legs separated; arms may be extended on armboards. Replace safety strap above the knees. Apply electrosurgical dispersive pad.

Skin Preparation

Begin on the dorsum of the penis extending from the umbilicus to the lower thighs, and down to the table at the sides.

Draping

Cuffed towel under the scrotum, folded towels around pubic region, and a laparotomy sheet

Equipment

Electrosurgical unit

Instrumentation

Basic/Minor procedures tray
Ruler and /or caliper
Andrews suction tip 9½"
Hegar dilators
Senn retractors (2) blunt
Metzenbaum scissors, long, 9"

Supplies

Blades (1) No. 10, (2) No. 15
Basin set
Needle magnet or counter
Electrosurgical pencil (needle tip)
Foley catheter
Dissectors (e.g., peanut)

Antibiotic solution and bulb syringe (optional)

Prostheses and necessary equipment (e.g., syringes, needles, connectors)

Special Notes

Check with the surgeon regarding the size and type of implant.

The prosthesis should be sterilized and handled in strict accordance with manufacturers recommendations. Extra precautions must be observed to avoid contamination of the prosthesis with lint, glove powder, and so on to minimize foreign body reaction.

Prepackaged sterile prostheses should not be opened until the surgeon confirms the size.

MARSHALL-MARCHETTI-KRANTZ PROCEDURE

Definition

Suspension of the bladder neck and proximal urethra to the symphysis pubis.

Discussion

This procedure is performed to correct urinary stress incontinence caused by weakness of the support of the bladder neck and proximal urethra. If there are other causes of incontinence, for example, neurological problems, this surgery is not appropriate. Elevation of the bladder neck restores continence.

Procedure

A Pfannenstiel incision is used. After displacing the muscles, a self-retaining retractor is employed. The prevesical space of Retzius is entered. The bladder is identified and reflected from the vagina. The urethra is exposed. Sutures are placed in the paraurethral tissues, suspending them to the periosteum at the symphysis pubis. At intervals, counterpressure is applied by a gloved hand vaginally. The space of Retzius may be drained. The wound is closed in layers.

Preparation of the Patient

The patient is in a modified lithotomy position; arms may be extended on armboards. Apply electrosurgical dispersive pad.

Skin Preparation

Begin at the incision (Pfannenstiel) extending from nipples to lower thighs, and down to the table at the sides. Follow this by a vaginal preparation beginning at the pubic symphysis and extending down over the labia. Cleanse each inner thigh. Prepare vaginal vault and cervix using spongesticks (three). The perineum and anus are prepared last, discarding each sponge after wiping the anus. A Foley catheter is inserted and connected to straight drainage.

Draping

Drape sheet under the buttocks, leggings, folded towels, and a transverse sheet (abdomen)

Equipment

Stirrups
Electrosurgical unit
Suction

Instrumentation

Major procedures tray
Self-retaining retractor (e.g., Balfour)
Hemoclip appliers (assorted sizes and lengths)
Heaney needle holders

Supplies

Basin set
Blades (2) No. 10, (1) No. 15
Electrosurgical pencil
Suction tubing
Hemoclips (assorted)
Drain (e.g., Penrose or Jackson-Pratt)

Special Notes

Stirrups are well padded to avoid nerve damage.

Lift both legs at the same time when putting the patient in stirrups to prevent postoperative lumbosacral strain.

Raise and lower legs slowly to prevent disturbances caused by rapid alterations in venous return.

Extra gloves are needed for the assistant who applies vaginal counterpressure.

HYDROCELECTOMY

Definition

Excision of a portion of the tunica vaginalis testis with evacuation of fluid contained therein.

Discussion

A hydrocele is an accumulation of serous fluid around the testis within the tunica vaginalis resulting from trauma or infection or occurring spontaneously. In children, indirect inguinal hernia may accompany the hydrocele.

Procedure

An inguinal or scrotal approach may be employed. In the inguinal approach the testis and spermatic cord are delivered into the inguinal wound. The hydrocele fluid is aspirated through a small incision or with a needle and syringe. Excessive sac wall is excised or may be wrapped around and sutured behind the epididymis. Hemostasis is achieved. If a hernia is present, it is repaired (see p. 67, adult; p. 531, pediatric). The incision is closed.

Preparation of the Patient

The patient is supine with legs apart; arms may be extended on armboards. Apply electrosurgical dispersive pad.

Skin Preparation

Scrotal Approach. Begin at the scrotum extending from umbilicus to lower thighs, and down to the table at the sides.

Inguinal Approach. Begin at the inguinal area on the affected side extending from the umbilicus to lower thighs, and down to the table at the sides.

Draping

Cuffed towel under the scrotum, folded towels around the pubic area, and a laparotomy sheet

Equipment

Electrosurgical unit

Instrumentation

Basic/Minor procedures tray (adult)
Pediatric minor procedures tray (child)

Supplies

Basin set
Blades (1) No. 10, (2) No. 15 (adult); (2) No. 15 (child)
Needle magnet or counter
Penrose drain, small (retraction)
Syringe (30 mL) and needle (20 gauge)
Scrotal suspensory support (adults)

VASECTOMY

Definition

Excision of a segment of the vas deferens with ligation of the distal and proximal ends.

Discussion

The procedure is done bilaterally for the purpose of male contraception or to prevent orchitis prior to prostatectomy. Occasionally the vas may be multiple or absent on either side.

Procedure

The vas is palpated through the scrotum before the anesthetic is administered. A scrotal incision is made, the vas is seized, and it is freed of surrounding tissue. A segment of vas is excised and the ends ligated. The severed ends may be cauterized or crushed with a clamp prior to ligation. The severed ends may be allowed to retract or may be buried within the scrotal connective tissue and sutured in place. The wound is closed. The procedure is repeated on the other side.

Preparation of the Patient

The patient is supine with legs apart; arms may be extended on armboards (or one arm may be tucked in at the side). The safety strap is fastened above the patient's knees. Apply electrosurgical dispersive pad.

Skin Preparation

Begin at the scrotum extending from above the pubic symphysis to the lower thighs. Prepare perianal area last, discarding each sponge after wiping over the anus.

Draping

Folded towels and a laparotomy sheet

Equipment

Electrosurgical unit

Instrumentation

Vasectomy tray

Supplies

Electrosurgical pencil
Blade (1) No. 15
Scrotal support
Small basin

Special Notes

Local anesthesia is frequently employed.

An ice pack may be applied to the scrotum immediately postoperatively.

In addition to the surgical permit, a sterilization permit may be required.

VASOVASOSTOMY

Definition

Anastomosis of the severed ends of the vas deferens.

Discussion

The procedure is performed to reestablish continuity of the vas deferens in the previously vasectomized patient to restore fertility.

Procedure

A scrotal incision exposes the vas deferens above and below site of the previous ligation. The scar tissue is excised from both ends of the vas. Under magnification sutures are placed in the mucosal lining of the lumen. Muscularis is approximated separately. The wound is closed.

Preparation of Patient, Skin Preparation, and Draping

See Vasectomy, p. 204.

Equipment

Electrosurgical unit
Loupes or microscope

Instrumentation

Basic/Minor procedures tray
Vasovasostomy microscopic instruments, for example,
  1 tissue forceps, 2 curved smooth forceps, 1 curved tying forceps, 1 Castroviejo needle holder, 1 vas holder

Supplies

Basin set
Blades (1) No. 15, (1) No. 11

Electrosurgical pencil with needle tip
Scrotal support

Special Notes

Check with the surgeon regarding use of loupes or microscope.
 Have ice pack ready (optional).

CUTANEOUS VASOSTOMY

Definition

Establishment of an opening of the vas onto the scrotal skin.

Discussion

Cutaneous vasostomy is performed to drain an infected epididymis or testis, in which an incised loop of vas is sutured to the scrotal skin. Vasography may be done by injection of contrast media into the severed end(s). The wound or wounds usually close spontaneously after the precipitating episode subsides.

Procedure

An incision is made over the vas, which is seized and freed of surrounding tissue. The vas is divided, and the severed ends are sutured to the scrotal skin.

Preparation of the Patient, Skin Preparation, Draping, Equipment, Instrumentation, and Supplies

See Vasectomy, p. 204.

SPERMATOCELECTOMY

Definition

Excision of a cystic swelling of the spermatic ductal system, usually at the epididymis.

Discussion

This condition is a benign cystic swelling of the sperm-conveying ductal system, usually of the epididymis. If fertility is a consideration and the excision of the cyst interrupts the duct, a side-to-side anastomosis of the epididymis and vas (epidymovasostomy) is performed to maintain continuity of the system.

Procedure

A scrotal incision is made and the pathology assessed. The cystic mass is excised. If an obvious interruption of the ductal system is created, anastomosis is performed using fine absorbable sutures with the aid of loupes or a microscope. The anastomosis may be tested for patency using a blunt needle (e.g., 20 gauge), syringe, and methylene blue dye. The incision is closed.

Preparation of the Patient, Skin Preparation, Draping, Equipment, Instrumentation, and Supplies

See Vasovasostomy, pp. 205 206.

ORCHIECTOMY

Definition

Removal of one or both testicles.

Discussion

The procedure is performed for endocrine control of prostatic carcinoma, primary tumors of the testes, severe testicular trauma, or irreversible vascular compromise after testicular torsion.

Procedure

For benign disease or endocrine control, the incision can be made transcrotally or inguinally. The testis is identified, the spermatic cord ligated, and the testis removed. The same procedure is repeated bilaterally as indicated. For primary testicular malignancy, high ligation of the spermatic cord is done. Radical lymphadenectomy may be performed through an abdominal incision or laparoscopically; lymph node–bearing fatty tissues from the level of the renal vessels, and about the aorta, to the level of the transsection of the spermatic cord, are removed. A testicular prosthesis may be placed at the time of orchiectomy, at a later date, or not at all.

Preparation of the Patient, Skin
Preparation, Draping, Equipment,
Instrumentation, and Supplies

See Hydrocelectomy, pp. 202–203.

Special Notes

In addition to the surgical permit, a sterilization form may be required.

CYSTOSCOPY

Definition

Endoscopic examination of the interior of the urethra, the bladder, and ureteral orifices.

Discussion

Cystoscopy is indicated for diagnosis of urinary tract symptoms (e.g., hematuria, pyuria), to catheterize the ureters, to obtain a biopsy specimen, to treat lesions, and for follow-up examination of an operative or endoscopic procedure.

Procedure

A well-lubricated cystoscope is inserted in the urethra; the urethra may be dilated initially with a sound. In the presence of a stricture, the urethra is dilated with filiform sounds. The urethra is inspected as the cystoscope is advanced into the bladder. The obturator is removed, and a urine specimen is obtained. The bladder is filled with irrigation fluid, and under direct visualization the bladder, ureteral orifices, bladder neck, and urethra are examined. A panendoscope, a resectoscope, or a ureteral catheterizing endoscope may be required.

Preparation of the Patient

The patient is usually on the cystoscopy table in the lithotomy position. Regional, general, or topical anesthesia may be employed. If a procedure in addition to cystoscopy is performed, apply electrosurgical dispersive pad.

Skin Preparation

Women. See Dilatation and Curettage, p. 157.
Men. Cleanse entire pubic area including scrotum and perineum.

Draping

Leggings and a fenestrated sheet

Equipment

Extra IV standard pole for hanging irrigation fluid
Fiberoptic light source
Electrosurgical unit (available)

Instrumentation

Cystoscope (telescope, obturator and sheath)
Fiberoptic light cord
Stopcock
Hemostat
Urethral sounds
Syringe (30 mL)
Medicine glass, syringe (10 mL), penile clamp (for topical anesthetic instillation)
Graduated pitcher (to measure residual urine)

Supplies

Topical anesthetic (e.g., lidocaine [Anestacon])
Lubricant

Irrigation solution (e.g., 2000 or 3000 mL distilled water)

Disposable cystoscopic irrigation tubing

Catheters (as requested)

Test tubes (for specimen collections)

Special Notes

Well-padded knee supports avoid pressure on neurovascular structures in the popliteal space.

The scrub person prepares the instrument table; a scrub person is usually not required during the procedure.

If a procedure in addition to cystoscopy is performed, irrigation solution should be nonelectrolytic and isotonic (e.g., glycine, sorbitol).

Particular care must be taken to position patients with hip problems carefully.

Care is taken not to damage lensed telescopes and fiberoptic light cords.

For bladder fulguration a resectoscope is needed; for lithopaxy add a lithotrite and corresponding scope; for ureteral catheterization add a catheterizing telescope and ureteral catheters.

Replace irrigation as necessary.

Instruments may be disinfected with a 2% aqueous glutaraldehyde solution (e.g., Cidex; rinse them very well).

CYSTOSTOMY

Definition

An opening is made into the bladder.

Discussion

Cystostomy is performed for purposes of urinary diversion to relieve obstruction and to "protect" the site of a more distal surgical procedure, such as vesicourethral anastomosis. This procedure may be done independently or as an adjunct to another procedure. The procedure may be performed as a suprapubic laparotomy or percutaneously with the bladder distended.

Procedure

A low vertical or transverse incision is used. The bladder may be distended by a urethral catheter (if a catheter can be inserted). The dome of the bladder is incised, and a Pezzer or Malecot catheter is inserted and secured with absorbable sutures to obtain a watertight closure. The catheter exits the main incision, or preferably a stab wound, and is secured to the skin with a stitch. The wound is closed; drainage is optional. Tube cystostomy may complement other open bladder procedures (e.g., lithotomy). A urethral catheter may be placed until the cystostomy tract matures to minimize leakage.

Preparation of the Patient

The patient is supine; arms may be extended on armboards. Trendelenburg may be requested. A suprapubic puncture approach is frequently performed under local anesthesia. Check with the surgeon regarding insertion of Foley catheter and instillation of irrigation or antiseptic fluids.

Skin Preparation

Males. Begin at the suprapubic region extending from 7.5 cm (3 inches) above the umbilicus to the lower thighs, and down to the table at the sides; the genitalia are included.

Females. Begin with the vaginal preparation (see Dilatation and Curettage, p. 157) after placing patient's legs in a froglike position. Return patient's legs to supine position. Replace safety strap above knees. Proceed with abdominal prep beginning at the suprapubic region.

Draping

Folded towels and a laparotomy sheet

Equipment

Electrosurgical unit
Suction

Instrumentation

SUPRAPUBIC LAPAROTOMY
Major procedures tray
Long instruments tray
Urethral sounds
Catheter stylet
Trocar (available)
Hemoclip appliers (assorted sizes and lengths)

PERCUTANEOUS APPROACH
Limited procedure tray
Catheter stylet, and trocar

Supplies

Basin set
Blades (2) No. 10, (1) No. 15, (1) No. 11
Needle magnet or counter
Electrosurgical pencil
Suction tubing
Foley catheter and sealed drainage unit
Irrigation solution and syringe (e.g., 30 ml with cone tip)
Hemoclips (small, medium, large)
Catheter for cystotomy (e.g., Pezzer, Malecot)

Special Notes

Irrigating solutions should be sterile, isotonic, and at body temperature.

The circulator may be requested to unclamp urethral catheter when the bladder is incised.

CYSTECTOMY

Definition

Removal of the urinary bladder.

Discussion

A partial cystectomy may be performed when the lesion is localized. Total radical cystectomy is performed depending upon infiltration of the lesion, evidence of metastases, and the ability of the patient to tolerate the procedure. Prior to cystectomy, a urinary diversion procedure, for example, bilateral ureterosigmoidostomy, ureteroileostomy (ileal-loop), or cutaneous ureterostomy must be performed.

This procedure is performed most often for malignancy primary to the bladder or in adjacent organs. Other indications include neurologic disorders, radiation injury, congenital defects, intractable infection, and severe trauma. When malignant disease is present, the depth of infiltration, presence of metastases, and general condition of the patient will dictate the extent of the procedure. Superficial bladder lesions are treated transcystoscopically by various modalities, with radiation therapy, or partial cystectomy. Total radical cystectomy is performed when an infiltrating lesion is restricted to the bladder and there are no distant metastases. In conjunction with cystectomy a urinary diversion procedure is performed, either a cutaneous ureterostomy or, preferably, an ileal conduit (ureteroileostomy) or colonic conduit (ureterocolostomy). Pelvic lymphadenectomy may be performed as well.

Procedure

A midline or low transverse incision is made, the operative field explored, and the extent of the pathology assessed. The bladder is dissected from its vascular supply. The prostate and seminal vesicles are included in the specimen. The distal ureters, urethra, and vasa are divided and ligated. In the female, hysterectomy (see Total Abdominal Hysterectomy, pp. 170–171) including the proximal vagina, urethra, and distal ureters are included in the specimen. Urinary diversion (see Ileal Conduit, pp. 228–229) is then performed or it may have been performed prior to cystectomy. A closed-system wound drain may be employed. The wound is closed in layers.

Preparation of the Patient

Males. The patient is supine; arms may be extended on armboards for a suprapubic approach.

Females. The patient is placed in a lithotomy position (while the urethra and bladder are mobilized), and then the patient is moved into a supine position for a suprapubic approach for the cystectomy.

Apply electrosurgical dispersive pad.

Skin Preparation

Suprapubic. Begin at the suprapubic area extending from nipples to lower thighs, and down to the table at the sides.

Vaginal. Begin at the pubic symphysis and extend downward over the labia. Cleanse each inner thigh. The vaginal vault is cleansed using spongesticks (three). The perineum and anus are cleansed with remaining sponges; discard each sponge after wiping the anus.

Draping

Suprapubic Approach.
Folded towels and a transverse sheet

Vaginal Approach.
Drape sheet under the buttocks, leggings, and a laparotomy sheet

Equipment

Electrosurgical unit
Suction

Instrumentation

SUPRAPUBIC APPROACH
Major procedures tray
Long instruments tray
Kidney procedures tray
Gastrointestinal procedures tray
Abdominal hysterectomy tray (available)

Self-retaining retractor (e.g., Balfour, O'Connor-O'Sullivan)
Hemoclip appliers (assorted sizes and lengths)

VAGINAL APPROACH
Basic/Minor procedures tray
Dilatation and Curettage (D & C) tray

Supplies

SUPRAPUBIC APPROACH
Basin set
Blades (2) No. 10, (1) No. 15, (1) No. 11, (1) No, 12
Needle magnet or counter
Suction tubing
Electrosurgical pencil
Dissectors (e.g., peanut)
Hemoclips (assorted sizes)
Urostomy or ileostomy pouch
Drain (e.g., Hemovac, Jackson-Pratt, Penrose)

VAGINAL APPROACH
Basin set
Blades (1) No. 10, (1) No. 15, (1) No. 11, (1) No. 12
Needle magnet or counter
Suction tubing
Electrosurgical pencil

Special Notes

Verify with blood bank that blood ordered is available.

An automatic stapling device may be used to perform the intestinal anastomosis; it may also be used in the construction of the ileal or colonic conduit.

TRANSURETHRAL RESECTION OF THE PROSTATE (TURP) AND/OR LESIONS OF THE BLADDER OR BLADDER NECK (TURB)

Definition

Transurethral resection is the piecemeal removal of prostatic tissue and/or lesions of the bladder or bladder neck transcystoscopically.

Discussion

The procedure is particularly desirable when the patient is a poor surgical risk, thereby eliminating the need for open prostatectomy. If carcinoma is present, following histologic studies of resected specimen, open prostatectomy may be indicated in the good-risk patient.

Procedure

The urethra may be dilated. Cystoscopy is performed to assess the hypertrophy and inspect the bladder. The resectoscope complete with sheath and obturator is passed. The irrigation tubing, fiberoptic light cord, and cautery cable are connected. The obturator is removed and the operating element with the foroblique telescope and cutting loop is inserted through the sheath. The bladder is continuously irrigated. The urethra and bladder trigone are reexamined. Electrodissection is employed to remove pieces of prostatic hypertrophied tissue. At intervals the fragments of tissue and blood clots are washed out of the bladder; the Ellik evacuator and Toomey syringe may be employed. Total removal of all fragments of tissue is desired. When resection is complete, the bladder and prostatic fossa are examined for residual unattached fragments of tissue. Adequate hemostasis is ensured, and the resectoscope sheath is removed. A Foley catheter (with 30-mL bag) is inserted into the bladder, filled with 5 to 10 mL of fluid, and then drawn into the prostatic fossa where an additional 12 to 25 mL of fluid is introduced to provide additional hemostasis.

Preparation of the Patient

The patient is in the lithotomy position on the cytoscopy table. Regional or general anesthesia may be employed. Apply electrosurgical dispersive pad.

Skin Preparation

Cleanse entire pubic area including scrotum and perineum.

Equipment

Electrosurgical unit
Fiberoptic light source
IV standard for irrigation fluid

Instrumentation

Resectoscope (complete with sheath, obturator), cutting loops, operating element, foroblique telescope, rotating contact, rubber tips, electrosurgical cord
Fiberoptic light cord
Evacuator (e.g., Ellik) and basin of glycine solution
Urethral dilators
Hemostat
Strainer or screen
Various collection devices
Stopcock
Toomey syringe
Syringe, 30 mL

Supplies

Lubricant
Isotonic (nonhemolytic) irrigant (e.g., sorbitol or glycine)
Disposable irrigation system
Foley catheter with 3-mL balloon and drainage unit

Special Notes

See Cystoscopy, p. 210.

OPEN PROSTATECTOMY

Definition

Excision of the prostate gland via surgical incision.

Discussion

Prostatectomy is usually performed to relieve urinary obstruction caused by benign or malignant disease. There are four approaches to prostatectomy.

1. *Transurethral prostatectomy* is performed most often; see Transurethral Prostatectomy, pp. 215–217.
2. *Suprapubic prostatectomy* is performed incising the bladder, which permits correction of associated conditions such as calculi and diverticula. This procedure is not used for malignancy.
3. *Retropubic prostatectomy* avoids entry into the bladder and allows good visualization of the field. Limited malignancies may be treated by this approach.
4. *Perineal prostatectomy* affords excellent visualization and access to the prostate and seminal vesicles and is useful for radical excision of the prostate, which includes the capsule, seminal vesicles, and portions of the vasa. The approach is inadequate to perform iliac node dissection. Perineal prostatectomy may result in impotency, and possible injury to the rectum is increased.

Some authorities advocate that, prior to radical prostatectomy, pelvic lymphadenectomy should be performed. If lymph node matastasis is present, a lesser resection (procedure) should be performed and/or palliative chemotherapy and radiotherapy instituted.

Bilateral vasectomy (see pp. 203–205) is usually performed in conjunction with prostatectomy to avoid retrograde infection.

Procedure

Suprapubic. The bladder is exposed through a transverse or vertical suprapubic incision. The dome of the bladder is incised, and the bladder is aspirated and explored for additional pathology. An incision is made in the bladder posteriorly over the prostate; the prostate is enucleated by finger dissection. Hemostasis is achieved. A transurethral Foley catheter is placed; a suprapubic catheter exits a stab wound incision in the bladder and abdominal wall. A drain may be placed in the prevesical space. The anterior bladder incision and the wound are closed.

Retropubic. A suprapubic incision is made; the

prostate and bladder neck are exposed in the prevesical space. The prostate capsule is incised and the gland enucleated by digital dissection. Hemostasis is achieved. A Foley catheter is positioned in the urethra, and the capsule is repaired. A drain may be employed. The wound is closed.

Perineal. A tractor is placed in the bladder transurethrally to displace the prostate toward the perineum; a curvilinear incision is made in the perineum. In benign disease the prostate is enucleated from its capsule. For malignancy the entire gland, its capsule, the seminal vesicle, and distal portion of the vasa are excised. Care is taken to avoid injury to the rectum. A urethrovesical anastomosis is performed after a transurethral Foley catheter is placed. The wound is drained and the incision is closed.

Preparation of the Patient

Suprapubic and Retropubic. The patient is supine with the legs separated and the arms extended on armboards. Shoulder braces are required when the patient is in the Trendelenburg position.

Perineal. The patient is in exaggerated lithotomy position with the knees touching the chest; arms may be extended on armboards. The buttocks are tilted and elevated (e.g., with folded bath towels). Shoulder braces are needed when patient is in the Trendelenburg position.

Apply electrosurgical dispersive pad.

Skin Preparation

Suprapubic and Retropubic. Begin at the suprapubic region extending from 7.5 to 10 cm (3 to 4 inches) above the umbilicus, to the lower thighs, and down to the table at the sides. Cleanse perineum and anus last, discarding each sponge after wiping the anus.

Perineal. Begin at the suprapubic region extending from the umbilicus to the lower thighs. Cleanse perineum and anus last, discarding each sponge after wiping the anus.

Draping

Suprapubic

Cuffed towel and a sheet under the scrotum (extending to the foot of the table), folded towels and a laparotomy or transverse sheet (depending on incision)

Retropubic

Folded towels, an impervious sheet from the scrotum to the foot of table, folded towel over the scrotum and penis (secured by towel clips), and a fenestrated sheet

Perineal

A sheet under the buttocks, leggings, towels around perineal area, and a fenestrated sheet

Equipment

Electrosurgical unit
Suction
Shoulder braces
Stirrups (for perineal approach)

Instrumentation

Major procedures tray
Long instruments tray
Open prostatectomy tray
Prostatic lobe forceps, prostatic enucleator
Boomerang suture passer
Heaney needle holders (2)
Lahey clamps (4)
Otis prostatic urethral sounds
Hemoclip appliers (assorted)

For Suprapubic, Add

Self-retaining abdominal retractor (e.g., Judd-Mason)

For Retropubic, Add

Millin retropubic bladder retractor

For Perineal, Add

Perineal prostatectomy retractors: lateral, anterior, bifurcated, and perineal self-retaining (e.g., Denis-Browne)

Supplies

Basin set
Blades (2) No. 10, (1) No. 15, (1) No. 11, (1) No. 12
Needle magnet or counter
Electrosurgical pencil
Suction tubing
Dissectors (e.g., peanut)
Hemoclips (assorted sizes and lengths)
Irrigation syringe, 30 mL with cone tip
Irrigation solution (e.g., saline)
Lubricant
Hemostatic catheter (e.g., No. 24 Foley with 30-mL balloon and drainage bag)
Suprapubic catheter (e.g., Malecot, Pezzer)
Penrose drain, 1″

Special Notes

Bladder irrigation fluid should be sterile, isotonic, and at body temperature.

If stirrups are used in positioning, they should be well padded to avoid nerve injury.

NEPHRECTOMY

Definition

Removal of a kidney.

Discussion

This procedure is performed for numerous conditions including hydronephrosis, pyelonephritis, renal atrophy, renal artery stenosis, trauma, and tumors of the kidney and ureter. When the major portion of the ureter is also excised, the procedure is termed nephroureterectomy.

Procedure

For benign disease a flank incision is made (with or without rib resection). Gerota's fascia is incised. The kidney and ureter are mobilized. The ureter is divided and the distal end ligated. The vascular pedicle is ligated. For malignant disease a radical nephrectomy is performed. A transperitoneal or anterior retroperitoneal incision is used; for large upper-pole lesions, a transthoracic approach may be employed. On the right side, the duodenum is protected with moistened laparotomy pads. The vascular pedicle is transsected and lymph-node-bearing tissue excised. Gerota's fascia is dissected from surrounding tissues. The ureter is divided, and the kidney and surrounding fat, adrenal gland, and fascia are removed en bloc. If tumor is present in the renal vein, the vena cava is mobilized and the tumor embolus removed. When the lower ureter is involved in the malignant process, ureterectomy is included. When a flank incision is used for the nephrectomy, a secondary lower flank or inguinal incision is used to expose the distal ureter extraperitoneally. The distal ureter is dissected free of surrounding tissues, and a small cuff of bladder is excised with the intramural portion of the ureter. The bladder incision is repaired, a suprapubic cystostomy catheter may be placed, and the distal ureter and bladder cuff are delivered into the flank wound and removed with the kidney. The flank incision may be closed with or without drainage. For trauma and some presentations of calculus disease involving only a portion of the kidney, a partial nephrectomy may be performed.

Preparation of the Patient

The lateral position is usually the position of choice when the approach is lumbar (flank) or transthoracic; the affected side is up. The patient's waist is over the middle break in the table; the table is flexed. The arm on the unaffected side is extended on an armboard; the arm on the affected side may be supported by a Mayo stand padded with a pillow (or a double armboard may be used). The torso may be stabilized by kidney rests (larger one in front) and/or pillows or sandbags. The leg on the unaffected side is extended, and the uppermost leg is flexed with a pillow between the legs; adequate padding is needed around the feet and ankles.

The position is secured by wide adhesive tape at the shoulder, thighs, and legs, fastened to the underside of the table.

For the abdominal approach the patient is supine; arms may be extended on armboards. The table is in a modified Trendelenburg position. The thorax on the affected side may be elevated for optimal exposure. When nephroureterectomy is performed, a flank incision and a secondary lower flank or inguinal incision are employed. The patient is turned from the lateral to the supine position. Particular care is taken to protect the first incision with sponges, towels, and/or drapes. Some surgeons use a single incision extending from beneath the twelfth rib to the suprapubic area. The thorax on the affected side may be elevated to achieve adequate exposure.

Skin Preparation

Lateral. Begin at the level of the 12th rib extending from the axilla to 2 to 3 inches below the iliac crest, and down to the table anteriorly and posteriorly.

Abdominal. Begin at the incision extending from the axilla to the midthighs, and down to the table at the sides. *Nephroureterectomy* (second incision): Carefully prepare from just below the first incision to the midthighs, and down to the table at the sides.

Draping

Nephrectomy
Folded towels and a transverse sheet
Nephroureterectomy
Folded towels, two transverse sheets, and additional drapes to cover the first (flank) incision when two incisions are used; folded towels and a transverse sheet which is cut for a single incision

Equipment

Pillows, kidney rests, and so on (for position support)
Suction
Electrosurgical unit

224 • Surgical Procedures Including Minimal Access Procedures

Instrumentation

Major procedures tray
Long instruments tray
Kidney tray
Thoracotomy tray, Vascular procedures tray, and Gastrointestinal procedures tray (available)
Hemoclip appliers (assorted sizes and lengths)

Supplies

Basin set
Blades (2) No. 10, (1) No. 15, (1) No. 11, (1) No. 12
Suction tubing
Needle magnet or counter
Asepto syringe
Hemoclips (assorted sizes)
Dissectors (e.g., peanut)
Penrose drains, long (2) 1″ (for retraction and drainage)
Wound suction drain, for example, Jackson-Pratt (available)
Chest tube (argyle) and a closed chest drainage unit, for example, Pleurevac (for transthoracic approach)
Suprapubic catheter (for nephroureterectomy), for example, Pezzer, Malecot, and drainage unit

Special Notes

The surgeon may request hypothermia measures (e.g., hypothermia mattress).

Have the patient's x-ray films in the room.

Verify with blood bank that blood is available as ordered.

Protect skin under adhesive tape with tincture of benzoin.

The scrub person needs to save all perirenal fat in a small basin of normal saline. The fat may be used as a bolster to stop bleeding.

When two incisions are employed, the patient is repositioned, reprepared, and redraped; an additional instrument tray is unnecessary.

UPPER TRACT UROLITHOTOMY (URETEROLITHOTOMY, PYELOLITHOTOMY, NEPHROLITHOTOMY)

Definition

Removal of calculi from the ureter, renal pelvis, and kidney.

Discussion

Numerous techniques are available in removing calculi from the urinary tract. If lithotriptic procedures (extracorporeal shock wave lithotripsy, ultrasonic, and other nephroscopic and transcystoscopic modalities) are unsuccessful or unavailable, or there are contraindications to these techniques, open surgery is required.

Procedure

Proximal Calculi. A flank incision is made with rib resection (twelfth) optional. For stones within the renal parenchyma (nephrolithotomy), temporary interruption of the renal circulation is achieved by occluding the main vessels atraumatically. After the position of the stone is ascertained, the parenchyma incised and the calculus removed, the kidney is repaired. Fatty tissue may be used to bolster the suture line. Stones in the renal pelvis (pyelolithotomy) or in the proximal ureter (ureterolithotomy) are extracted through incisions overlying the stones. Atraumatic clamps, tapes, or vessel loops occlude the distal ureter to prevent migration of fragments. The collecting system is irrigated and sutured closed.

Distal Calculi. Calculi in the distal ureters are approached retroperitoneally by inguinal, lower midline abdominal, or transverse oblique incision. The stone is palpated, noting that the ureter proximal to it may be dilated. Control of the ureter proximal and distal to the stone is achieved with vessel loops or atraumatic clamps. The ureter is opened and the stone retrieved. Irrigation may be employed, and the ureter is closed.

Drainage may be employed in any of these approaches. The wound is closed in layers.

Preparation of the Patient

The position of the patient is lateral if the stone is in the kidney or proximal ureter, see Nephrectomy, pp. 222–223. The patient is supine for stones in the distal ureter. Apply electrosurgical dispersive pad.

Skin Preparation

Lateral Approach. See Nephrectomy, p. 223.
Abdominal Approach. Begin at the incision extending from axilla to midthighs, and down to the table at the sides.

Draping

Folded towels and a transverse sheet (for lateral or abdominal approach)

Equipment

Kidney rests, pillows, and so on (for position support)
Suction
Electrosurgical unit

Instrumentation

Major procedures tray
Long instruments tray
Kidney tray
Thoracotomy tray, Vascular procedures tray, and Gastrointestinal procedures tray (available)
Hemoclip appliers (assorted sizes and lengths)

Supplies

Blades (2) No. 10, (1) No. 15, (1) No. 11, (1) No. 12
Suction tubing
Electrosurgical pencil
Needle magnet or counter
Asepto syringe
Hemoclips (assorted sizes)

Vessel loops and umbilical tapes
Dissectors (e.g., peanut)
Penrose drain, 1″ (retraction)

Special Notes

Have the patient's x-ray films in the room.

Have nephroscope and fiberoptic light source available.

To facilitate calculus extraction, the surgeon may inject a mixture of calcium chloride, thrombin, and cryoprecipitate to form a "clot" around the calculus and prevent its migration.

CUTANEOUS URETEROSTOMY

Definition

Establishment of a ureteral stoma on the abdominal wall.

Discussion

Cutaneous ureterostomy is a form of urinary diversion performed for distal ureteral obstruction caused by tumor, radiation injury, fibrosis, and intractable infection. The procedure is usually temporary, later incorporating the stoma into an ileal-loop conduit or the anastomosing of the affected ureter to the opposite ureter (ureteroureterostomy).

Procedure

Depending upon the level of the obstruction, a flank incision is made. The ureter is exposed and dissected free. The obstruction may or may not be dealt with at this time (depending on the condition of the patient). The ureter, transsected as far distally as possible, exits out a stoma site and is matured (sutured) to the abdominal skin. A urostomy pouch is placed. The incision is closed.

Preparation of the Patient

The patient is supine; arms may be extended on armboards. Apply electrosurgical dispersive pad.

Skin Preparation

Begin at the incision extending from nipples to midthighs, and down to the table at the sides.

Draping

Folded towels and a laparotomy sheet

Equipment

Electrosurgical unit
Suction

Instrumentation

Major procedures tray
Long instrument tray
Self-retaining abdominal retractor (e.g., Balfour)
Hemoclip appliers (various sizes and lengths)
Iris scissors and fixation forceps (ureteroureterostomy)

Supplies

Basin set
Blades (2) No. 10, (1) No. 15, (1) No. 11, (1) No. 12
Needle magnet or counter
Suction tubing
Electrosurgical pencil
Dissectors (e.g., peanut)
Hemoclips (assorted)
Splinting catheter (usually Silastic)
Urostomy pouch

Special Notes

For the ureteroureterostomy anastomosis, the ureter is prepared using iris scissors and fixation forceps.

ILEAL CONDUIT

Definition

An isolated segment of ileum into which the ureters are implanted exiting as a urostomy stoma on the abdominal wall.

Discussion

This procedure is performed in conjunction with cystectomy (see pp. 212–213). Creation of an ileal conduit has superseded ureterosigmoidostomy and cutaneous ureterostomy, avoiding the potential of ascending urinary infection, diarrhea, skin problems, and so on. Most often the ileal segment is brought out as a urostomy stoma, but a continent pouch with a nipple valve may be constructed (Koch). In selected cases when urinary sphincter function remains intact, the ileal segment may be anastomosed as a bladder substitute to the proximal urethra, preserving urinary function. An isolated loop of the sigmoid colon may be used instead of ileum.

Procedure

See Cystectomy, pp. 212–213. The ileal conduit may be constructed prior to or after the bladder is excised. The distal ileum is exposed; a segment (approximately 15 cm) is divided from the ileum, maintaining its mesentery. The continuity of proximal and distal ileum is reestablished. The mesentery is closed over the intervening mesentery of the isolated loop to avoid internal herniation. The proximal end of the isolated loop is closed. The ureters are dissected and anastomosed to the ileal loop. The distal end of the ileal loop is brought out to the stoma site (right lower quadrant of the abdomen). The stoma is sutured to the skin, and a urostomy pouch is applied. The abdominal wound is closed. Drainage is optional. Stapling devices may be employed to perform the intestinal anastomoses and closure of the proximal end of the isolated loop.

Preparation of the Patient

The patient is supine; arms may be extended on armboards. Apply electrosurgical dispersive pad.

Skin Preparation

Begin cleansing at the incision (check with the surgeon). Extend preparation from the nipples to midthighs, and to the table at the sides.

Draping

Folded towels and a laparotomy sheet

Equipment

Electrosurgical unit
Suction

Instrumentation

Major procedures tray
Gastrointestinal procedures tray
Long instruments tray
Self-retaining abdominal retractor (e.g., Balfour)
Hemoclip appliers (assorted sizes and lengths)
Ruler
Automatic stapling device (optional)

Supplies

Basin set
Blades (2) No. 10, (1) No. 15, (1) No. 11, (1) No. 12
Needle magnet
Suction tubing
Electrosurgical pencil
Dissectors (e.g., peanut)
Hemoclips
Ureteral stent (e.g., Silastic ureteral catheter)
Urostomy pouch
Staples (optional)
Drain (e.g., Penrose, optional)

ADRENALECTOMY

Definition

Excision of either or both of the adrenal glands.

Discussion

This procedure is done to excise primary tumors of the adrenals, benign or malignant (usually unilaterally), or to modify an endocrine-dependent tumor, as in breast or prostatic malignancy. During the entire perioperative period, corticosteroid replacement must be administered. Small fragments of the adrenal cortex may be implanted in the patient's thigh musculature so that some glandular function is preserved.

Adrenalectomy can be performed employing an anterior or posterior approach. The posterior approach is less traumatic to the patient, but it does not permit exploration of the abdomen, concomittant oophorectomy when indicated, or other coincidental intra-abdominal procedures. The anterior approach also affords the opportunity to search for ectopic adrenal tissues.

Procedure

Posterior Approach. The patient may be in the lateral position if unilateral adrenalectomy is performed. For bilateral adrenalectomy the patient is prone. An incision is made from the lower ribs (the 12th rib is resected after the muscles are separated) to the posterior iliac crest. The fascia is incised and Gerota's capsule exposed. The adrenal gland is identified and excised, taking care not to injure the kidney. The left adrenal vein is divided from the renal vein, and the right adrenal vein is divided from the inferior vena cava. Careful hemostasis of the fragile vasculature is required; clips may be employed. The incision is closed in layers. If the pleura was entered, drainage may be necessary.

Anterior Approach. An upper abdominal longitudinal incision is made. The peritoneal cavity is explored, and additional procedures are performed as indicated. The retroperitoneal space is entered on the right after reflecting the duodenum, and on the left through the lesser sac. Precautions are taken to assure that hemostasis is maintained, as noted above. The adrenal gland (one or both) is excised, and the wound is closed in layers.

Preparation of the Patient

The patient is in the lateral position with the affected side up for unilateral adrenalectomy.

For a bilateral adrenalectomy, the abdominal or posterior approach may be employed. For the abdominal approach the patient is supine; arms may be extended on armboards. For the less frequently employed posterior approach, the patient is prone. Following insertion of an intravenous line and endotracheal intubation (while the patient is on the gurney), the patient is carefully rolled over to the prone position onto the table. The arms are extended on armboards angled toward the head of the table with the hands pronated. Chest rolls are placed under the patient from the acromioclavicular joint to the level of the iliac crests to facilitate breathing. Female breasts and male genitalia are protected. A pillow(s) is placed in front of the ankles. Pads may be placed under the elbows and knees. The safety strap is secured across the patient's thighs.

Skin Preparation

Lateral Position. Begin cleansing at approximately the level of the twelfth rib extending from the axilla from 5 to 7.5 cm (2 to 3 inches) to below the iliac crest, and down to the table at the sides.

Abdominal Approach. Begin cleansing for a right paramedian incision extending from the axilla to midthighs, and down to the table at the sides.

Prone Position. Begin cleansing for bilateral curvilinear incisions that begin at the level of the tenth rib and extend to the superior border of the iliac crests. Prepare from the axilla to the upper thighs, and down to the table at the sides.

Draping

Folded towels and a laparotomy sheet (for lateral or abdominal)

Folded towels and a transverse sheet that may be cut to accommodate the incisions (for prone)

Equipment

Pillows, kidney rests, and so on (for positioning)
Electrosurgical unit
Suction

Instrumentation

Major procedures tray
Long instruments tray and kidney tray
Thoracotomy tray, Vascular procedures tray, and Gastrointestinal procedures tray (available)
Hemoclip appliers (assorted sizes and lengths)

Supplies

Basin set
Blades (2) No. 10, (1) No. 15, (1) No. 11, (1) No. 12
Suction tubing
Electrosurgical pencil
Needle magnet or counter
Asepto syringe
Dissectors (e.g., peanut)
Penrose drain, 1″ (for retraction)
Hemoclips (assorted, optional)

Special Notes

Ask the surgeon which approach will be used.

Check with the surgeon and anesthetist regarding need for vasodilating drugs such as phentolamine.

Hormones such as hydrocortisone may be requested.

EXTRACORPOREAL SHOCK WAVE LITHOTRIPSY (ESWL)

Definition

Disintegration of upper urinary tract calculi by means of precisely directed shock waves delivered to a patient immersed in a water bath.

Discussion

The ESWL unit (e.g., Dornier HM3) makes possible the removal of most upper urinary tract calculi without surgery. Multiple shock waves produced by an electrode beneath the immersed patient pass from the water into the body, pulverizing the calculus into sandlike particles that are eliminated in the urine. The shock waves selectively fragment the stone, which is of a higher density than the surrounding area, thus sparing significant injury to surrounding soft tissues and bone, which are more resilant.

A modular lithotripter developed by the manufacturers of the currently employed ESWL system has recently become available. The new lithotripter (Dornier HM4) does not require immersion of the patient. This bath-free unit employs a self-contained water cushion that couples to the patient's body. Patient positioning is achieved by a computer-controlled guidance system that permits focus on the calculus with an even greater degree of accuracy than the existing system. This precision positioning with placement of the x-ray source beneath the treatment table and actuation of the triggering mechanism by the EKG and respiratory motion may decrease the number of shock waves required and reduces radiation exposure to the patient and staff. Sedation of the patient without need for anesthesia is an additional advantage of this newer modification.

Procedure

The patient is safety-strapped onto the "gantry" stretcher, which is then lowered into the immersion tub. The water level should be approximately 5 cm (2 inches) below the overflow outlet. Image intensifiers on either side of the patient are rotated into place. X-ray "window" balloons are inflated to improve the quality of the image (there being less distortion of the beam through air as compared to water). The physician positions the stone on the crosshairs of both monitors by adjusting the gantry. The previously placed waterproofed EKG leads are double-checked, noting that the release of the shock waves must appropriately coincide with the cardiac cycle to avoid arrhythmias. The shock waves are then released at the physician's discretion. The patient is repositioned as necessary to maintain the calculus in the crosshairs of the monitors as it is being disintegrated. The voltage is read continuously and altered to change the intensity of the shocks. The total number of shock waves required depends upon the size, composition, and location of the calculus, as well as the physique of the patient. Stones begin to fragment after 1200 (sometimes fewer) shocks have been delivered; 2400 shocks is generally considered the maximum dose.

For calculi located in the proximal portion of the ureter (superior to the pelvic brim), the surgeon may attempt to reposition the calculus back into the kidney (renal pelvis) in order to achieve the maximum effect of ESWL. Transcystoscopically under fluoroscopic control, a ureteral catheter is positioned in the ureter immediately distal to the calculus. The ureter is then filled with a lidocaine mixture (e.g., 2% Xylocaine jelly and sterile water 3:1). If the calculus cannot be repositioned into the renal pelvis, the physician may elect to perform ESWL with the stone in the ureter. In that case, two or three additional ureteral catheters may be positioned beside the stone and just distal to the stone to prevent its premature passage while still intact, thereby preventing possible injury to the ureter. The ESWL procedure is then performed. Alternatively, the physician may try to shatter the calculus using ultrasonic lithotripsy transureteroscopically (see Ultrasonic Lithotripsy, pp. 242–243).

Preparation of the Patient

The ESWL procedure may be performed under general or block (spinal, epidural) anesthesia. The patient may be prepared in an anesthesia holding area or the ESWL room. If cystoscopy or ureteroscopy precedes ESWL, the patient may be anesthetized in the cystoscopy room. Following the administration of anesthesia, the patient is transferred to the gantry stretcher and strapped in for safety and to counter the effects of buoyancy.

Skin Preparation

None is required. Following the immersion of the patient in the tub, the circulator wipes his or her hand along the skin surface area overlying the affected kidney to release air bubbles that could accumulate, thereby reducing the efficiency of the shock waves.

Draping

None, required.

Equipment

If cystoscopy, retrograde pyelography, or ureteroscopy are performed prior to ESWL:

> X-ray cassettes
> Fiberoptic light source for cystoscope
> Extra IV standards for irrigation fluid

Dornier ESWL system components:

1. Special tub and frame
2. Localization system
   a. X-ray generator, high-voltage generator, control cabinet
   b. Control panel
   c. Two x-ray tube housing assemblies (under tub)
   d. Two image intensifiers
   e. Two TV monitors
3. Shock wave generation unit
   a. Capacitor charging unit
   b. Pulse generator
   c. Shock wave generator
   d. EKG trigger unit
   e. Ellipsoid reflector
   f. Underwater electrode
4. Patient positioning unit: Guideway and gantry stretcher
5. Hydraulic supply system
   a. Suspended telescopic cylinder (vertical)
   b. Two cylinders (horizontal)
   c. Hydraulic supply unit
   d. Accumulator
6. Water treatment system
7. Control cabinet

Supplies

When cystoscopy, retrograde pyelography, or ureteroscopy precedes ESWL:

Specimen bottles, culture tubes
Ureteral catheters and adaptors (to attach to drainage system)
Lubricant
Foley catheters

For ESWL:
Underwater electrode
X-ray cassettes

Instrumentation

None required for ESWL
Cystoscope, ureteroscope, or ultrasonic wand (see Ultrasonic Lithotripsy, pp. 242–243) may be requested prior to ESWL procedure

ESWL UNIT USE PROCEDURE

1. Patient data recorded
2. Gantry stretcher adjusted without patient
3. Patient placed and secured on gantry stretcher
4. Gantry stretcher adjusted with patient
5. Patient prepared (reiterate to the patient what will be happening)
6. Gantry stretcher and patient moved into tub
7. Image intensifiers swung into place with balloons inflated
8. X-ray unit adjusted
9. Monitors adjusted
10. ECG triggering unit adjusted
11. Kidney stone located
12. X-ray window ventilated
13. Capacitor charging unit adjusted
14. Shock waves released
15. Shock circuit switched off
16. Image intensifiers moved backward and swung out
17. Patient lifted out of tub
18. Water drained
19. Used electrode removed, new electrode inserted
20. Tub cleaned and disinfected

Special Notes

A lithotripter supervisor is essential to the well-run lithotripsy unit. The supervisor is responsible for checking and preparing the lithotripsy equipment and assisting the physician and the anesthetist.

It is absolutely essential for the circulator working with the lithotripsy patient to be thoroughly familiar with the ESWL unit.

The epidural catheter (if used) needs to be protected in the water bath. A partially split 2″ × 2″ sponge may be placed at the base of the catheter. The catheter tubing may then be protected by a sterile, plastic adhesive drape that seals it from the water.

Care is required in positioning the patient on the gantry stretcher to avoid undue pressure, particularly on the limbs.

The water temperature of the tub should be maintained at 36°C (97°F). Temperatures below 35°C (95°F) or above 37°C (99°F) should be adjusted.

X-ray balloons ("windows") must be inflated when x-rays are taken and are usually deflated when radiography is completed.

Lead aprons are worn by personnel when x-rays are taken.

The underwater electrode generally needs to be replaced after every 700 to 800 shocks. The plastic sleeve must be removed from the electrode; if the generator is moved forward with the plastic sleeve, the mechanism will be damaged.

Towels and blankets are kept in a warmer to dry and cover the patient following immersion in the tub.

Additional charting information is required for the operative procedure report including:

Water temperature
Shock wave voltage
Electrode series
Total number of shock waves delivered
Fluoroscopy time

EXTRACORPORAL SHOCKWAVE LITHOTRIPSY WITHOUT WATER BATH

Definition

Disintegration of upper urinary tract calculi by means of precisely directed shock waves generated by an electromagnet through water-filled cushions that couple with the patient.

Discussion

The "second-generation" ESWL unit (e.g., Lithostar by Siemens) has x-ray tubes in a retractable overhead position, one at 90° and the other at 30° (both anterior and posterior views), while also having fluoroscopy imaging capabilities. The unit has two retractable shockheads that come up from inside the table top to couple with the patient. The shockhead to be used depends upon the location of the stone.

This newer lithotripter delivers low-pressure shockwaves that are able to break the stone without being painful to the patient. Patients may be treated in the supine or prone position with the head of the patient at either the head or the foot of the table, depending upon the patient's body structure and the location of the stone.

The Lithostar lithotripter, unlike the Dormier HM3 lithotripter, has no disposable electrodes. Shockwaves for the Lithostar are generated by an electromagnet. The shockheads are replaceable, but generally they will last through 1 million blasts. It also has the capability of taking standard x-ray films while the patient is on the table.

The Lithostar for clinical purposes is a low-energy machine that pulverizes a stone by direct action without any explosion. It works on both ureteral and renal stones. After approximately every 100 shocks, fluoroscopy is used to locate the remaining stone. Adjustments are then made in repositioning the patient before continuing the treatment. Using the machine to its maximum advantage by trying to crack and pulverize a stone in only one session, up to 10,000 blasts may be administered.

Procedure

If the patient has a renal stone, the patient is positioned in the supine position with his head at the "correct" end of the table. A kidney-ureter-bladder (KUB) film is taken with the shockhead down and the table in its lowest position. The KUB film is reviewed. Then the panel under the right side of the patient (for a right-sided stone) is removed, which alerts the computer that the right shockhead will be used. The centering button on the computer is activated, and the fluoroscopy pedal is depressed until the stone is visualized on plane I. The patient is then moved on the table so that the stone is very close to the crosshairs. The automatic positioning system is used to bring the stone to the crosshairs on plane II. The computer grid can be seen when it is activated; the cursor/track ball is active, and the blast path is seen as small white dots. The cursor is placed on the stone with the track ball.

At the completion of the treatment, the shockhead is lowered, the table is brought down to its lowest level, and a KUB film is taken to determine the size and location of the stone fragments.

Preparation of the Patient

The position of the patient is determined by the location of the stone and body habitus. Ultrasound gel is put on the shockhead and on the patient's skin. The shockhead is raised to the patient. The patient is then alerted that the shocks are going to start.

Skin Preparation

Ultrasound gel is applied to the patient's skin in the area in which the shockhead will be placed.

Draping

The patient may be covered with a sheet or blanket.

Equipment

Pillow
Pulse oximeter
Automated blood pressure cuff
Special lithotripter table, computer with a main control panel (with the ability to trace the stone, take KUB films, take snapshots, and more), 2 shockheads, one 90° angle x-ray tube, and one 38° x-ray table

Supplies

Foley catheter and drainage bag
EKG patches
Medications

Cipro. Preoperatively 500 mg by mouth (Cipro is a broad-spectrum antibiotic.)

Toradol. 30 mg intramuscular injection (Toradol is a nonsteroidal anti-inflammatory drug.)

Sublimaze. 1–2 mL intravenously (Sublimaze is a potent narcotic analgesic.)

Phenergan. Given in varying amounts (Phenergan is an antihistaminic, sedative, and antiemetic.)

Versed. Individualized dosage (Versed is a short-acting central nervous system depressant.)

Special Notes

A lithotripter supervisor is responsible for checking and preparing the lithotripsy equipment, assisting the surgeon, watching out for the patient's well-being, and administering medications. (An anesthetist is rarely present.)

All personnel working with the lithotripsy unit must be thoroughly familiar with it.

Care is taken to position the patient correctly and comfortably.

Additional charting information is required as each hospital policy dictates.

Be certain to tell the patient when shocks are to begin so that the patient will not jump when feeling the first shock.

Monitor patient's blood pressure, heart rate, respirations, EKG, and oxygen saturation.

ULTRASONIC LITHOTRIPSY

Definition

Disintegration of urinary tract calculi located in the ureter by means of ultrasonic waves delivered by a probe inserted transureteroscopically.

Discussion

The ultrasonic lithotripter generates ultrasonic waves that shatter a calculus within the ureter. The pulverized particles are eliminated in the urine. This procedure may be extended to include stones in the renal pelvis that are approached by percutaneous nephrostomy. Extracorporeal shock wave lithotripsy (ESWL) is the preferred method for the disintegration of stones in the renal pelvis when applicable.

Procedure

Cystoscopy is performed, and a guide wire is passed into the affected ureter. Under fluoroscopic control a ureteroscope is passed into the ureter over the guide wire. It may be necessary to dilate the ureter using graduated-sized catheters or a dilating pressure balloon catheter. Once the ureter is sufficiently dilated, the ureteroscope is passed over the guide wire. The ultrasonic wand is passed through the ureteroscope, and the stone is either shattered or dislodged by ultrasonic waves and removed by suction.

Preparation of the Patient, Skin Preparation, and Draping

See Cystoscopy, p. 209.

Equipment

Ultrasonic lithotripter unit, foot switch, and power cord
Fiberoptic light source for cystoscope
Extra IV standard for irrigation fluid

Instrumentation

Cystoscopy instruments including light cord
Ureteroscope, light cord, alligator forceps
Ultrasonic wand
Bridge adaptor (accommodates ultrasonic wand)

Supplies

Surgical jelly lubricant
Irrigating solution
Suction tubing
Disposable irrigation system
Coated movable core guidewire (e.g., $0.035'' \times 150$ cm)
Ureteral catheters and adaptors to connect to drainage
Xylocaine jelly, 2%
Foley catheter and drainage unit
Syringe, 10 mL
Test tubes for specimen collection
Ureteral stent (e.g., double-J stent to avoid obstruction
  from large calculi)

Special Notes

Connect suction to lithotripter wand.
   Irrigating solution may be water, normal saline, or
lactated Ringer's solution.

ELECTROHYDRAULIC LITHOTRIPSY

Definition

Fragmentation of urinary tract calculi found in the
bladder by means of electrohydraulic shock waves delivered by a probe inserted transcystoscopically.

Discussion

An electrohydraulic lithotripter releases a series of
high-voltage sparks that when placed in a 0.15% or
(⅙ normal) saline solution, produce a series of sharp,
high-amplitude shock waves that crack and fragment
the bladder calculi. The fragments may then be eliminated in the urine. These shock waves have no adverse

244 • Surgical Procedures Including Minimal Access Procedures

effect on tissue because of tissue flexibility. Only a few surgeons have extended this procedure to include ureteral stones.

Procedure

Cystoscopy is performed. The electrohydraulic lithotripter probe is passed through the cystoscope so that the electrode tip lies 1 to 2 mm from the calculus and 1 to 2 mm from the tip of the cystoscope. The stone is then cracked and fragmented by the hydraulic shock waves.

Preparation of the Patient, Skin Preparation, and Draping

See Cystoscopy, p. 209.

Equipment

Electrohydraulic lithotripter unit, power cord, foot switch, cable
Fiberoptic light source for cystoscope
Extra IV standard for irrigation fluid

Instrumentation

Cystoscopy instruments including fiberoptic light cord (see Cystoscopy, p. 209)
Extender cable
Disposable probes
Alligator forceps, Wappler forceps, Ellik evacuator, Toomy syringe (for fragments)

Supplies

Lubricant
Irrigation solution 0.15% (⅙ normal) saline
Disposable irrigation system
Foley catheter and drainage unit

Special Notes

Do not reuse electrode.
  Sterilize lithotripter extender cable with ethylene oxide gas *only*.

Do not use the electrohydraulic lithotripter on any patient with a pacemaker.

The surgeon may request the irrigating solution to be kept at room temperature.

The irrigating solution of 0.15% (⅙ normal) saline may be prepared in the operating room by adding 500 mL of normal saline to a 3-L bag of sterile distilled water from which 500 mL have been discarded. Alternatively, 6 mL of concentrated sodium chloride solution (23.4%) can be added to each liter of sterile water.

Chapter 13

Thoracic Procedures

BRONCHOSCOPY

Definition

Endoscopic visualization of the trachea, main bronchi and their openings, and most of the segmental bronchi.

Discussion

This procedure is performed for aspiration of secretions, biopsy, or removal of a foreign object. Rigid and flexible fiberoptic bronchoscopes are used. An advantage of the flexible scope is that more peripheral subdivisions may be inspected; a disadvantage is that foreign objects and copious, viscid mucous cannot be removed through its lumen.

Procedure

Rigid. The head is lowered, and a well-lubricated scope is inserted into the mouth. The epiglottis is elevated with the tip of the bronchoscope, and the scope is passed into the trachea. The scope is advanced into the bronchi. Bronchoscopy washings, biopsy, and so on may be obtained. A foreign body may be removed. Laser may be employed; see Appendix, pp. 619–624, for precautions. The patient is well suctioned, and the scope is removed slowly.

Flexible. Following intubation, the well-lubricated

bronchoscope is inserted through the adaptor into the endotracheal tube (secured by the anesthetist) and advanced as necessary. Bronchoscopy washings, biopsy taken with forceps or brush, and so on may be obtained. The patient is well suctioned, and the scope is removed slowly.

Preparation of the Patient

General Anesthesia. The patient is supine; the anesthetist moves to the patient's side, and the surgeon is at the head of the table. The patient's shoulders are just above the top break in the table so that the head may be lowered.

Topical Anesthesia. The patient is usually sitting up at the edge of the table facing the surgeon while the circulator or the scrub person helps support the patient from behind. (A foot stool is needed.)

Skin Preparation

None.

Draping

The patient may be covered with a drape sheet. A drape sheet covers the back table. Gloves are worn.

Equipment

Suction
Fiberoptic light source (scope)
Foot stool (for patient during topical anesthesia)
Fiberoptic headlight and light source)

Topical Anesthesia. Topical anesthetic tray on a Mayo stand. Have available:

- Laryngeal mirrors
- Lingual spatula
- Anesthetic spray
- Laryngeal syringe with straight and curved cannulas
- Medicine cups (for drugs of preference)
- Emesis basin
- Luer lock syringe, 10 mL with 22-gauge needle
- Tissues

Instrumentation and Supplies

Rigid Bronchoscopy
Rigid fiberoptic bronchoscope (check size)
Endotracheal adaptor (for anesthetist)
Fiberoptic telescope
Fiberoptic light cords (2)
Suction cannulas
Suction tubing
Specimen collectors (e.g., Lukens tubes)
Sponge carriers (2) (loaded with bronchoscopy sponges)
Biopsy forceps
Grasping forceps
Lubricant
Bronchoscopy sponges
Small basin with sterile saline and syringe (for washings)
Telfa and 25-gauge needle (for removing specimen)
Laser may be employed; see Appendix, pp. 619–624 for precautions

Flexible Bronchoscopy
Flexible fiberoptic bronchoscope
Endotracheal adaptor (for anesthetist)
Fiberoptic light cord
Biopsy forceps
Brush (and slides and alcohol to collect specimen)
Culture jar for biopsy specimen
Small basin with sterile saline and syringe (for washings)
Suction tubing
Specimen collector (e.g., Lukens tube)
Lubricant
Telfa and 25-gauge needle (for removing specimen)

Special Notes

Prior to the procedure be certain there is an endotracheal adaptor for the anesthetist.

Antifogging solution may be applied to the lens before use and wiped off to prevent fogging (e.g., Ultrastop, pHisoHex).

The room lights may be turned off and x-ray view boxes turned on.

The patient's upper lip and teeth may be protected with a plastic mouth guard or a damp sponge.

Have a sitting stool for the surgeon.

Hold specimen collector upright, and pinch off suction tubing after specimen is obtained or it will be aspirated into the suction unit.

Keep syringe filled with saline ready for washings.

Pass biopsy forceps with tips closed.

Guide forceps and other instruments into the scope as necessary.

Take care not to crush specimens; use a needle only to remove specimen and place it on Telfa.

Specimens must be dispatched promptly.

MEDIASTINOSCOPY

Definition

Endoscopic visualization of the mediastinum (tracheobronchial junction, bronchi, aortic arch, and regional lymph nodes).

Discussion

This procedure is performed when a malignancy is suspected. Tissue may be biopsied.

Procedure

A transverse incision is made over the suprasternal notch and extended down to the pretracheal fascia. Hemostasis is achieved. Using blunt dissection, the superior mediastinum is entered. The scope is passed. Care is taken to avoid injury to nearby blood vessels. Lymph node tissue may be biopsied. Needle aspiration is employed to identify a nonvascular structure. A specimen may be obtained using biopsy forceps. Hemostasis is achieved. The scope is removed, and the wound is closed.

Preparation of the Patient

General anesthesia is administered and an endotracheal tube is inserted. The patient is supine with the neck extended by a rolled towel under the shoulders. The anesthetist moves to patient's side, and the surgeon operates at the head of the table. Apply electrosurgical dispersive pad.

Skin Preparation

Begin at the suprasternal notch; include the entire neck and shoulders down to the table, extending from chin to nipples.

Draping

Folded towels and a sheet with a small fenestration

Equipment

Electrosurgical unit
Suction
Fiberoptic light source

Instrumentation

Mediastinoscopy tray

Supplies

Basin set
Blade (1) No. 15
Telfa and 22-gauge needle (for specimen removal)

Special Notes

Approach is both endoscopic and surgical.

A sponge count is taken before scope is removed and at closure of wound.

Remove specimen from biopsy forceps with a needle only to avoid damage to cells.

SEGMENTAL RESECTION OF THE LUNG

Definition

Excision of anatomic subdivisions of the pulmonary lobes; only segments containing diseased tissue are removed (lesion must have a segmental distribution).

Discussion

Indications for this procedure include bronchiectasis, cysts or blebs, benign or metastatic tumors, and tuberculosis.

Procedure

The affected lung is exposed through a posterolateral incision. The diseased segment is identified. The visceral pleura is dissected free from blood vessels and bronchi of the appropriate bronchiopulmonary segment. The segmental pulmonary vein and segmental branches of the pulmonary artery are ligated. The segmental bronchus is isolated, doubly clamped, and transsected; suctioning of the area prior to clamping prevents blood and fluid from entering the unaffected lung. The bronchial stump is sutured or stapled. The suture line is tested for air leaks. The pleural space is irrigated. Hemostasis is achieved. A chest tube (one or more) is inserted. The wound is closed in layers. The chest tube is connected to a sealed drainage unit.

Preparation of the Patient

The patient is usually in the lateral position with the affected side uppermost. The arm on the unaffected side is positioned on an armboard, and the arm on the affected side is supported by a Mayo stand padded by a pillow (or a double armboard may be used). The torso may be stabilized by kidney rests, and/or pillows or sandbags. The leg on the unaffected side is extended, and the leg on the affected side is flexed, with a pillow between the legs and adequate padding around the feet and ankles. The position is secured by wide adhesive tape at the shoulder, hip, and legs anchored to the underside of the table. Slanting the upper section of the table downward encourages drainage to the trachea. Check with the surgeon regarding insertion of a Foley catheter. Apply electrosurgical dispersive pad.

Skin Preparation

Begin cleansing for a posterolateral incision extending from the shoulder and arm to the iliac crest, and down to the table anteriorly and posteriorly.

Draping

Folded towels and a transverse sheet (a sterile, adhesive plastic drape and drape sheets may be requested)

Equipment

Items for positioning: Pillows, kidney rests, sandbags, beanbags, Mayo stand, extremity padding
Electrosurgical unit
Suction
Fiberoptic light source (if headlight is used)
Scale (to weigh sponges)

Instrumentation

Major procedures tray
Thoracotomy tray
Vascular procedures tray
Hemoclip appliers, assorted sizes, long-handled
Long Pean clamps
Stapling devices (optional)
Cushing vein retractors

Supplies

Basin set
Suction tubing
Electrosurgical pencils (2)
Needle magnet or counter
Blades (3) No. 10, (1) No. 15
Dissectors (e.g., peanut)

Asepto syringes (2)
Magnetic instrument pad (optional)
Staples (optional)
Hemoclips (assorted sizes)
Vessel loops, umbilical tapes
Chest drainage tube(s) (e.g., Argyle)
Connector, for example, straight or large Y (if 2 tubes are used)
Sealed drainage unit (e.g., Pleurevac)

Special Notes

Have the patient's x-ray films in the room.
Ascertain that blood is available as ordered.
Have second suction immediately available.
Weigh sponges.
Keep accurate record of irrigation fluid used.

WEDGE RESECTION OF THE LUNG

Definition

Excision of a small wedge-shaped section of the periphery of the lung.

Discussion

This procedure is performed to remove a limited pulmonary lesion, either for diagnostic or therapeutic purposes.

Procedure

The affected lung is usually exposed through a posterolateral thoracotomy. The lesion is identified. A wedge of peripheral lung tissue containing the lesion is excised over clamps (a linear stapler may be used). The lung tissue held in the clamps is sutured. The suture line is tested for air leaks. Additional sutures may be required to achieve hemostasis and check air leaks. A chest tube is inserted. The wound is closed in layers. The chest tube is connected to a sealed drainage unit.

Preparation of the Patient, Skin
Preparation, Draping, Equipment,
Instrumentation, and Supplies

See Segmental Resection of the Lung, pp. 251–253.

PULMONARY LOBECTOMY

Definition

Excision of one or more lobes of the lung.

Discussion

This procedure is usually performed when the lesion is
limited to the lobe.

Procedure

The affected lung is exposed through a posterolateral
incision. The diseased lobe is identified. The visceral
pleura is dissected free from the hilus. The pulmonary
artery and vein of the diseased lobe are ligated and divided. The bronchus is isolated, doubly clamped, and
transsected; suctioning of the area prior to clamping
prevents blood and fluid from entering the nonaffected
bronchus. The bronchial stump is sutured; more frequently a stapling device may be employed. The suture
line is tested for air leaks. The pleural cavity is irrigated. Hemostasis is achieved. Chest tubes are inserted. The chest is closed in layers. Chest tubes are
connected to a sealed drainage unit.

Preparation of the Patient, Skin
Preparation, Draping, Equipment,
Instrumentation, and Supplies

See Segmental Resection of the Lung, p. 251–253.

PNEUMONECTOMY

Definition

Removal of the lung.

Discussion

The chief indication for pneumonectomy is bronchogenic carcinoma; among other indications are extensive unilateral tuberculosis, some benign tumors, bronchiectasis, and multiple lung abscesses. At the completion of this procedure, the affected pleural cavity is empty and the mediastinal structures are liable to shift position, causing central circulatory compromise. Special measures may be employed to stabilize the mediastinum at the end of the procedure.

Procedure

The affected lung is exposed through a posterolateral thoracotomy. The chest is explored, and the feasibility of the procedure is determined. Advanced metastases contraindicate resection, in which case chest tubes are inserted, the wound is closed, and chest tubes are connected to a sealed drainage unit. The mediastinal pleura is dissected free. The bronchus, pulmonary artery, and superior and inferior pulmonary veins are isolated. Care is taken to avoid injury to the vagus nerve. The pulmonary artery and veins are ligated. The bronchial stump is clamped, transsected, and sutured or stapled; suctioning prevents blood and fluid from entering the unaffected lung. Lymph-node–bearing tissues are excised as necessary. Hemostasis is achieved. The chest is closed in interrupted layers.

Preparation of the Patient, Skin Preparation, Draping, Equipment, Instrumentation, and Supplies

See Segmental Resection of the Lung, pp. 251–253.

Special Notes

Ask the surgeon if a chest tube or large syringe with a large-bore needle will be necessary postoperatively to create a slightly negative pressure in the affected pleural space and stabilize the mediastinum.

DECORTICATION OF THE LUNG

Definition

The stripping of a restrictive membrane on the visceral pleura that interferes with respiration.

Discussion

Some indications for decortication of the lung are chronic empyema, clotted hemothorax, and tuberculosis.

Procedure

The affected lung is exposed through a posterolateral incision; rib resection may be indicated for adequate exposure. The fibrous membrane is carefully peeled away from the visceral pleura. Hemostasis may be difficult. Chest tubes are inserted. The wound is closed in layers. Chest tubes are connected to a sealed drainage unit.

Preparation of the Patient, Skin
Preparation, Draping, Equipment,
Instrumentation, and Supplies

See Segmental Resection of the Lung, pp. 251–253.

INSERTION OF TRANSVENOUS
ENDOCARDIAL PACEMAKER

Definition

Placing of an electrode lead in the endocardium through the cephalic, subclavian, or jugular vein and attaching the lead to a pulse generator.

Discussion

A permanent pacemaker is necessary when a heart block exists.

Types
Asynchronous. Stimulates ventricular contraction when a specified rate of pacing is required.

Demand. Initiates ventricular contraction only when the heart rate falls below a preset rate.

Physiologic. Synchronizes atrial and ventricular activity to improve cardiodynamics.

Procedure

A cut down is performed to expose the subclavian, cephalic, or external jugular vein; the right side is preferred. Through a venotomy, a pacing electrode is inserted and advancd (under fluoroscopy) into the right ventricle. The electrode is attached to an external pacemaker for testing. An incision is made in the chest wall and deepened down to the fascia, creating a "pocket" for the pulse generator. A tunneling instrument is used to make a path for the electrode, which is attached to the pulse generator. The pulse generator is placed in the pocket. Both incisions may be irrigated with antibiotic solution and closed.

Preparation of the Patient

The patient is supine; the head may be turned to the left. Usually the left arm is restrained at the side (check pressure point at the elbow), and the right arm is extended on an arm table. The procedure is often performed under local anesthesia. The patient is monitored continuously. An anesthetist is usually present. Apply electrosurgical dispersive pad.

Skin Preparation

Begin cleansing the right chest, including right axilla, shoulder, and arm to the elbow. Extend preparation from the chin to lower ribs; prepare well beyond the midline on the left border, and down to the table on right side.

Draping

The hand is grasped in a tube or an impervious stockinette. A large sheet is draped over the hand table and tucked under the shoulder. Folded towels and a fenestrated sheet or individual drape sheets complete the draping.

Equipment

Electrosurgical unit
Hand table
Image intensifier and C-arm (x-ray department)
External pacemaker

Instrumentation

Pacemaker tray
Hemoclip appliers (small and medium)

Supplies

Basin set
Tube or impervious stockinette
Blades (2) No. 10, (1) No. 15, (1) No. 11
Needle magnet or counter
Electrosurgical pencil
Local syringe and needle (e.g., 10-mL control syringe, 25-gauge, 1½″ needle)
Vessel loops
Antibiotic irrigation and bulb syringe (optional)

Special Notes

Lead aprons are worn for protection during fluoroscopy.

Make the patient as comfortable as possible as the procedure may be lengthy.

Check with the surgeon regarding availability of the generator and leads (usually brought by a pacemaker company representative).

X-ray equipment can be set up in the room on the patient's left side.

The scrub person positions the back table on the patient's right side and assists the surgeon side to side.

Complete the forms from the manufacturer. Chart serial numbers.

CORRECTION OF PECTUS EXCAVATUM

Definition

The correction of pectus excavatum, or funnel chest, refers to the straightening of a deformity of the anterior chest wall in which there is a depression of the sternum and costal cartilages.

Discussion

This procedure may be performed to alleviate circulatory or respiratory symptoms, although it is most frequently performed for cosmetic reasons. Variations of the procedure are performed according to the extent of the deformity. The patient is often a child.

Procedure

Approach is through a vertical presternal incision. The origins of the pectoral muscles are reflected. Rib cartilages are separated from the sternum. The xiphoid process is transsected from the sternum. An incision is made into the anterior mediastinum, and the pericardium is dissected from the sternum. According to the extent of the deformity, the sternum is reshaped by a wedge-shaped osteotomy, or reversed, and the sternum and costal cartilages are trimmed as necessary. The sternum is fixed in place with sutures. Previously detached muscles are resutured to their points of division. Drains are placed, or chest tubes are inserted if the pleural cavity has been entered. The wound is closed. Chest tubes, if used, are attached to a sealed drainage unit.

Preparation of the Patient

The patient is supine and the chest is slightly elevated, for example, with a rolled sheet. Arms may be extended on armboards. Apply electrosurgical dispersive pad.

Skin Preparation

Begin at the midline, extend from the chin, to below the umbilicus, and down to the table at the sides.

Draping

Folded towels and a laparotomy sheet

Equipment

Electrosurgical unit
Suction
Power source for saw (e.g., Stryker)

Instrumentation

Minor orthopedic procedures tray
Bone holding instruments tray
Thoracotomy tray and Vascular procedures tray (available)
Gigli saw set
Power saw, for example, Stryker (with circular blade)
Lebsche sternal knife
Mallet
Bone tenacula (2) single-hook
Awl with fenestration
Pliers

Supplies

Basin set
Blades (2) No. 10, (1) No. 15
Electrosurgical pencil
Suction tubing
Needle magnet or counter
Bone wax
Drains (optional)

Special Notes

Children require padded extremity restraints, smaller drapes and instruments, and so on; see pp. 518–520 for Pediatric General Information.

THYMECTOMY

Definition

Removal of the thymus gland.

Discussion

This surgery is performed in an attempt to alleviate myasthenia gravis or to remove benign or malignant tumors. The thymus gland is largest in infancy and atrophies in adulthood.

When a thymectomy is performed to treat myasthenia gravis, the possibility of respiratory compromise must be anticipated. Prolonged endotracheal intubation or a tracheostomy may be necessary with the concomitant administration of neostigmine methyl sulfate (Prostigmin).

Procedure

Approach is usually through a sternal splitting incision. The mediastinal fat pad is incised and the thymus gland dissected from it and the underlying pericardium. Vascular attachments are ligated. Care is taken to avoid the great vessels and the parathyroid glands. Hemostasis is achieved. A drain may be inserted. If either pleural space has been entered, a chest tube(s) and a sealed drainage unit may be necessary.

Preparation of the Patient

The patient is supine; arms may be extended on armboards. Apply electrosurgical dispersive pad.

Skin Preparation

Sternal Splitting Incision. Begin at the midline extending from the chin to below the umbilicus, and down to the table at the sides.

Draping

Folded towels and a fenestrated sheet

Equipment

Electrosurgical unit
Suction
Power source for saw (e.g., Stryker, Sarns)

Instrumentation

Thoracotomy procedures tray
Vascular procedures tray
Basic/Minor procedures tray
Tracheostomy tray (available)
Lebsche sternal knife
Mallet
Sternal saw (e.g., Stryker, Sarns)
Rake retractors (4- and 6-prong)

Supplies

Basin set
Blades (2) No. 10, (1) No. 15 adult; (2) No. 15 children
Electrosurgical pencil
Suction tubing
Drain (e.g., ¼″ Penrose) (optional)
Umbilical tape (for retraction)
Dissectors (e.g., peanut)
Needle magnet or counter
Bone wax
Chest tube(s), connector, and sealed drainage unit (op-
  tional)

Special Notes

Sternal sutures (e.g., wire) are available.

THORACOSCOPY

Definition

Endoscopic visualization of the pleural space(s).

Discussion

Thoracoscopy is currently performed employing a
video-assisted system (video-assisted thoracoscopic
surgery: VATS). This reintroduced modality can be
used for diagnosis and treatment of numerous pleural
and intrapleural conditions including diseases of the
pleura, mediastinum, pericardium, esophagus, lungs,
and assessment of thoracic trauma. Tissue sampling,

drainage of fluid collections, and diverse surgical procedures can be performed. Definitive treatment of lung masses (wedge resection, lobectomy, pneumonectomy) have been accomplished as well as procedures for pneumothorax (secondary to pulmonary blebs and empyema). Dissection of the esophagus for benign and malignant conditions as in hiatal herniorrhaphy, vagotomy, or transhiatal esphagectomy have been described. Esophagomyotomy, creation of a pericardial window, thymectomy, sympathectomy (for hyperhidrosis and for various vasospastic syndromes), and excision of mediastinal cysts are examples of this expanding capability. In light of rapidly evolving instrumentation and expertise, many procedures currently performed only through open thoractomy will be managed thoracoscopically.

Thoracoscopy is indicated when noninvasive or minimally invasive diagnostic procedures (x-rays, scans, bronchosopy, and so on) have not yielded sufficient information and particularly for treatment of patients with reduced pulmonary function for whom the risk of formal thoracotomy is great. When a thoracoscopic approach can be accomplished, postoperative morbidity is greatly diminished as compared with open thoracotomy. Also, in contrast to a limited open thoracotomy, thoracoscopy permits inspection of the entire hemithorax under excellent illumination and magnification. Controversial, however, are the procedures requiring an ancillary incision (as for specimen retrieval) in light of improved open techniques and postoperative epidural analgesia especially with respect to the high cost of the endoscopic technology.

The risks of thoracoscopy include hemorrhage, air embolism, diaphragmatic injury, injury to adjacent organs, and so on, in which case prompt conversion to open thoracotomy is required. Contraindications include lesions in proximity to major central vessels and patients in whom the anesthetist cannot safely maintain unilateral pneumothorax. In postoperative cardiac patients in an anticoagulated status, thoracoscopic drainage of pericardial effusion may be preferable to a repeat sternotomy approach.

Procedure

Thoracoscopy is usually performed under general anesthesia although a limited procedure may be performed employing local anesthesia at the port site, the patient receiving basal sedation. The ability to perform thoracoscopy is enhanced by the use of a double-lumen endotrachial tube so that the nonoperative lung can be ventilated while permitting pneumothorax on the operative side. When this tube cannot be inserted (e.g., small trachea), pneumothorax on the operative side can be increased by judicious insufflation of carbon dioxide, in which case ports with pneumatic seals (as for laparoscopy) are used.

An initial port is established at the fourth to seventh intercostal space midaxillary to posterior axillary line (according to pathology and the surgeon's preference). Prior to insertion of the port, digital exploration confirms clear entrance into the pleural cavity. The telescope is inserted, the situation assessed, and the feasibility of the thorascopic procedure is determined. Two or three additional ports are established according to the location of the lesion. When excision of a larger specimen is anticipated, a limited ancillary incision is made, for example, submammary, 6 cm. Endoscopic instruments are deployed to retract, dissect, ligate, and excise and suture the tissues. Laser (Nd:YAG noncontact), suction/irrigation/cautery devices are utilized when the ancillary incision is employed; standard thoracotomy instruments may be used. The laser is particularly useful to excise smaller lesions not amenable to stapling. Upon completion of the definitive procedure, specimens are retrieved in a specimen bag to avoid seeding of malignant cells or infectious materials through a 12 mm port. Larger specimens are retrieved through the ancillary incision usually without a need to spread the ribs. A chest tube is inserted through an appropriate port and connected to a closed drainage unit. The incisions are closed in the usual manner. Particularly after a lesser procedure, the chest tube may be removed prior to the patient's leaving the operating room or in the recovery room.

Preparation of the Patient

General anesthesia is administered through a double-lumen endotrachial tube. The patient is usually in the lateral position with the affected side uppermost. The arm on the unaffected side is placed on an armboard, and the pressure points are padded. An axillary roll may be placed under the patient's dependent arm. The arm on the affected side is angled toward the head and supported by a Mayo stand padded with a pillow (or a double armboard may be used). The torso is stabilized with kidney rests and/or pillows, sandbags, or a bean-bag. The leg on the unaffected side and pressure points at the knee, ankle, and foot are padded. The leg on the affected side is flexed with a pillow(s) between the legs, ankles, and feet. The position may be secured by wide adhesive tape at the shoulder, hip, and legs, which is anchored to the underside of the table. Check with the surgeon regarding the insertion of a Foley catheter. Apply electrosurgical dispersive pad.

Skin Preparation

Begin cleansing at the nipple extending from the shoulder and underarm to the iliac crest and down to the table anteriorly and posteriorly.

Draping

Folded towels and a laparoscopy sheet (or laparotomy or transverse sheet); a sterile, adhesive plastic drape and additional drape sheets may be requested. Camera cord cover (plastic with ties)

Equipment

Pillow(s) and padding for positioning
Electrosurgical unit
Suction
Light source (e.g., Xenon 300 W)
Video monitors (2)
VCR
Mavigraph (video printer, optional)

Argon beam coagulator (optional)
Nd:YAG noncontact laser (optional)

Instrumentation

Thoracotomy tray (open)
Major procedures tray
Vascular procedures tray
Trocars (2) 10 to 11 mm blunt, (2) 10 to 12 mm sharp,
   usually disposable
Reducers
0° and 30° telescopes and cords
Camera and cord
Light cord
Cushing vein retractors
Pean clamps, long (available)
Lung retractor (patch spreader)
Clip appliers
Monopolar electrosurgical cord
Modified ring forceps
Endoscopic instruments:
   Hook and/or spatula dissector
   Graspers, (1) toothed, (1) serrated, (1) blunt
   Dissecting forceps
   Suture carrier
   Suture ligator
   Scissors, (1) hook, (1) micro, (1) straight
   Electrosurgical/suction/irrigator with spatula or
      right-angle tip
   Pennington clamps (2)
   Allis clamps (2)
   Babcock clamps (2)
   Tonsil clamps (2)
   Lung retractor (e.g., Naticoke)
   Clip appliers
   Thorascopic endostapler with safety lock (optional)

Supplies

Basin set
Suction tubing
Electrosurgical pencil (hand control)

Blades (1) No. 10, (1) No. 15
Disposable trocars (optional)
Camera cord cover
Lens defogger (e.g., Elvis or Fred)
Peanut sponges
Vessel loops and umbilical tapes (available)
Magnetic instrument pad
Clip cartridges
Chest drainage tube (e.g., Argyle No. 28)
Local anesthetic (e.g., Marcaine) and syringe
Sealed drainage unit with connector (e.g., Pleurevac)
Ligation sutures
Foley catheter (optional)
Staple cartridges (disposable, GIA)
Adhesive skin closure strips (e.g., Steristrips)

Special Notes

After the patient is in the room, position the monitors.

Have the patient's x-ray films in the room.

Following draping, the scrub person passes off the camera cable, light cord, suction tubing, and electro-cautery cord.

Connect and turn on the light source and white balance camera.

The circulator turns on the VCR (to record) if requested.

Recheck the position of monitors so they can be easily viewed.

The circulator connects the remaining items: irrigation tubing, suction tubing, and electrosurgical cord.

Keep the lens clean as necessary.

The circulator positions electrosurgical unit. (Usually the surgeon uses a foot pedal.)

Always be prepared for Thoracotomy with the instrument tray open.

Ascertain that blood is available as ordered.

Camera, scopes, and cords may be soaked for 30 minutes in a periacetic solution, for example, Steris, to achieve sterilization.

If the opposite side is also to be operated upon, the patient is repositioned, reprepped, and redraped; the anesthetist repositions endobronchial tubes accordingly.

Be prepared for possible emergency thoracotomy.

THORACOSCOPIC WEDGE RESECTION OF THE LUNG

Definition

Thoracoscopic excision of a wedge-shaped section of the periphery of the lung.

Discussion

This procedure provides a large biopsy specimen when diffuse pulmonary disease is present or may totally excise an isolated lesion that is anatomically amenable to this relatively atraumatic technique while sparing the patient a formal thoracotomy. Primary benign and malignant lesions or metastatic malignant lesions or localized infectious lesions or bullae may be treated by this modality.

Procedure

General anesthesia is established with a double-lumen endotrachial tube. An initial 10/12 mm port is established at the fifth or sixth intercostal space (ICS); and at the fourth or fifth ICS anterior axillary line and the seventh or eighth ICS midaxillary line. After the pathology is assessed, the affected site is grasped, and a staple line placed to give an appropriate margin of clearance to the lesion, alternating grasper and stapler through different ports if necessary. A second or third staple line completes the wedge and the specimen is retrieved (using an endoscopic specimen bag through a 12 mm port or ancillary small incision). Hemostasis is ascertained and air leakage checked by partially inflating the collapsed lung. A noncontact Nd:YAG laser may be used to achieve local hemostasis and seal air leaks, and whereas the same can be used to excise the specimen altogether, the stapler is faster and gives more satisfactory hemostasis and control. A chest tube is placed through a port site and the incisions closed.

Preparation of the Patient, Skin
Preparation, Draping, Equipment,
Instrumentation, Supplies, and Special
Notes

See Thoracoscopy, p. 265–268.

VIDEO-ASSISTED THORACOSCOPIC PNEUMONECTOMY

Definition

Transthoracoscopic excision of the lung.

Discussion

The indications for this procedure, when technically
feasible, are the same as for pneumonectomy through
thoracotomy, pp. 265–268.

Procedure

Three ports are established, lower at the posterior and
anterior axillary lines and an upper at the posterior axillary line; in addition a 6 cm submammary incision is
made. After assessment of the pathology, the lung tissue is seized with grasping or modified sponge forceps,
and the lung is retracted anteriorly and inferiorly. Major vessels are dissected, stapled, and divided. (Prior to
division of major vessels a vascular clamp is loosely
placed proximal to the site of division in case of mechanical failure of the staple line.) Division of the inferior pulmonary ligament permits exposure of the inferior pulmonary vein. The main stem bronchus is
exposed, peribronchial nodes removed, and the
bronchus stapled and divided. The superior pulmonary
vein is divided, periaortic nodes excised, and the specimen removed through the inframammary incision.
During the procedure standard instruments may be introduced through this incision. The incisions are closed
after placement of a chest tube through the lower posterior port site. Measures are taken to stabilize the mediastinum.

Preparation of the Patient, Skin
Preparation, Draping, Equipment,
Instrumentation, Supplies, and Special
Notes

See Thoracoscopy, pp. 265–268.

VIDEO-ASSISTED THORACOSCOPIC ESOPHAGOGASTROMYOTOMY

Definition

Division of the longitudinal and circular muscles of the
distal esophagus.

Discussion

This procedure is performed to treat achalasia of the
esophagus, a neuromuscular disorder with failure of
the lower esophageal sphincter to relax. Initial symptoms include dysphasia, and later, as the esophagus dilates above this functional obstruction, regurgitation
and weight loss. After thorough investigation and failure of pharmacologic agents and balloon dilation, surgical division of the distal esophageal muscle fibers
gives lasting relief. This procedure (modified Heller,
long or short segment, depending upon physiologic
studies) is performed transabdominally or transthoracically and now by thoracoscopic approach. Propo-
nents of this approach believe that the technology of
high magnification and illumination provide a more
complete visualization of the operative field with less
trauma to surrounding structures than the open procedure. The laparoscopic approach may be used, but thoracoscopy is more direct and probably less destructive
to the structures about the esophageal obstruction.

Procedure

After anesthesia is established with a double-lumen
endotrachial tube, a fiberoptic gastroscope is passed
that aids in the identification of the esophagus for traction and manipulation minimizing the extent of dissec-

tion. At the completion of the procedure, its effect can be directly visualized. The patient is turned to the right lateral decubitus position. Five ports are employed: seventh intercostal space (ICS) posterior axillary line, third or fourth ICS midaxillary line, fourth ICS posterior axillary line, seventh ICS anterior axillary line, and sixth ICS anterior axillary line. The lung is retracted and the inferior pulmonary ligament divided; the esophagus is identified, and the outer longitudinal and inner circular muscle fibers are divided using a hook cautery (or cautery scissors) from the level of the inferior pulmonary vein to the diaphragm. Care is taken to avoid injury to the mucosa (which may be suture repaired); hence prophylactic antibiotics are administered immediately prior to surgery. Pressure on the diaphragm reveals the esophagocardiac junction, and the final division of fibers is continued onto the cardia of the stomach.

The divided muscle is bluntly separated to 40 percent of the circumference of the esophagus to prevent adherence in the healing process. The esophageal hiatus may be repaired as necessary. The endoscopist can then assess the adequacy of the myotomy. Careful hemostasis is necessary throughout the procedure especially if periesophagitis resulting from prior dilatations is present. A chest tube is placed through a lower port, and the incisions are closed.

Preparation of the Patient, Skin Preparation, Draping, Equipment, Instrumentation, Supplies, and Special Notes

See Thoracoscopy, pp. 265–268.

Chapter 14

Cardiovascular Surgery

CAROTID ENDARTERECTOMY

Definition

Excision of intimal plaque from the carotid artery.

Discussion

This procedure is done to restore carotid artery blood flow and enhance cerebral circulation in order to relieve transient cerebral ischemia or prevent stroke.

Procedure

An incision is made along the anterior border of the sternomastoid muscle. The carotid sheath is exposed and incised. Care is taken to identify and prevent injury to cranial nerve branches. Proximal and distal control of the carotid artery and its bifurcation is achieved with vascular clamps and/or umbilical tapes, and vessel loops. Arteriotomy is made with a No. 11 blade and Pott's scissors. An intraluminal shunt from the common carotid artery to the internal carotid artery may be inserted and secured with tourniquets or shunt clamps. Plaque is freed from the arterial wall. Care is taken to extract all plaque and debris to prevent subsequent embolization. If an intimal flap has developed, it is tacked to the vessel wall with fine

sutures to prevent dissection when blood flow is restored. The arterial lumen may be flushed with heparin solution. The arteriotomy is closed primarily, or
if the lumen appears stenotic, a patch graft (autogenous or synthetic) may be employed. Prior to placement of final sutures, the shunt, if used, is removed,
and the lumen is flushed to remove any residual debris or air bubbles. The wound is closed in layers. A
drain may be employed.

Preparation of the Patient

The patient is supine with the head slightly extended
and turned toward the opposite side. Excessive rotation
of the head and extension of the neck is avoided because this significantly decreases blood flow to the
carotid-vertebral artery system. The head may be supported by a doughnut. A rolled towel may be placed between the scapulas. Apply electrosurgical dispersive
pad.

Skin Preparation

Begin at the neck on the affected side extending from
the infra-auricular border to the axilla, and down to the
table at the sides.

Draping

Folded towels and a fenestrated sheet

Equipment

Head rest (e.g., doughnut)
Electrosurgical unit
Suction
Scales (weigh sponges)

Instrumentation

Basic/Minor procedures tray
Shunt tray
Hemoclip appliers, short (small and medium)

Supplies

Basin set
Blades (2) No. 10, (1) No. 15, (1) No. 11
Electrosurgical pencil
Suction tubing
Umbilical tapes, vessel loops
Dissectors (e.g., peanut)
Heparinized saline
Graduate and disposable syringe
Hemostatic agents (e.g., Avitene, Surgicel)
Hemoclips (small, medium)
Shunt (e.g., Javid)

Special Notes

Have the patient's x-rays in the room.

The anesthetist usually records the time the carotid artery is clamped.

Every effort is made by the surgical team to minimize the amount of time the carotid artery is clamped; organization of equipment, efficiency of movement, and attention to the wound site by the scrub person is extremely important.

Retractors must have dull teeth to avoid injury to blood vessels.

Moistened umbilical tapes and vessel loops are passed on a clamp (e.g., tonsil).

A shunt may be fashioned out of a 5 to 7.5 cm (2 to 3 inch) piece of vinyl tubing or a commercially prepared shunt (e.g., Javid) may be used.

Check with the blood bank that blood is available as ordered.

Weigh sponges.

Keep an accurate record of irrigation used.

ABDOMINAL AORTIC PROCEDURES (ABDOMINAL AORTIC ANEURYSMECTOMY, ABDOMINAL AORTIC ENDARTERECTOMY) WITH AORTOILIAC GRAFT

Definition

Aortic Aneurysmectomy is the excision and/or internal bypass of an attenuated widening of the aortic wall (aneurysm) that requires the insertion of a prosthetic graft to reestablish vascular continuity; if the aortic bifurcation is involved an aortoiliac Y-graft is employed.

Aortic Endarterectomy is the removal of intimal plaque with the insertion of a tubular graft or patch to restore the integrity of the aorta.

Discussion

These lesions most often result from arteriosclerosis. The aortic wall weakens and dilation occurs; thrombus fills most of the increased lumen, a potential source of emboli. Infection also may lead to weakening of the wall and aneurysm formation (mycotic aneurysm). In the absence of an aneurysm, it may be possible to spare the aorta by resecting plaque and repairing the aorta and/or its major branches or by bypassing the diseased segment (aortoiliac or aortofemoral graft).

Aortic aneurysm surgery is usually performed as an elective procedure. If an aneurysm ruptures incompletely, dissection of the aortic wall by blood and clot will occur, resulting in an acute surgical emergency.

Procedure

The abdominal aorta is approached by a long midline incision. The intestines are mobilized and packed out of the field. The posterior parietal peritoneum is incised, and the aorta is exposed taking care to protect the inferior vena cava and ureters. When the aneurysm involves the inferior mesenteric artery, the artery may be sacrificed (or preserved if backflow is brisk). Proximal and distal control is obtained with vascular forceps. The aneurysm is opened and the clot evacuated. The lumbar vessels are suture-ligated, leaving the posterior portion of the aneurysm in situ. The aorta and usually the common iliac arteries are transsected and anastomoses made using a prosthesis. When appropriate, the inferior mesenteric artery (distally), or renal artery (proximally), may require reimplantation. Special prostheses (grafts) are available. Control clamps are removed and the anastomoses tested for leakage. The shell of the aneurysm may be closed over the prosthesis for reinforcement. In endarterectomy the aorta and iliac vessels are incised, the plaque removed, and the vessels repaired with or without prosthetic patches. In aortic bypass, the aorta is connected to the iliac or femoral vessels according to their degree of patency, eliminating the need for extensive endarterectomy. Various combinations of these techniques can be employed. Local anticoagulation with heparinized saline may be used. Prior to closure of the anastomoses, clots are flushed out by transient release of the control clamps. The posterior peritoneum is closed, and the wound is closed.

Preparation of the Patient

The patient is supine with arms extended on armboards. Apply electrosurgical dispersive pad. Check with the surgeon regarding insertion of a Foley catheter.

Skin Preparation

Begin at the midline extending from axillae to midthighs, and to the table at the sides.

Draping

Folded towel (thirds lengthwise) over pubic area, folded towels around the operative site, sterile, plastic adhesive drapes (2), optional, and a laparotomy sheet (which may be cut) or individual drape sheets

Equipment

Electrosurgical unit
Suction (2 units)
Scales (weigh sponges)
Headlight and fiberoptic light source (optional)
Doppler (optional)

Instrumentation

Major procedures tray
Vascular procedures tray
Balfour retractor

Weitlaner retractors (2)
Harrington retractors (2)
Extra towel clips
Hemoclip appliers (various sizes and lengths)

Supplies

Basin set
Blades (2) No. 10, (1) No. 15, (1) No. 11
Needle magnet or counter
Suction tubings (2)
Electrosurgical pencil
Penrose drains, umbilical tapes, vessel loops
Dissectors (e.g., peanut)
Hemostatic agent (e.g., Avitene, Surgicel, Thrombo-
    stat)
Needle 18-gauge (to vent, to prevent air embolus)
Graft (type and size of choice)
Hemoclips (various sizes)
Heparin (anticoagulant) and heparinized saline (di-
    luted to preference)
Protamine sulfate (neutralizes heparin)
Antibiotic (intravenous or for irrigation, optional)
Graduate and syringes

Special Notes

Have the patient's x-rays in the room.
    Check with the surgeon regarding the type and size
of graft, and prepare the graft for use according to surgeon's directions.
    Mark pedal pulses before preparing the skin so that
if a pulse check is requested, it can be found immediately.
    Have a variety of Fogarty catheters (irrigation and
embolectomy) in the room.
    Check urinary output as requested.
    Do *not* cut double-armed sutures.
    Check with the blood bank that blood is available as
ordered.
    Weigh sponges.
    Keep an accurate record of amount of irrigation used.

Moistened umbilical tapes and vessel loops are passed on a clamp (e.g., tonsil).

FEMOROPOPLITEAL BYPASS

Definition

The interposition of a graft from the common femoral artery to popliteal artery in order to bypass an occluded segment of the superficial femoral artery.

Discussion

The graft may be the patient's own saphenous vein (autogenous) or a synthetic prosthesis. Patency of the popliteal artery must be determined prior to the surgery by angiography. When the popliteal artery is occluded, shunting the blood flow to a more distal artery becomes necessary.

Procedure

A vertical incision is made from above the inguinal ligament over the course of the greater saphenous vein; there may be several interruptions in the incision. The saphenous vein is harvested for a graft by dividing and ligating its multiple branches. The segment is flushed with a heparinized saline and tested for leakage. The common femoral artery and its bifurcation are exposed. The distal popliteal artery is exposed, retracting or excising the gastrocnemius and soleus muscles posteriorly and adductor muscles anteriorly. The posterior tibial nerve is protected. A tunneling instrument is used to make a passage from the femoral triangle to the popliteal space under the sartorius muscle. The femoral artery is controlled with a vascular clamp and heparinized. The graft is sutured to the common femoral artery, making certain that the distal portion of the vein is used, that is, reversed anatomical position. Endarterectomy and patch angioplasty may be performed at the origin of the deep femoral artery. The graft is passed through the tunnel (avoiding kinking or tension) and anastomosed to the popliteal artery. Prior to placing the final sutures, the graft is flushed with blood controlled by pressure or further sutures. Intra-operative angiography may be done. The incisions are closed. If vessels distal to the popliteal artery are used, similar maneuvers are performed.

Preparation of the Patient

The patient is supine with the affected thigh externally rotated and abducted, and the knee flexed. Arms may be extended on armboards. Check with the surgeon regarding insertion of Foley catheter. Apply electrosurgical dispersive pad.

Skin Preparation

Both legs may be prepared for harvesting saphenous vein(s). Check with the surgeon.

Unilateral. Begin at the groin on the affected side extending from the umbilicus to the toes (including front and back of thigh, leg, and entire foot). Prepare down to the table on affected side and well beyond midline on opposite side.

Bilateral. Prepare both groin regions extending from the umbilicus to the toes (including front and back of thighs, legs, and feet). Two persons are required to complete the preparation, or a leg holder may be used.

Draping

Unilateral. The affected extremity is held up and abducted. A large sheet is draped over the end of the table. A towel (folded in thirds, lengthwise) is placed over the pubic area. A split sheet is draped under the thigh. Two towels are placed on the table, the foot is lowered onto the towels, and the towels are fashioned into a boot and clipped. A large sheet is draped over the top of the patient's body. The affected leg may be passed through a laparotomy sheet and lowered to the table, or individual drape sheets complete the draping.

Bilateral. The legs are held up and abducted. A large drape sheet is placed over the end of the table. A towel (folded in thirds, lengthwise) is placed over the pubic area. Sheets are draped along the sides of the patient and fastened. A large sheet is draped under the thighs. Two towels for each foot are placed on the table, the feet are lowered onto the towels, and the towels are fashioned into boots and clipped. Another large sheet is draped over the top of the patient.

Equipment

Leg holder (optional)
Electrosurgical unit
Suction

Instrumentation

Basic/Minor procedures tray
Vascular procedures tray
Hemoclip appliers, short (small, medium, large)
Tunneling instrument

Supplies

Basin set
Suction tubing
Electrosurgical dispersive pencil
Blades (2) No. 10, (1) No. 15, (1) No. 11
Umbilical tapes, Penrose drains, vessel loops
Heparin and heparinized saline (diluted to surgeon's preference)
Protamine sulfate (neutralizes heparin)
Needle magnet or counter
Dissectors (e.g., peanut)
Antibiotic (intravenous or for irrigation), optional
Graduate and syringes
Hemostatic agents (e.g., Gelfoam, Surgicel, Thrombostat, Collastat, Oxycel, and Avitene)
Graft (type and size of choice)

Special Notes

Have the patient's x-ray films in the room.
    Check with the surgeon regarding type and size of graft and its preparation.

Do *not* cut double-armed sutures.

The surgeon may choose to perform intraoperative angiography. Notify the x-ray department. Check with the surgeon for type of catheters needed; have available syringes and contrast medium. Observe x-ray safety precautions, see p. 21.

A glove may be placed over the distal portion of the foot instead of a boot.

GREATER SAPHENOUS VEIN LIGATION AND STRIPPING

Definition

Excision of the greater saphenous vein and its tributaries.

Discussion

This procedure is indicated in patient's with varicose vein disease secondary to venous valvular incompetence. Another indication is superficial thrombophlebitis of the lower extremities. The lesser saphenous vein system may also be excised as indicated.

Procedure

An oblique incision is made in the groin overlying the saphenofemoral junction. The superficial fascia is incised and the proximal portion of the saphenous vein is mobilized, divided, and ligated close to the saphenofemoral junction. Tributaries are divided and ligated as indicated. A transverse incision is made over the saphenous vein distally anterior to the medial malleolus; tributaries are exposed, divided, and ligated. The probe end of the internal stripper is inserted into the distal end of the saphenous vein and threaded proximally. A ligature is tied about the distal end, securing the vein about the acorn end of the stripper. The stripper (with vein attached) is gently pulled out through the proximal incision as the assistant applies pressure with a folded towel over the course of the vein in the leg and thigh. The vein may be removed segmentally, or sections of it may be removed with external strippers. Saphenous vein branches and perforating veins (usually marked by the surgeon preoperatively) are stripped, excised, or ligated. This might entail numerous small incisions. The lesser saphenous vein (posterior aspect of the leg) may require similar treatment. All incisions are closed, dressed, and wrapped with an elastic bandage.

Preparation of the Patient

The patient is supine; arms may be extended on armboards. The affected thigh is externally rotated and abducted, and the knee is flexed. The patient is secured to the table with the safety belt fastened over the unaffected thigh. Apply electrosurgical dispersive pad.

Skin Preparation

Unilateral. Begin at the groin on the affected side extending from the umbilicus to the toes (including front and back of thigh, leg, and foot). Prepare down to the table on the affected side and well beyond the midline on the opposite side.

Bilateral. Prepare both groin regions extending from the umbilicus to the toes (including front and back of thighs, legs, and feet). Two persons are required to complete the preparation, or a leg holder may be employed.

Draping

Unilateral. The affected extremity is held up and abducted. A large sheet is draped over the end of the table. A towel (folded in thirds, lengthwise) is placed over the pubic area. A split sheet is draped under the leg. Two towels are placed on the table, the foot is lowered onto the towels, and the towels are fashioned into a boot and clipped. A large sheet is draped over the top of the patient's body. The affected leg is passed through a laparotomy sheet and lowered to the table or individual drape sheets may complete the draping.

Bilateral. The legs are held up and abducted. A large drape sheet is placed over the end of the table. A towel (folded in thirds, lengthwise) is placed over the pubic area. Sheets are draped along the sides of the patient and fastened. A large sheet is draped under the legs. Two towels for each foot are placed on the table, the feet are lowered onto the towels, and the towels are fashioned into boots and clipped. Another large sheet (or more) is draped over the top of the patient.

Equipment

Leg holder
Electrosurgical unit
Suction

Instrumentation

Basic/Minor procedures tray
Vascular procedures tray
Internal and external vein strippers
Hemoclip appliers, short (small, medium, large)
Weitlaner retractor, sharp

Supplies

Basin set
Marking pen
Blades (2) No. 10, (1) No. 15
Needle magnet or counter
Suction tubing
Electrosurgical pencil
Elastic bandages

Special Notes

A glove may be placed over the distal portion of the foot instead of a boot.

The scrub person should remove the vein from the internal stripper by cutting the suture in order to have it available for continued use.

PORTASYSTEMIC SHUNT

Definition

Diversion of portal venous blood to the systemic venous system.

Discussion

This procedure is performed to relieve elevated portal venous pressure (portal hypertension), which can result in bleeding from esophageal or gastric varices, ascites, and hepatic failure. The primary cause is cirrhosis. The portal blood may be shunted into the inferior vena cava from the portal vein (end to side or side to side), from the splenic vein (with splenectomy), from the distal splenic vein (retaining the spleen), or from the superior mesenteric vein (with or without an interposing prosthetic graft). The particular type of shunt is determined by the patient's condition and the surgeon's preference. Preoperative angiography (splenoportagram) is useful for diagnosis.

Procedure

A portacaval shunt will be described. A long right subcostal incision is usually employed; less often a thoracoabdominal incision is made. Careful dissection is performed because even minor vessels may bleed significantly. The duodenum is reflected, exposing the inferior vena cava. The hepatoduodenal ligament is incised, protecting the common bile duct and hepatic artery. The portal vein is exposed from the porta hepatis to the superior border of the pancreas. Portal pressure is measured for a reference through a needle inserted in a small mesenteric vein. Partial occlusion of the vena cava and the portal vein are obtained with vascular clamps. Anastomosis is made side-to-side after excising a generous window in either vein. For end-to-side anastomosis the portal vein is transsected at the porta hepatis, ligating the proximal stump securely. The distal end is anastomosed to the side of the vena cava. Repeat manometry is done. The wound is closed in layers.

Preparation of the Patient

The patient is supine with the right side elevated by a folded sheet; arms may be extended on armboards. Check with the surgeon regarding insertion of Foley catheter. Apply electrosurgical dispersive pad.

Skin Preparation

Begin in the subcostal region, extending from the axillae to the upper thighs, and down to the table at the sides.

Draping

Folded towels and a laparotomy sheet

Equipment

Electrosurgical unit
Suction
Spinal manometer
Scale (for weighing sponges)

Instrumentation

Major procedures tray
Vascular procedures tray
Hemoclip appliers (assorted sizes and lengths)

Supplies

Basin set
Blades (2) No. 10, (1) No. 15, (1) No. 11
Electrosurgical pencil
Suction tubing
Needle magnet or counter
Three-way stopcock, polyethylene tubing (e.g., angiocath), and syringe
Hemoclips (assorted sizes)

Special Notes

To measure portal pressure, polyethylene tubing inserted into a jejunal mesenteric vein is attached to a three-way stopcock and a spinal manometer.

Portal pressure is measured again following the portacaval anastomosis to determine if the shunt is functioning.

Weigh sponges.

Measure irrigation fluids accurately.

Check with the blood bank that blood is available as ordered.

ARTERIOVENOUS SHUNT, ARTERIOVENOUS FISTULA

Definition

Establishment of a communicating prosthetic loop (shunt) or a direct communication between an artery and vein (fistula).

Discussion

Arteriovenous shunt and arteriovenous fistula are usually performed under local, anesthesia. The procedure is performed to provide easy access for venipuncture with a large-bore needle for purposes of renal dialysis and infusion chemotherapy. Several varieties of arterial venous communication may be achieved employing a buried synthetic prosthesis, an arteriovenous fistula, or an external prosthesis (least often used).

Procedure

Incisions are made over selected arterial and venous sites (often the radial artery and cephalic vein of the proximal forearm). Use of the nondominant forearm is preferable; lower extremities can be used if forearm sites cannot be used for some reason such as previous surgery. Vascular clamps or bulldogs control the vessels. An incision is made into the lumen of the artery, which may be dilated with coronary artery dilators. The venous side is ligated distally. A shunt (e.g., bovine artery prosthesis) is anastomosed to the artery and vein. Heparin solution is instilled into the graft. If a fistula is to be performed, the selected artery is anastomosed to an adjacent vein. The wound is closed and a protective dressing placed.

Preparation of the Patient

The patient is supine with the nondominant forearm extended on a hand table; the other arm may be extended on an armboard.

Skin Preparation

Begin at the proposed site of the shunt on forearm; include entire forearm and hand from fingertips to several centimeters (inches) above the elbow.

Draping

The hand is held up in a tube or an impervious stockinette. A large cuffed sheet is draped over the table and under the arm. A folded towel is wrapped around the arm and clipped. A drape (or split) sheet is draped under the arm and clipped. A drape sheet covers the shoulder and is clipped under the arm. Either a fenestrated sheet or additional drape sheets complete the draping.

Equipment

Electrosurgical unit
Hand table
Loupes (optional)
Sitting stools (2) for surgeon and scrub person

Instrumentation

Shunt tray
Coronary artery dilators

Supplies

Basin set
Electrosurgical pencil
Needle magnet or counter
Blades (1) No. 10, (1) No. 15, (1) No. 11
Silastic cannula(s)
Teflon tips (2)
Shunt connector
Heparinized saline (diluted to surgeon's preference)
Graduate (for heparin solution) and syringe
Heparin
Shunt clamps (2)

Special Notes

If an external shunt is performed, two shunt clamps are to be secured to the gauze dressing when the procedure is completed. Should the cannula become separated from the connector, both ends of the cannula must be clamped immediately.

CARDIAC PROCEDURES

Definition

Involves the correction of congenital anomalies, acquired diseases of the heart, pericardium, and great vessels (including repair and replacement of diseased valves, resection of ventricular aneurysm, pericardiectomy, pulmonary embolectomy, and replacement of segments of the great vessels) and the revascularization of ischemic myocardium.

Discussion

Three representative cardiac procedures will be described. Pediatric cardiac surgery, procedures to correct congenital anomalies, cardiac transplantation, and the employment of artificial cardiac devices will not be discussed. Insertion of an intra-aortic balloon catheter will be covered briefly.

1. *Aortic valve replacement:* Involves the excision and replacement of the diseased aortic valve
2. *Mitral valve replacement:* Involves the excision and replacement of the diseased mitral valve
3. *Coronary artery bypass:* Refers to the grafting of the internal mammary artery or segments of autologous saphenous vein to bypass coronary artery obstruction

Cardiac surgery often necessitates the use of cardiopulmonary bypass. To fully comprehend cardiac abnormalities and the function of cardiopulmonary bypass, knowledge of anatomy and the circulation is mandatory.

Cardiopulmonary Bypass. Cardiopulmonary bypass is the technique by which the patient's blood is diverted, oxygenated, and reperfused. This artificial means of oxygenating and circulating the blood is employed for intracardiac, coronary artery bypass, and procedures of intrathoracic major vessels.

Prior to instituting cardiopulmonary bypass, the patient is anticoagulated with heparin. For patients with heparin intolerance ancrod/Arvin may be used. This status is reversed following the procedure with protamine sulfate. Protamine sulfate can cause catastrophic pulmonary vasoconstriction in some patients undergoing cardiopulmonary bypass; therefore, it is advisable to have prostaglandin E on hand to reverse the reaction.

Cardiopulmonary bypass may be either total or partial. For *total bypass* (used for intracardiac procedures as valve replacements, septal defects, major anomalies, and ventricular aneurysm resection), all the blood is diverted from the heart, except intrinsic cardiac circulation, by completely occluding the vessels about the bypass cannulae. *Partial bypass* (used for coronary artery surgery, thoracic aortic aneurysms, and so on) allows a portion of the blood flow to pass through the heart by limiting the degree of occlusion about the cannulae.

There are several anatomical sites at which cardiopulmonary bypass can be established. The femoral vein, inferior vena cava, and right atrium are examples of sites from which blood is diverted from the patient to the pump. Blood is returned to the patient through the femoral artery, subclavian artery, or the ascending aorta. The preference of the surgeon, nature of the surgery, and condition of the vessels will determine the sites chosen for each patient.

A commonly used configuration is the cannulation of the right atrium by a single multiholed cannula, the tip of which inserts into the inferior vena cava, transporting the venous return from the patient to the pump. A cannula inserted in the ascending aorta returns blood to the patient from the pump.

During cardiac surgery the patient's hemodynamics and other physiologic functions are monitored continuously. In addition to those monitors employed for most major surgeries, such as the electrocardiogram, pulse oximeter, urimeter, and so on, invasive hemodynamic catheters are placed. These include an arterial line to measure blood pressure directly and to serve as a ready access for blood gas determination sampling, and a central venous pressure (CVP) or Swan-Ganz line to measure intracardiac pressures. The electroencephalogram may be monitored.

Hypothermia and/or pharmacologic agents may be employed when it is necessary to slow or arrest the heart. Hypothermia can be induced by using a hypothermia mattress, the direct application of iced saline, and/or by cooling the blood being returned to the patient from the pump oxygenator. Pharmacologic agents used to produce cardioplegia contain a potassium solution that induces hyperkalemia, resulting in electromechanical cardiac arrest. Body temperature is restored, and the potassium preparation is flushed out, at the conclusion of the cardiac procedure. The heartbeat may resume spontaneously, or electrical cardioversion may be employed to restore effective activity to the heart in its state of arrest or ventricular fibrillation. Pacemaker wires are often inserted at the completion of cardiopulmonary bypass.

Intra-aortic Balloon Catheter. An increasingly performed adjunct to cardiopulmonary bypass is the insertion of an intra-aortic balloon catheter. This procedure can also be performed independent of cardiopulmonary bypass following myocardial infarction. The purpose of the intra-aortic balloon catheter is to increase coronary artery flow and to assist peripheral perfusion. This procedure is indicated following myocardial infarction or cardiopulmonary bypass when left ventricular function is inadequate. The cylindrical balloon catheter, which is inserted through the femoral artery, is positioned in the descending aorta distal to the level of the left subclavian artery and attached to an intra-aortic balloon pump unit. The femoral arteriotomy site is reinforced with prosthetic graft material. The pump is coordinated with the patient's electrocardiogram so that the balloon inflates during diastole, forcing blood retrogradely to better perfuse the coronary arteries, and antegradely into the distal aorta, and its branches. This improves oxygenation of the myocardium and increases peripheral blood flow, thus diminishing the workload of the heart. When counterpulsation assist is no longer necessary, the catheter is removed by opening the arteriotomy site.

Procedures

Aortic Valve Replacement. Approach is through a median sternotomy. Cannulation for total cardiopulmonary bypass is achieved. The aorta is occluded distal to the valve. A cardioplegic solution is infused through the aortic root into the coronary arteries. Aortotomy is performed. The valve is excised. The annulus is measured, and the appropriate size prosthesis is inserted and sutured into place. The aortotomy is closed. Air is vented from the left ventricle and the aorta. The aorta is unclamped. Cardiopulmonary bypass is discontinued. The wound may be irrigated with an antibiotic solution. Temporary pacemaker electrodes are sutured to the heart. Mediastinal drains are inserted. The wound is closed.

Mitral Valve Replacement. Approach is through a median sternotomy. Cannulation for total cardiopulmonary bypass is achieved. The ascending aorta is occluded. A cardioplegic solution is infused through the aortic root into the coronary arteries. A left atriotomy is performed to expose the mitral valve. The valve is excised, the annulus measured, and the appropriate prosthesis is inserted and sutured into place. The aortic cross-clamp is removed, and air is aspirated from the aorta. Cardiopulmonary bypass is discontinued. The wound may be irrigated with an antibiotic solution. Temporary pacemaker electrodes are sutured to the heart. Mediastinal drains are inserted. The wound is closed. There are many types of cardiac valve prostheses available, including preserved biological valves (porcine) or totally fabricated prostheses of various sizes, shapes, and mechanics. More than one valve may require replacement.

Coronary Artery Bypass Graft. Approach is through a median sternotomy. The internal mammary artery directly, free segments of the saphenous vein, or a combination of these will be grafted. The internal mammary artery is dissected to obtain maximal length and is evaluated for adequate blood flow. If saphenous vein segments are to be used, they are harvested and tested for leaks. Cannulation for partial cardiopulmonary bypass is achieved. The aorta is occluded, and the cardioplegic solution is infused. A coronary artery is isolated, and dilators may be inserted. The graft is anastomosed to the coronary artery and tested for leaks. Multiple grafts may be necessary. The grafts may be placed sequentially, that is one graft segment can be anastomosed to more than one coronary artery. The aortic cross-clamp is released, and a portion of the aorta is then occluded. The grafts are measured, cut, and anastomosed to the aorta. The clamp on the aorta is removed. (Some surgeons prefer to perform the aortic anastomoses on bypass prior to the coronary artery anastomoses. The sequence of anastomoses varies with each surgeon, particularly if multiple grafts are performed.) Grafts are again inspected for leaks. All sources of air bubble accumulation are vented. Cardiopulmonary bypass is discontinued. The wound may be irrigated with an antibiotic solution. Temporary pacemaker electrodes are sutured to the heart. Mediastinal drains are inserted. The wound is closed. Coronary artery bypass may be performed in conjunction with a valve replacement procedure.

Preparation of the Patient

The patient is supine. (For coronary artery bypass a pillow is placed under the knees to maintain slight flexion, which provides access to the proximal greater saphenous veins.) After the vascular access lines are placed in the upper extremities, the arms are padded and tucked in at the patient's sides. A Foley catheter is inserted and connected to a urimeter. Apply electrosurgical dispersive pad.

Skin Preparation

Valve Replacement. Begin at the midline of the chest, extending from the chin to midthighs, and down to the table at the sides. The genitalia are prepped last.

Coronary Artery Bypass. The preparation is best performed by two persons, or a leg holder may be used. Begin at the midline of the chest extending from the chin to the pubic symphysis, and down to the table at the sides. The thighs and legs are prepared front and back including the feet. The genitalia are prepared last.

Draping

Valve Replacement. A drape sheet is placed over the end of the table. A towel (folded in thirds, lengthwise) is placed over the genitalia. A sheet is draped over the thighs and legs. Towels folded longitudinally are placed along the patient's sides and across the sternal notch. Sterile, adhesive plastic drapes may be applied across the chest and abdomen. Large drape sheets are placed at the sides and across the top of the patient.

Coronary Artery Bypass. Two circulators lift and abduct the legs as a large drape sheet is placed on the end of the table. A towel (folded in thirds, lengthwise) is placed over the genitalia. A split sheet is placed under and around both legs. Two towels for each foot are placed on the table. The feet are lowered onto the towels, and the towels are fashioned into boots and clipped. Towels are folded longitudinally and placed along the patient's sides and across the sternal notch. Sterile, adhesive plastic drapes may be applied across the chest and abdomen. Large drape sheets are placed at the sides and across the top of the patient.

Equipment

Extra IV standards
Suctions (4)
Cell Saver
Hypothermia mattress
Temperature probe

Cardioverter
Electrosurgical unit

Instrumentation

Cardiac procedures tray
Oscillating saw (cordless or with cord, as available)
Hemoclip appliers (assorted sizes and lengths)

Supplies

Supplies for vascular lines, CVP and/or Swan-Ganz
    lines, and a cardioplegia administration set
Basin set
Knife blades (2) No. 10, No. 15, No. 11
Beaver blade
Large graduate pitchers (2)
Heparinized saline
Assorted syringes and needles
Sterile, adhesive plastic drapes (2)
Electrosurgical pencils (2) (1 spatula, 1 needle point)
Electrosurgical pencil holders (2) (optional)
Needle magnets or counters
Suction tubing
Cell Saver suction tubing
Asepto (or bulb) syringes (2)
Foley catheter tray
Urimeter
Hemostatic agents (e.g., Gelfoam or Surgicel)
Teflon felt strips and pledgets
Suture boots
Bone wax
Pacemaker wires
Elastic bandages (for saphenous vein grafts)
Mediastinal drains (2) with Y-connector
Intrapleural sealed drainage unit (e.g., Pleurevac)
Defibrillator paddles
Hemoclips (assorted sizes)

Special Notes

The circulator(s) and scrub person(s) must be thoroughly familiar with the routine of the surgeon and the
"open heart" team.

Pad the patient's arms to protect hemodynamic monitoring lines.

The scrub person should keep instruments free of blood clots, plaque, and tissue debris.

A bag fashioned out of a Mayo stand cover may be fastened to the head of the table for the defibrillator paddles.

Fibrin "glue" (mixture of thrombin, calcium, and cryoprecipitate) may be injected over bleeding site (e.g., graft site).

Several liters of iced saline may be needed when going on the pump.

Measure urine every 15 minutes while on the pump.

A separate tray of instruments may be used for saphenous vein removal.

Warm saline may be used coming off the pump.

Check with the blood bank that blood is available as ordered.

Weigh sponges.

Keep track of irrigation fluid used so that blood loss can be determined accurately.

Follow hospital policy regarding the insertion of a prosthesis for valve replacements.

Chapter 15

Orthopedic Surgery

OPEN REDUCTION OF A CARPAL BONE FRACTURE

Definition

Realignment and fixation of fractures (or fracture dislocation) of the bones of the wrist through an operative incision.

Discussion

Most fractures of the wrist are treated by closed reduction and immobilization (cast). Surgery is required when the fracture is displaced or dislocated or when there is a nonunion. Fixation may be achieved with a number of devices including pins, wires, and a compression plate and screws. Persistent nonunion may necessitate a bone graft from a bone in the forearm or the iliac crest. More severe injuries may require excision of carpal bones and/or the radial or ulnar styloid process to prevent arthritis. Arthrodesis of the wrist may be preferable in patients who engage in manual labor. Numerous permutations of fractures and dislocations occur. The most common fracture is of the scaphoid (navicular) bone.

Procedure

The approach is determined by the fracture site and the preference of the surgeon. For fracture of the scaphoid, an incision may be made on the dorsum of the wrist distal to the radiocarpal joint. Tendons and nerve roots are protected. Small bone fragments are excised; larger fragments are aligned and fixed with wires or pins, or by bone graft pegs (obtained with a tubular gouge). If a graft is employed, an additional incision is made to expose the radial styloid from which a bone graft may be taken. In some cases of nonunion as necrosis, larger fragments or the entire bone may be excised. The wound is closed. A splint or cast is applied.

Preparation of the Patient

The patient is supine with the affected arm extended on a hand table; the other arm may be extended on an armboard. Sheet wadding and a tourniquet are applied to the affected arm. Apply electrosurgical dispersive pad.

Skin Preparation

Begin at the wrist and cleanse the hand (including fingers and interdigital spaces) and forearm (front and back), extending 5 to 7.5 cm (2 to 3 inches) beyond the elbow.

Draping

The extremity is held up in a tube (or impervious) stockinette; the hand table is covered with a drape sheet. A cuffed sheet is draped under the arm. A folded towel is wrapped around the arm and clipped. A drape (or split) sheet covers the shoulder and is clipped under the arm. A fenestrated sheet or additional drape sheets completes the draping.

Equipment

Suction
Electrosurgical unit
Tourniquet and insufflator
Sitting stools (3) (surgeon, assistant, scrub person)
Power source for power drill (available)
Cast cart

Instrumentation

Minor orthopedic procedures tray
Hand drill or power drill and cord, drill bits
Kirschner wires
Tubular gouge (for bone graft peg)

Supplies

Basin set
Sheet wadding (unsterile for tourniquet)
Esmarch bandage
Blades (1) No. 10, (2) No. 15
Tube (or impervious) stockinette
Needle magnet or counter
Bulb syringe
Graduate
Suction tubing
Electrosurgical pencil
Antibiotic irrigation (optional)

Special Notes

Have x-ray films ready in the room.

Do not allow preparation solutions to pool under tourniquet.

Place tourniquet as high on extremity as possible.

Wrap sheet wadding around extremity smoothly. Tourniquet ends must overlap at least 5 cm (2 inches). Do not apply the tourniquet at the elbow. Setting for an adult is approximately 300 mm Hg for the upper extremity. Monitor tourniquet time and setting. Tourniquet must be released after 2 hours to avoid injury.

Be prepared to assist the surgeon in applying a splint or cast.

Protective goggles may be worn.

EXCISION OF GANGLION

Definition

Removal of a cystic dilation of the capsule of a joint or tendon sheath that contains synovial fluid.

Discussion

The most frequent site of origin is the dorsum of the carpus. Careful complete excision makes recurrence rare.

Procedure

A transverse incision is made over the ganglion. Soft tissue dissection to expose the ganglion is done. Care is taken to avoid injury to nerve branches. The ganglion is mobilized and excised (including a generous border at its base). The wound may be irrigated. The tendon sheath is repaired as necessary. The wound is closed. An elastic bandage is applied.

Preparation of the Patient, Skin Preparation, and Draping

See Open Reduction of a Carpal Bone Fracture, p. 297.

Equipment

Electrosurgical unit
Tourniquet and insufflator
Suction (available)
Sitting stools (2) (surgeon and scrub person)

Instrumentation

Minor orthopedic tray
Hay's metacarpal retractors, pediatric Deaver retractor (available)

Supplies

Basin set
Sheet wadding (unsterile for tourniquet)
Blades (2) No. 15
Tube (or impervious) stockinette
Esmarch bandage
Needle magnet or counter
Bulb syringe
Electrosurgical pencil
Suction tubing (optional)
Elastic bandage

Special Notes

For tourniquet precautions, see Open Reduction of a Carpal Bone Fracture, p. 298.

CARPAL TUNNEL RELEASE

Definition

Decompression of the median nerve on the volar surface of the wrist.

Discussion

Symptoms of carpal tunnel syndrome (compressed median nerve) such as numbness and tingling of fingers and weakness of intrinsic thumb muscles are usually relieved by division of the deep transverse carpal ligament.

Procedure

A curved incision is made parallel to the thenar crease and angled toward the ulnar side of the wrist. Care is taken to avoid injury to sensory branches of the median nerve. After the skin and subcutaneous tissue are excised and reflected, the transverse carpal ligament (flexor retinaculum) is divided. The skin is closed. A compression dressing and a splint may be applied.

Preparation of the Patient

The patient is supine with the affected arm extended on a hand table; the other arm may be extended on an armboard. Sheet wadding and a tourniquet are applied to the affected arm. Apply electrosurgical dispersive pad.

Skin Preparation

Cleanse the hand (begin at the palm, including fingers, nails, and interdigital spaces), the wrist, and the forearm to the elbow.

Draping, Equipment, Instrumentation, and Supplies

See Excision of a Ganglion, p 299.

Special Notes

For tourniquet precautions see Open Reduction of a
Carpal Bone Fracture, p. 298.

ARTHROSCOPIC CARPAL TUNNEL RELEASE

Definition

Decompression of the median nerve on the volvar surface of the wrist using an arthroscope.

Discussion, Preparation of the Patient, Skin
Preparation, Draping and Equipment

See Carpal Tunnel Release, p. 300.

Procedure

The skin is marked at the wrist, and the tourniquet is
inflated. A skin incision is made at the wrist, and the
trocar is inserted. The lens is then exchanged within
the trocar. With the use of probes and endoscopic
knives, the release is performed. The incision is closed.
A soft dressing and a splint may be applied.

Instrumentation

Have available a 2.7 mm scope and endoscopic knives
and probes. Also necessary is a hand and foot tray in
case the procedure becomes an open one.

OPEN REDUCTION OF THE HUMERUS

Definition

Realignment and fixation of a fracture of the arm employing an operative incision.

Discussion

A variety of fractures of the humerus may occur. When
closed reduction and immobilization are unsatisfactory
or when there is a nonunion, fixation may be achieved
with rods and a compression plate and screws.

Procedure

An appropriate incision is made over the fracture site avoiding neurovascular structures. If malunion has occurred, osteotomy is performed to restore alignment. Generally the fracture is fixed with screws and a compression plate; for condylar fractures threaded Kirschner wires or screws may be employed. The wound is closed. The arm is immobilized.

Preparation of the Patient

The patient is supine with affected arm in a comfortable position (possibly across the chest); the other arm may be extended on an armboard. A sandbag or rolled sheet may be placed under the shoulder on the affected side. In distal fractures, a tourniquet may be used. Apply electrosurgical dispersive pad.

Skin Preparation

Begin with the arm and hand; extend from the fingertips to the shoulder. Cleanse the axilla well; extend to the table posteriorly, beyond the midline of the chest anteriorly, and down to the level of the lower ribs.

Draping

The extremity is held up in a tube (or impervious) stockinette. A large drape sheet is tucked under the patient's shoulder. A towel is folded longitudinally and towel-clipped around the top of the arm (the stockinette is brought up to the shoulder). A drape (or split) sheet is draped under the arm and clipped at the shoulder. A drape sheet covers the shoulder and is clipped under the arm. A fenestrated sheet or additional individual drape sheets complete the draping.

Equipment

Suction
Electrosurgical unit
Power source for drill
Tourniquet and insufflator (for distal fractures)
Cast cart

Instrumentation

Basic orthopedic procedures tray
Bone holding instruments tray
Bone hooks, drill bits, Bennet retractors
Fixation device, for example, Rush rods (with awl, driver, and extractor), screws and plates, compression set (with drill sleeve), Steinmann pins
Power drill and cord

Supplies

Basin set
Sheet wadding (unsterile)
Blades (2) No. 10
Electrosurgical pencil
Suction tubing
Needle magnet or counter
Graduate
Bulb syringe
Tube (or impervious) stockinette
Esmarch bandage
Antibiotic irrigation (optional)

Special Notes

Have x-ray films in the room.

Check level of gas in tank for power drill.

For tourniquet precautions see Open Reduction of a Carpal Bone Fracture, p. 298.

Be prepared to assist the surgeon in applying a cast or splint.

Protective goggles may be worn.

OPEN REDUCTION OF THE RADIUS AND/OR ULNA

Definition

Realignment and fixation of fractures of the forearm employing an operative incision.

Discussion

When closed reduction is unsatisfactory or when a nonunion exists, fixation may be achieved with a variety of devices including rods, intramedullary nails, and long screws.

Procedure

An appropriate incision is made depending on the location of the fracture. Neurovascular structures are identified and protected. Radial head fractures (in adults) may require excision; all fragments and debris are removed including excess periosteum. A splint is applied. Radial shaft fractures are repaired with compression plates, or a triangular medullary nail (Sage) is inserted via the radial styloid. Proximal ulna or olecranon fractures are treated by fixation with long screws or wires for smaller fragments. Fixation for distal wrist fractures may be achieved with screws or Kirschner wires, or specially shaped plates (e.g., T-plates) may be used. A splint or bivalve cast is applied.

Preparation of the Patient

The patient is supine; the affected arm is positioned across the chest or extended on a hand table; the other arm may be extended on an armboard. Sheet wadding and a tourniquet are applied to the affected arm. Apply electrosurgical dispersive pad.

Skin Preparation

Begin with the forearm, include the hand, fingers, and interdigital spaces. Next scrub the elbow up to the level of the tourniquet.

Draping

The extremity is held up in a tube (or impervious) stockinette, and a large drape sheet is draped under the arm (and over the hand table if one is used). A folded towel is wrapped around the arm and clipped, and the tube stockinette is brought up over the towel. A drape (or split) sheet is draped under the arm and clipped. A drape sheet covers the shoulder and is clipped under the arm. A fenestrated sheet or additional drape sheets complete the draping.

Equipment

Hand table (optional)
Suction
Electrosurgical unit
Tourniquet and insufflator
Power source for drill
Cast cart

Instrumentation

Basic orthopedic procedures tray
Small-bone holders, nail set, drill bits, awl
Power drill and cord
Fixation device, for example, screws and plates, com-
   pression set (and drill sleeve), Steinmann pins,
   Kirschner wires, long screws, intramedullary nails,
   Rush rods (with awl, driver, and extractor)

Supplies

Basin set
Sheet wadding
Blades (2) No. 10
Tube (or impervious) stockinette
Esmarch bandage
Needle magnet or counter
Graduate
Bulb syringe
Suction tubing
Electrosurgical pencil
Antibiotic irrigation (optional)

Special Notes

See Open Reduction of the Humerus, p. 303

OPEN REDUCTION OF AN OLECRANON PROCESS FRACTURE

Definition

Realignment and fixation of fractures of the elbow employing an operative incision.

Discussion

When fragments are separated, open reduction and internal fixation are indicated. Small fragments may be removed and the triceps tendon reattached to the ulnar shaft. Large fragments may be fixed with a figure-of-eight wire loop, Kirschner wires, screws, and/or intramedullary pins (e.g., Steinmann).

Procedure

See Open Reduction of the Radius and/or Ulna, p. 304.

Preparation of the Patient

The patient is supine with affected extremity on a hand table or flexed across the chest; the other arm may be extended on an armboard. Sheet wadding and a tourniquet are applied to the affected arm. Apply electrosurgical dispersive pad.

Skin Preparation

Begin at the elbow extending from the tourniquet to the fingertips (including fingers and interdigital spaces).

Draping

See Open Reduction of the Radius and/or Ulna, p. 304.

Instrumentation

Basic orthopedic procedures tray
Drill bits, awl
Hibbs and Bennet retractors
Fixation device: Wire and/or screws, Kirschner wires, intramedullary pins (e.g., Steinmann)
Wire tightener
Bone holders
Power drill and cord

Supplies

Basin set
Sheet wadding
Blades (2) No. 10

Tube stockinette
Esmarch bandage
Needle magnet or counter
Wire (e.g., 18 gauge or 20 gauge stainless steel)
Graduate
Bulb syringe
Suction tubing
Electrosurgical pencil
Penrose ¼" (retraction for ulnar nerve)
Antibiotic irrigation (optional)

Special Notes

See Open Reduction of the Humerus, p. 303.

WRIST ARTHROSCOPY

Definition

Introduction of an arthroscope into the wrist joint for the purposes of diagnosis and treatment.

Discussion

Wrist arthroscopy is in a developmental stage. It is used to clarify diagnoses that are inadequately defined by arthrograms or MRI scans. Most commonly the diagnoses of synovitis, disruption of ligamentous structures, and loose bodies can be detected and treated. When treatment can be accomplished, usually as an outpatient, postoperative morbidity is reduced as compared to an open procedure.

Procedure

On the dorsum of the wrist after anesthesia is administered and the operative field is prepared, the landmarks are palpated and several portal entry sites are marked. The primary radial carpal portal is 1 cm distal to the dorsal radial tubercle between the extensor pollicis longus laterally and the extensor digitorum communis tendons between the radius and the lunate bone. Additional portals can be established distal to the ulnar head on either side of the extensor carpi ulnaris tendon and in the midcarpal area proximal to the capitate, lateral to the third metacarpal and an additional site in line with the fourth metacarpal proximal to the capitate hamate joint. The sites provide visualization of the local structure with diminished risk of nerve and blood vessel injuries. An 18 gauge needle is inserted through the portal adjacent to the pollicis longus tendon. The radial carpal joint is distended with 5 to 7 mL of lactated Ringer's solution. The needle is removed, the puncture incision is enlarged, and a blunt trocar and cannula are inserted to penetrate the joint. The flow of fluid indicates that the joint has been entered. An arthroscope, 2.7 mm, is inserted. The various structures are visualized as the scope is advanced to the ulnar side of the wrist. An 18 gauge needle is inserted medial to the extensor carpi onaris tendon and used as an inflow site with the additional flow necessary to maintain clear visualization without air bubbles and extravisation. Under direct visualization, additional portals are established at the sites noted above. After the systematic examination of the joint is completed by direct visualization and by palpation and sensation with the usual articular probe, the arthroscope and other instrumentation as probes and joint shaver, cartilaginous soft tissue lesions can be excised or debrided, and loose bodies can be removed.

Procedures include shortening of the ulnar head, synovectomy, and repair of the scapholunate disruptions have been described and additional procedures are currently being developed.

Preparation of the Patient

The patient is prepared and draped as for any wrist procedure. The arm is abducted free of the table. An overhead traction device, a forearm stabilizer, and a felt cuff over the upper arm and two finger traps are used to position the limb and to open joint spaces during surgery. The wrist stabilizer has protective padding. The hand is suspended over a loop of traction rope that connects to a hook on the overhead device above, to the finger traps below. All parts beneath the hook are sterile. Eight to ten pounds of traction are applied.

Proper distention of the wrist should prevent excessive bleeding, but a tourniquet may be applied to the upper arm to be utilized, if necessary.

Skin Preparation and Draping

See Open Reduction of the Radius and/or Ulnar, p. 304.

Equipment

Overhead traction device with hook
Felt cuff (upper arm)
Tourniquet
Finger traps (2)
Wrist stabilizer with protective padding
Loop of traction rope
Traction weight (8 to 10 pounds)
Video monitor
VCR (optional)
Mavigraph (optional)
Shaver system
Camera control unit
Xenon light source

Instrumentation

Same as for Arthroscopy of the Knee except that scopes are 2.7 mm and 4.0 mm; see p. 339.

Supplies

Basin set
Blades (2) No. 15
Graduate
Needle, 18 gauge
Suction
Electrosurgical pencil
Soft padding and cast (available)

Special Notes

Check that all equipment works prior to surgery.
White balance the camera.
Position the monitor on the side opposite the affected elbow.

All instruments must be carefully washed (if not disposable) and then flash sterilized except the arthroscope. Steris 20 soaking solution is recommended for sterilizing the arthroscope.

REPAIR OF RECURRENT ANTERIOR DISLOCATION OF THE SHOULDER

Definition

Strengthening of the anterior joint capsule and musculotendonous support of the shoulder.

Discussion

There are many procedures and modifications of procedures for the repair of recurrent anterior dislocation; posterior dislocations are rare.

Types

Bankart. The glenoid labrum and the anterior part of the capsule (which should cushion and support the humeral head) are reattached to the rim of the glenoid cavity.

Putti-Platt. The subscapularis tendon and the capsule are detached from the humerus and sutured laterally on the humeral neck in order to strengthen anterior supporting structures and to prevent excessive external rotation of the shoulder.

Bristow. The coracoid process and attached muscles are detached, inserted into the neck of the scapula, and fixed. The transferred muscular origins serve as a buttress across the anterior and inferior aspect of the joint and also anchor the lower half of the subscapularis.

Procedure

An anterior incision is made over the pectoral groove. The joint capsule is exposed and the extent of the injury inspected. The coracoid process, with its muscular attachments, is osteotomized from the scapula. The subscapularis tendon is reattached to the coracoid process with a screw (or transferred to the anterior neck of the scapula). The lateral portion of the subscapularis tendon may be resutured to the joint capsule, and the medial edge of the subscapularis resutured to the rotator cuff or at the bicipital groove, overlapping the layers of the joint (Putti-Platt). The osteotomized coracoid tip may be transferred to the neck of the glenoid under the fibers of the subscapularis using a screw (Bristow). The soft tissues are repaired and the incision closed. A sling and swathe or Velpeau dressing is applied.

Preparation of the Patient

The patient is supine with the affected shoulder elevated with a sandbag or folded sheet. The arm on the affected side is flexed over the chest; the other arm may be extended on an armboard. Apply electrosurgical dispersive pad.

Skin Preparation

Begin at the anterior aspect of the shoulder extending from the submandibular region to the inferior costal margin. Hold up and prepare the arm. Cleanse the axilla well. Prepare the back of the shoulder and the back of the arm down to the table. Cleanse forearm and hand.

Draping

The extremity is held up in a tube (impervious) stockinette. A large, cuffed drape sheet is tucked under the patient's shoulder. The tube stockinette is brought up over the shoulder. A split sheet is draped under the arm and clipped. A large drape (or split) sheet is draped over the shoulder and clipped below. The arm may be passed through a fenestrated sheet, or individual drape sheets may be used to complete the draping.

Equipment

Sandbag or folded sheet (positioning)
Suction
Electrosurgical unit
Power source(s) for saw and drill

Instrumentation

Basic orthopedic procedures tray
Retractors (eg., Hibbs, Bennett, Bankart)
Osteotomes
Steinmann pins
Power drill, cord, drill bits
Power saw and cord
Fixation devices: for example, screws, staples (and in-
    strumentation)

Supplies

Basin set
Blades (2) No. 10, (1) No. 15
Needle magnet or counter
Suction tubing
Electrosurgical pencil
Tube (impervious) stockinette
Bulb syringe
Graduate
Antibiotic irrigation (optional)
Sling and swathe or Velpeau dressing

Special Notes

Have x-ray films in the room.
    Check levels in tanks for power equipment.
    Do not allow preparation solution to pool under the
patient's shoulder.
    Check with the surgeon regarding the immobiliza-
tion of the shoulder following the procedure.
    Protective goggles may be worn.

ARTHROSCOPY OF THE SHOULDER

Definition

Endoscopic visualization of the shoulder joint.

Discussion

Diagnosis and treatment of shoulder joint pathology
has been difficult until the arthroscope came into use.
With the arthroscope, extensive visualization of the

intra-articular aspect of the shoulder joint is possible. Indications for this procedure include removal of loose bodies, lysis of adhesions, synovectomy, bursectomy, biopsy of the synovium, stabilization of dislocation, correction of rotator cuff tears, and decompression of the subacromial area.

Procedure

The bony anatomical landmarks are outlined. Three portals are generally employed; the precise points are modified by the patient's size. The posterior portal is made 2 centimeters inferior and 1 centimeter medial to the posterolateral corner of the acromium. The anterior portal is determined arthroscopically inferior to the biceps tendon under direct vision. A transarticular guide rod is inserted into the arthroscopic cannula through the anterior capsule tenting the skin at approximately 2 centimeters below the anterior edge of the acromium. A stab wound is made, and an additional arthroscopic cannula is inserted over the rod into the joint. The lateral portal is established 2 centimeters distal to the lateral border of the acromium. The trocar is passed through the deltoid muscle to the greater tuberosity. A cannula is then directed into the bursal cavity beneath the anterior third of the acromium. The scope is then manipulated to inspect all aspects of the shoulder joint and to assess the pathology. Appropriate therapeutic measures are performed accordingly; the facilitation of a "mini open" or a formal open procedure can likewise be performed employing the most direct and least traumatic modalities.

Preparation of the Patient

Following the administration of general anesthesia and the insertion of an endotrachial tube, the patient is placed in either a modified Fowler's (beach chair) position or a lateral decubitus position.

Modified Fowler's Position. Align the patient's body over the breaks in the table. The back of the table is elevated while the hips and knees are flexed. A doughnut may be used to support the patient's head. The patient can be secured to the table with adhesive

tape across the forehead (which is protected by a
4″ × 4″ pad). The nonoperative arm is placed in the patient's lap on a pillow, or it may be well padded and
tucked in at the patient's side, taking care not to injure
the fingers. A pillow is placed under the knees and legs
to prevent pressure on the patient's heels. A blanket is
placed over the patient's lap, and the patient is secured
with the safety strap. A U-drape may be placed proximally to protect the patient's face from fluids. Apply
electrosurgical dispersive pad.

Lateral Decubitus Position. The patient is placed
on a beanbag (on the table) on the nonoperative side. A
foam headrest is used to support the head and neck and
to protect the dependent ear. An axillary roll is placed
beneath the dependent thorax near the axilla to protect
the brachial plexus. A pillow is placed between the legs,
and the knees and ankles are protected by foam pads.
Kidney rests are used to help support the body in position. The nonoperative arm is flexed on a well-padded
armboard. The lateral side of the face is protected with
padding from inadvertent pressure during surgery. A
plastic U-drape is used to protect the face from fluids.
Apply electrosurgical dispersive pad.

Skin Preparation

Begin at the anterior aspect of the shoulder extending
from the submandibular region to the inferior costal
margin. Hold up the arm, and cleanse the axilla well.
Prepare the back of the shoulder down to the table.
Cleanse the arm, forearm, and hand.

Draping

A large drape sheet is used to cover the lower half of the
body. A "shoulder pack" specifically made for this purpose includes a plastic "U" and a top drape with a collecting pouch. Two drainage tubes are attached to the
connectors on the pouches of the drape and then inserted into a gravity reservoir. The patient's arm is secured in a sterilized foam traction boot. The arm is supported in a position of approximately 70° of abduction
and 10° of flexion.

Equipment

Beanbag, kidney rests, pillow(s), headrest and padding
   for positioning
Light source
Video monitors (2)
VCR (optional)
Mavigraph (optional)
Sterilized foam traction unit
Fluid standard (adjustable with sensors)
Suction
Arthroscopic pump
Weight for traction unit (usually 10 pounds)
Electrosurgical unit
Waste reservoir
Surgical power system

Instruments

Arthrotomy tray
Shoulder retractors
Arthroscope, camera and light cord, large irrigation
   cannula with blunt obturator, switching stick or orthopedic guide rod, arthroscopic sheath or appropriate bridge adaptor, plastic operating cannula with
   diaphragm and side port, rotator cuff liberator-
   elevator, high-speed power burr, gauge punch (3),
   circular rasp, suture passer, motorized shaver system with appropriate blades, acromionizer burr, full
   radius shaver blade, small outflow cannula with
   blunt obturator, conical ("Christmas tree") adaptor
   (for outflow cannula)

Supplies

Marking pen
Glycine or nonconductive isomotic glycerol solution (in
   3000 mL bags)
Electrosurgical pencil with subacromial electrode
Graduate
Knife blades No. 10 (1), No. 11 (1)
10 mL and 60 mL syringes
Extension tubing
Disposable tubing and connector

Spiral needle No. 18 × 3½
Sterile plastic bag to hold VCR control (optional)
Skin closure strips
Soft dressing
Special shoulder brace

Special Notes

Check that all equipment works prior to surgery.
  White balance the camera.
  Position the monitors.
  Keep fluid replacement bags ready at all times.
  All instruments may be carefully washed and then flash sterilized except the arthroscope and camera. Steris 20 soaking solution is recommended for sterilizing them.

OPEN REDUCTION OF FRACTURE OF THE HUMERAL HEAD (INCLUDING HUMERAL HEAD PROSTHESIS)

Definition

Realignment and fixation of the humeral head through an operative incision.

Discussion

Most of these fractures are not treated surgically. They are often associated with dislocations, and in children the epiphyses may be involved. Fixation may be achieved with wire and/or special plates. A severely comminuted fracture may require replacement of the humeral head with a prosthesis.

Procedure

For an avulsion fracture of the tuberosities, a deltopectoral approach is used. The fracture fragment is repaired with wire. The soft tissue injury (e.g., rotator cuff) is repaired. When the humeral head is fractured as well, additional wire and a T-compression plate may be required to achieve compression. Severely comminuted fractures may require a humeral head prosthesis.

The deltoid muscle is detached. Attachments of major tendons are preserved with adequate bone fragments. Loose fragments and debris are irrigated away. The prosthesis is driven into the humeral shaft and the bone fragments are attached to the prosthesis with wire sutures. Methylmethacrylate may be used in seating the prosthesis. The rotator cuff and soft tissue are closed over the wire sutures. The long head of the biceps tendon, previously detached, may be sutured to the repaired rotator cuff or implanted into the bicipital groove. The deltoid muscle is reattached. The incision is closed. A sling and swathe are placed.

Preparation of the Patient

The patient is supine with arms extended on armboards. For insertion of a prosthesis, the patient is supine with the knees over the lower break in the table. Following the administration of anesthesia, the sitting position is employed by raising the head of the table from the middle break. The foot of the table is lowered. A padded footboard supports the feet. The unaffected arm is placed on the patient's lap on a pillow secured with a padded restraint. The affected arm is usually supported by a sling. Apply electrosurgical dispersive pad.

Skin Preparation

Begin at the anterior aspect of the shoulder extending from the submandibular region to the inferior costal margin. Hold up the arm, and cleanse the axilla well. Prepare the back of the shoulder and the back of arm down to the table. Cleanse the arm and hand.

Draping

The extremity is held up in a tube stockinette. A large, cuffed drape sheet is tucked under the patient's shoulder. The tube stockinette is brought up over the shoulder. A drape (or split) sheet is draped under the arm and clipped. A large drape (or split) sheet is draped over the shoulder and clipped below. The arm may be passed through a fenestrated sheet, or individual drape sheets complete the draping.

Equipment

Footboard (padded), padded arm restraint, pillow
Electrosurgical unit
Suction
Power sources for drill and saw
Instrumentation
Basic orthopedic procedures tray
Osteotomes, Bennett and Hibbs retractors, threaded pins, wire tightener
Power drill, cord, and drill bits
Power saw and cord (optional)
Fixation devices, for example, wire (stainless steel No. 20), T-compression plate, screws
Prosthesis, with instrumentation, for example, Neer I and Neer II (total shoulder joint replacement) and rasps, impactor, extractor, and so on

Supplies

Basin Set
Blades (2) No. 10
Needle magnet or counter
Suction tubing
Electrosurgical pencil
Graduate
Bulb syringe
Tube (or impervious) stockinette
Methylmethacrylate kit
Antibiotic irrigation (optional)
Sling and swathe

Special Notes

Have x-ray films in the room.
  Check levels in tanks for power equipment.
  Protective goggles may be worn.

ARTHROSCOPY OF THE ELBOW

Definition

Arthroscopic visualization of the elbow joint.

Discussion

Arthroscopy of the elbow joint is currently in the developmental stage. When various noninvasive diagnostic techniques suggest the presence of loose bodies, posttraumatic adhesions, osteophytes, osteochondral fractures, osteochondritis dissecans, synovitis, and so on, elbow arthroscopy can be employed, under direct visualization, to establish and/or treat these entities. The nature and extent of local fractures can be evaluated; pyarthrosis can be drained and irrigated. Severe posttraumatic injuries and alkylosis are contraindications to this modality. Caution must be exercised in this small operative field to avoid injuring structures such as the brachial artery, median and ulnar nerves, and main branches of the radial nerve.

Procedure

Bony landmarks (radial head, lateral and medial epicondyles, olecranon tip) are palpated and marked on the skin. Commonly used portals include anterolateral, anteromedial, lateral, posterolateral, and posterior. Videoarthroscopes 2.7 mm and 4.0 mm are employed. The lateral portal is entered with an 18 gauge needle and distended with 25 to 30 mL of saline (or Ringer's lactate) by syringe. The anterolateral portal is then established first by needle puncture to ascertain position within the joint followed by insertion of a trocar and videoarthroscope. Inspection is begun, and additional portals are established under direct vision to avoid neurovascular injury. Removal of loose bodies or osteophytes and smoothing the areas of excision with a motorized burr or excision of soft tissue can be performed. The portal incisions are closed, and a pressure dressing is applied.

Preparation of the Patient

The patient is placed in supine position. Following the administration of general anesthesia, an overhead shoulder holder or similar suspension device is used to suspend the arm from a wrist gauntlet, with the arm balanced by a 5-pound weight. The arm is positioned to hang free of the edge of the table, with the shoulder in neutral rotation and abducted to 90°, and the elbow flexed to 90°. Maximum relaxation is achieved in this position. The balanced suspension permits elbow flexion and extension during the procedure.

Skin Preparation

Begin cleansing at the elbow, and include the arm, forearm, and hand.

Draping

See Open Reduction of the Radius and/or Ulna, p. 304.

Equipment

Pillow(s) for positioning
Overhead shoulder holder with wrist gauntlet and 5-pound weight
Tourniquet (optional)
Xenon light source
Video monitors (2)
VCR (optional)
Mavigraph (optional)
Suction
Power source for power equipment
Stools (available)

Supplies

Needles, No. 18, 1½″, and spinal, 3½″
Silastic tubing (2)
Sterile plastic bag to hold VCR (optional)
Pressure dressing
Splint (optional)

Special Notes

Check that all equipment works prior to surgery.
    White balance the camera.
    Check with the surgeon regarding the type of the suspension device.
    Position the monitors.

All instruments must be meticulously washed and then flash-sterilized except the scope and camera, which can be sterilized by soaking in Steris 20 solution.

INTERNAL FIXATION OF THE HIP

Definition

Stabilization of an intracapsular fracture of the femoral neck or an extracapsular fracture of the intertrochanteric region.

Discussion

The procedure is usually indicated in even the "poor-risk" patient to enable early postoperative patient mobilization. The procedure can even be performed under local anesthesia in some instances. Fixation may be achieved with a nail, pin, or screw across the fracture site, sometimes in conjunction with a plate along the femoral shaft.

Procedure

A fracture table may be employed. After anesthesia is induced, the fracture is reduced and checked by x-ray in two planes. Following skin preparation and draping, a lateral (less often an anterior) incision is made to expose the fracture site. The appropriate nail with plate, threaded pins, or a compression screw is placed after guide wires are inserted temporarily to check alignment. A drill is used to facilitate placement of the plate screws. X-ray check again is performed. The wound may be irrigated with an antibiotic solution. The wound is closed.

Preparation of the Patient

Determine if the fracture table is to be used. The patient is in the supine position either on the fracture table or the regular operating table (prepared for image intensifier). Adequate padding is needed to protect extremities and bony prominences. A sterile, plastic adhesive drape may be used to drape the perineum out of the field before preparing. Apply electrosurgical dispersive pad.

Skin Preparation

Begin over the greater trochanter extending from the nipple to the toes. Prepare beyond the midline of the abdomen anteriorly, and down to the table on the affected side. The preparation should include the entire leg and foot, which are held up and abducted.

Draping

Fracture table: Folded towels, a sterile, plastic adhesive drape, and a laparotomy sheet. *Regular table:* The leg is abducted and the foot grasped in a towel (which is clipped) and then covered with a tube (or impervious) stockinette. A large, cuffed drape (or split) sheet is draped under the thigh. Towels are secured around site of the incision. A large sheet is draped proximal to the inferior costal margin. The stockinette is rolled up over the extremity proximal to the iliac crest and fixed anteriorly and posteriorly. The leg is brought through a large fenestrated sheet. An opening is made in the stockinette over the site of the incision and is covered by a sterile, plastic adhesive drape.

Equipment

Fracture table (e.g., Stryker or Chick) or image intensifier extension
Electrosurgical unit
Suction
Power source for power drill

Instrumentation

Basic orthopedic procedures tray
Bone holding instruments tray
Hip retractors tray
Power drill, cord, and drill bits
Fixation device: Pins, (Knowles, Deyerle, Hagie), nail (Jewett, Smith-Petersen), or Richards compression

screw (lag screw, barrel, plate) and instrumentation particular to each device
Guide pins

Supplies

Basin set
Suction tubing
Electrosurgical pencil
Blades (4) No. 10
Bulb syringes (2)
Graduate
Tube (or impervious) stockinette if regular table is used
Sterile, plastic adhesive drapes (2) (optional, for perineum and operative site)
Antibiotic irrigation (optional)

Special Notes

Have x-ray films in the room.

Some surgeons prefer to double-glove and remove the first pair following completion of draping.

Notify the x-ray department when the patient is being positioned on the table. (Fluoroscopy will give views of fracture, guide pins, and position of nailing device.)

Observe x ray precautions, see p. 21.

Protective goggles may be worn.

FEMORAL HEAD PROSTHETIC REPLACEMENT

Definition

Substitution of the femoral head with a prosthesis made of vitallium or similar inert metal.

Discussion

This procedure is indicated in nonunion of femoral neck fractures, avascular necrosis of the femoral head, or in degenerative changes of the hip postfracture or from arthritis (primarily fractures that cannot be expected to heal retaining the femoral head). One advantage of this procedure is that immediate weight bearing is permitted; it is more extensive and entails more risks than procedures retaining the femoral head. Several protheses are used including Moore, Müller, Thompson, and Bateman.

Procedure

Several incisions and approaches are employed. A posterior incision may be made over the gluteus maximus superiorly and paralleling the proximal femur. The muscle fibers are split. The sciatic nerve is protected. The external rotators of the hip are freed from the femur, and the joint capsule is incised. Flexion, adduction, and internal rotation of the thigh are employed to dislocate the hip. The femoral head is removed and measured so that a similar-sized prosthetic head can be used. The medullary canal is reamed with a special rasp. The neck is shaped to receive the prosthesis without rotation, leaving enough of the calcar medially. After checking the size of the prosthesis in the actual acetabulum, the prosthesis is seated using special driving instruments for that particular prosthesis. Excess bone fragments are trimmed. Care is taken not to fracture the usually thinned femoral shaft. Methylmethacrylate may be used in seating the prosthesis into the femoral shaft. The incision is closed.

Preparation of the Patient

Usually a posterior approach is used with the patient in the lateral position with sandbags, Vac Pac, or kidney rests supporting the torso. The arm on the unaffected side is extended on an armboard, and the other arm is flexed over the chest, with a pillow between the arms, and secured by a padded restraint (or a double armboard may be used). The unaffected leg is extended, and the affected leg is flexed over it (or both legs may be flexed). A pillow is placed between the legs. Adequate padding around feet, ankles, and bony prominences must be taken into consideration. The position is secured by wide adhesive tape at the shoulder anchored to the underside of the table and by the safety strap over the unaffected leg. A sterile, plastic adhesive drape may be used to drape the perineum out of the field. Apply electrosurgical dispersive pad.

Skin Preparation

Begin over the greater trochanter extending from the nipple to the toes. Prepare beyond the midline of the abdomen anteriorly, and down to the table posteriorly. The preparation should include the entire leg and foot.

Draping

The leg is abducted, and the foot is grasped in a towel (which is clipped) and then covered with a tube (or impervious) stockinette. A large sheet is draped over the end of the table. A large drape sheet (cuffed) or a split sheet is draped under the leg. Towels are secured around site of the incision. A large sheet is draped proximal to the inferior costal margin. The stockinette is rolled up over the extremity proximal to the iliac crest and fixed anteriorly and posteriorly. The leg is brought through a fenestrated sheet. An opening is made in the stockinette over the site of the incision and covered by a sterile, plastic adhesive drape.

Equipment

Sandbags, Vac Pac, pillows, kidney rests, and padded
    restraints (for positioning)
Electrosurgical unit
Suction
Power sources for power drill and saw
Pillows (for positioning postoperatively)

Instrumentation

Basic orthopedic procedures tray
Hip retractors tray
Osteotomes, bone hooks
Drill bits (including ¼″ and ½″)
Extra guide pins
Power drill and cord
Power saw and cord

Femoral head extractor, acetabular knife, hip skid, femoral rasps, caliper, driver

Prosthesis (e.g., Moore, Bateman) and specific instrumentation

Supplies

Basin set

Blades (3) No. 10

Needle magnet or counter

Suction tubing

Electrosurgical pencil

Sterile, plastic adhesive drapes (2) (perineum and operative site)

Bulb syringes (2)

Graduate

Tube (or impervious) stockinette

Methylmethacrylate kit (optional)

Special Notes

Have x-ray films in the room.

Notify the x-ray department of the times films are to be taken.

Observe x-ray precautions, see p. 21.

Protect skin under adhesive tape with tincture of benzoin.

Some surgeons may prefer to double-glove and remove the first pair following draping.

Protective goggles should be worn.

Follow hospital policy for recording insertion of a prosthesis.

TOTAL HIP REPLACEMENT

Definition

Substitution of the femoral head with a prosthesis and the reconstruction of the acetabulum with the placement of an acetabular cup, both of which may be fixed with methylmethacrylate.

Discussion

Disorders of the hip joint for which this procedure may be indicated are rheumatoid arthritis, degenerative disease (e.g., osteoarthritis, posttraumatic conditions), avascular necrosis, damage caused by infection, and failed reconstruction. Numerous modifications of prostheses are employed, such as different alloys, porous coating, ceramics, or use of a bipolar cup. Some, but not all of these, require methylmethacrylate to seat the prosthesis. Prostheses requiring methylmethacrylate to ensure stability include Bechtol, OPTI-FIX, Spectron, Charnley, Charnley-Müller, Aufranc-Turner, Harris Precoat, and Ob. The noncemented technique may be employed when the prosthesis can be tightly fitted into healthy strong bone (i.e., not usually for use in the elderly). The press-fit type (Judet, Lord), porous metal (Harris/Galante, Lanceford, Bias, Engh), bipolar cup (Bateman), and ceramic (Mittelmeir) are varieties of noncemented prostheses. The hip is weight bearing within several days postoperatively when a cemented prostheses is used. When a noncemented prosthesis is used, the hip is not weight bearing for up to 3 months. The noncemented prosthesis has the advantage, however, of relatively easy removal should that become necessary. The long-term efficacy of the noncemented type (versus cemented) has not yet been assessed. The "Charnley type" cemented total hip cup prosthesis remains the standard.

Procedure

One of several techniques may be employed. In the lateral approach a longitudinal incision is made proximal to the greater trocanter and distally along the proximal femoral shaft. The fascia is incised, and the muscle fibers are separated. Scar tissue is freed. The insertions of the rotator muscles of the hip are divided (and tagged for later reapproximation). The hip joint capsule is exposed. By adduction and internal rotation, the hip is dislocated as gently as possible. If this maneuver is difficult, scar tissue and/or additional tendons may be divided. The femoral neck is osteotomized and the femoral head extracted. The proximal femur is trimmed and the medullary canal reamed to accept the prosthesis. The acetabulum is then exposed, any remaining labrum is excised, and the capsule is detached from the anterior and inferior margins. Cartilage and soft tissues are curetted from the acetabulum. Acetabular reamers are employed to prepare the acetabulum to accept the cup prosthesis. Anchoring holes are drilled in the acetabulum. The proper position and angulation of the cup are determined. Methylmethacrylate is prepared and applied, and the cup is positioned. Excess methylmethacrylate is trimmed. The femoral prosthesis is inserted, and test relocation is performed, making any corrections to provide proper seating of the prosthesis. The prosthesis is then removed and seated again after methylmethacrylate has been placed in the medullary canal; excess methylmethacrylate is trimmed. When the methylmethacrylate is set, the hip is relocated. The previously incised soft tissue and osteotomized (or tendon) attachments are replaced using nonabsorbable sutures. The wound is closed. A closed drainage system may be employed. Pillows are placed postoperatively to prevent adduction of the thighs.

Preparation of the Patient, Skin Preparation, and Draping

See Femoral Head Prosthetic Replacement, pp. 324–325.

Equipment

Laminar airflow (if available)
Sandbags, Vac Pac, kidney rests, pillows, and/or padded restraints (for positioning)
Electrosurgical unit
Suction
Power sources for drill and saw
Scales (to weigh sponges)
Pillows (for positioning postoperatively)

Instrumentation

Basic orthopedic procedures tray
Hip retractors tray
Hip gouges, hip skid, rasps, femoral head extractor, acetabular reamer, acetabular knife, caliper
Extra guide pins

Osteotomes, curettes, bone hooks
Power drill, cord, and drill bits (including ¼″ and ½″)
Trial prosthesis
Total hip implant and specific instrumentation

Supplies

Basin set
Suction tubing
Electrosurgical pencil
Blades (4) No. 10
Needle magnet or counter
Asepto or bulb syringes (2)
Graduate
Tube (or impervious) stockinette
Sterile, plastic adhesive drapes (2) (perineum and operative site)
Gelfoam and thrombin (available)
Abduction pillow
Antibiotic irrigation (optional)
Methylmethacrylate kit
Closed drainage unit (e.g., Hemovac)

Special Notes

Have x-ray films in the room.
Laminar airflow may be used.
Protect skin under adhesive tape with tincture of benzoin.
Have all instrumentation for specific prosthesis sterile.
Keep movement and conversation in the room to a minimum.
Some surgeons will double-glove and discard first pair after draping.
Keep accurate record of irrigation.
Check with the blood bank that blood ordered is available.
Check levels in tanks for power drill and saw.
Notify x-ray department of time films will be needed.
Observe x-ray precautions, see p. 21.
Be prepared to change suction apparatus and tubing if it becomes clogged.

Follow hospital policy for recording insertion of a prosthesis.

Protective goggles should be worn.

OPEN REDUCTION OF THE FEMORAL SHAFT

Definition

Realignment and fixation of a fracture of the femur through an operative incision.

Discussion

Surgical intervention may be indicated in certain fractures of the femur in the adult patient. Fractures of the femur in children and young adults are treated with traction followed by immobilization. Intramedullary nails include Hansen-Street, Küntscher, Lottes, Rush, Schneider, Enders, and Zickel. If a compression plate is used, it must have at least three holes above and below the fracture.

Procedure

Use of the fracture table is desirable. Temporary traction devices are removed prior to skin preparation. A posterolateral incision is made over the fracture site. The medullary canal is reamed with special medullary reamers. A guide pin is driven from the fracture site proximally to emerge subcutaneously just proximal to the greater trochanter. A small counterincision is made over the prominence of the emerging guide pin. The cortical opening can be enlarged with a drill. An appropriate length and diameter Küntscher rod is seated over the guide pin with the extractor eye oriented posterolaterally. The rod is then introduced into the now reduced distal segment and seated securely into the condylar region. The proximal end should protrude no more than 2.5 cm. If the fracture site is comminuted, wire loops are placed about the fragments. X-ray control is used as necessary to avoid creating false passages, malalignment, or fracture of the nail. The wound is closed.

Preparation of the Patient

The patient is usually positioned on the fracture table in the lateral position. The arm on the unaffected side is extended on an armboard, and the other arm is flexed across the chest; it may be positioned on a Mayo stand padded with a pillow (or a double armboard may be used). Adequate padding around feet, ankles, and bony prominences must be taken into consideration, particularly because the fracture table is very hard. If the fracture table is not used, the unaffected leg is extended and the affected leg is flexed over it. A pillow is placed between the legs, and the feet and ankles are padded. The patient is held in position by wide adhesive tape at the shoulders and by the safety strap over the unaffected thigh. A sterile, plastic adhesive drape may be used to drape the perineum out of the field before preparing. Apply electrosurgical dispersive pad.

Skin Preparation

Begin over the fracture site extending from the umbilicus to below the knee, well beyond the midline anteriorly (or to the sterile, plastic adhesive drape), and down to the table posteriorly. If the leg is draped free (i.e., the fracture table is not used), the leg and foot are completely prepared. A leg holder may be used.

Draping

The incisional site is draped with folded towels and a sterile, plastic adhesive drape (optional). Four sheets may be draped around the perimeter of the site; a fenestrated sheet covers the field. If the fracture table is not employed, see Femoral Head Prosthetic Replacement, p. 325.

Equipment

Fracture table (e.g., Stryker, Chick, as requested)
Leg holder (optional)
Suction
Electrosurgical unit
Power source for drill

Instrumentation

Basic orthopedic procedures tray
Hip retractor tray
Bone holding instruments tray
Drill bits, including ¼" gauge
Power drill and cord
Extra guide pins, screw set
Fixation device: Rods or nails (e.g., Hansen-Street, Küntscher, Rush) or compression set and instrumentation particular to that device

Supplies

Basin set
Suction tubing
Electrosurgical pencil
Needle magnet or counter
Sterile, plastic adhesive drapes (2) (perineum and operative site)
Blades (2) No. 10
Asepto or bulb syringes (2)
Graduate
Tube (or impervious) stockinette, 6" (if fracture table not used)

Special Notes

Have x-ray films in the room.

Protect skin under adhesive tape with tincture of benzoin.

Some surgeons prefer to double-glove and remove the first pair following completion of draping.

Notify the x-ray department when the patient is being positioned on the table for preliminary films.

Observe x-ray precautions, see p. 21.

Protective goggles may be worn.

ARTHROTOMY OF THE KNEE

Definition

Incision into the knee joint.

Discussion

A variety of injuries can occur about the knee joint. These include fractures, meniscal tears, and ligamentous injuries related to torsion or tearing of the ligaments. Synovectomy may be performed for chronic synovitis, for posttrauma, or after infectious conditions, in addition to rheumatoid arthritis, hemangioma, and villonodular changes. Arthroscopy may be employed for some presentations of these conditions. Others require arthrotomy; there is a wide variety of procedures. Some of these include:

Open Reduction of Femoral Condyle and Tibial Plateau Fractures. Alignment and stabilization of the articular surfaces of the distal femur and proximal tibia to provide joint stability.

Menisectomy. Excision of a torn meniscus and either/or both semilunar fibrocartilages.

Patellectomy. Excision of all or a portion of the patella.

Synovectomy. Excision of all or a portion of the synovial membrane of the knee.

Collateral or Cruciate Ligament Repair. Repair of damaged ligaments of the knee, restoring them as closely as possible to the original anatomy.

Procedure

Open Reduction of Fractures of Femoral Condyles and Tibial Plateau. A longitudinal incision is made exposing the fracture site. Debris and minor bone fragments are irrigated out. Temporary reduction may be achieved with Kirschner wires, which are removed following the insertion of Knowles pins, cancellous bone screws or bolts, and so on, with penetration of the opposite cortex. "T-fractures" of the femoral condyles may be stabilized with a plate or screws. In tibial plateau fractures the joint is explored after reflecting the iliotibial band and/or additional muscular attachments. Ligamentous and cartilaginous injuries are repaired. The fracture is reduced and fixed with hardware, as above. Cancellous bone from the proximal tibia may be packed into the fracture site. The wound is closed. A posterior splint may be applied.

Lateral Menisectomy. An anterolateral incision is made from the level of the patella to the upper tibia. The quadriceps aponeurosis and joint capsule are incised. The meniscus is grasped and excised taking care to avoid injury to the popliteus tendon, fibular collateral ligament, and vascular structures. A secondary posterolateral incision may be necessary to visualize and excise the posterior horn of the meniscus. The incisions are closed. A bulky compression dressing is applied.

Open Reduction of Fractures of the Patella and Patellectomy. A transverse prepatellar incision is made. The patellar tendon and joint are explored (and suture-repaired during closure). The fracture site is exposed. Debris and small fragments are irrigated from the joint. Major fracture fragments are approximated and repaired through a variety of techniques using wire and/or screws. Lesser fragments and the severely comminuted entire patella can be excised with shortening of the patellar tendon. The wound is closed, and a splint is applied.

Synovectomy. An anteromedial incision is made. The synovial membrane is excised from medial, lateral, and anterior aspect of the joint including prepatellar fat pad and menisci (if they are degenerated). Using a sponge or curette, pannus is removed from the femoral condyles. By flexing the knee, posterior synovium is excised. Optimal hemostasis is achieved. The wound is closed over a suction drain. The leg is immobilized.

Medial Collateral Ligament Repair. A medial longitudinal incision is made. The greater saphenous vein and sensory branches of the saphenous nerve are protected. The deep fascia is incised, and the sartorius muscle is retracted with the knee flexed. The tibial insertion of the medial collateral ligament is inspected. The joint capsule is incised, and the cruciate ligaments, menisci, and adjacent articular surfaces are inspected. Capsular tears and other ligamentous injuries are repaired; menisci, if injured, are excised. The joint is closed, and the medial collateral ligament and posterior oblique ligament are repaired by sutures in their midportion or by staples or sutures to bone at their origins or insertions. Tendons may be transferred if further strengthening is required. Hemostasis is achieved. A long leg cast is applied.

Preparation of the Patient

The patient is supine with the knees over the lower break in the table; arms may be extended on armboards. The patient is secured with the safety belt over the thigh of the unaffected extremity. Sheet wadding and a tourniquet are applied to the top of the thigh of the operative leg. Apply electrosurgical dispersive pad.

Skin Preparation

Begin at the knee extending from immediately below the tourniquet (on the thigh) to the ankle.

Draping

The leg is abducted and held up in a tube (or impervious) stockinette. A sheet is draped over the end of the table. A drape sheet (cuffed) or a split sheet is draped under the thigh. A folded towel (in thirds, lengthwise) is wrapped around the top of the thigh, and the tube stockinette is brought up over the folded towel. A U-shaped sheet is draped proximal to the knee and clipped below. Then a fenestrated sheet with a rubberized extremity hole completes the draping. An additional sheet will be necessary if the foot of the table is lowered (in order to flex the knee) during the procedure.

Equipment

Suction
Electrosurgical unit
Tourniquet and insufflator
Power source for drill (for fracture of patella)
Cast cart

Instrumentation

Basic orthopedic procedures tray
Knee arthrotomy tray

Power drill, cord, drill bits (fracture of patella)
Staples and instrumentation (ligament repair)
Kirschner wires
Fixation devices and instrumentation (as required)

Supplies

Sheet wadding
Basin set
Blades (2) No. 10, (1) No. 15
Wire, for example, stainless steel No. 18 (fracture of patella)
Suction tubing
Electrosurgical pencil
Needle magnet or counter
Asepto or bulb syringe
Tube (or impervious) stockinette, 6″
Esmarch bandage

Special Notes

Have x-ray films in the room.

Protective goggles may be worn.

Be sure knees are over lower break in the table.

Do not allow preparation solution to pool under the tourniquet.

Place tourniquet as high on the extremity as possible.

Wrap sheet wadding around the extremity smoothly.
Tourniquet ends should overlap about 7.5 cm (3 inches).

The setting for an adult is approximately 400 mm Hg for the lower extremity.

Monitor tourniquet time and setting.

Tourniquet must be released after 2 hours to avoid injury.

ARTHROSCOPY OF THE KNEE

Definition

Endoscopic visualization of the knee joint.

Discussion

By direct visualization of the intra-articular structures, diagnoses, as well as specific surgeries such as menisectomy, synovectomy, shaving of the patella, excision of loose bodies, and reconstruction or replacement of the anterior cruciate ligament can be performed.

Indications for arthroscopy of the knee (as well as in other joints) include confirmation of radiographic studies, diagnostic and therapeutic procedures, which, when feasible, minimize postoperative morbidity as compared to formal arthrotomy. By direct visualization of intra-articular structures, anatomical diagnosis is ascertained. Therapeutic procedures include menisectomy, repair of meniscus, synovectomy, patellar shaving, prosthetic repair of ligaments (synthetics versus allografts and homografts), and so on. Loose bodies may be removed directly or by irrigation. Biopsy specimens for conditions such as rheumatoid arthritis, and chondromalcia may be obtained.

Numerous synthetic materials are used for ligamentous grafting. Autografts, for example, from the central portion of the patellar tendon, or allografts are preferred by some surgeons. When the latter are employed, serologic testing of the tissue donor (for hepatitis, viral strains, human immunovirus [HIV], and syphilis) as well as antibiotics and cryopreservation are employed. The grafts are thawed immediately prior to use.

Procedure

The knee joint is examined under anesthesia. Range of motion and stability are ascertained. A tourniquet is applied but not inflated. The knee joint is distended with Ringer's lactate through an inflow cannula inserted laterally into the suprapatellar pouch adjacent to the superior pole of the patella. A 3 mm incision is made according to the surgeon's preference over the anterolateral aspect of the joint. A trocar and sheath are inserted; an obturator replaces the trocar in the sheath, and the obturator is advanced into the joint. The obturator is removed and replaced by the arthroscope with the attached camera. Inflow and outflow irrigation tubings are attached. Currently a fluid management system, for example, Intellijet, with the capability to automatically maintain the appropriate degree of distension, is used to provide a clear field and obviate the need for inflation of the tourniquet. The knee joint is thoroughly examined. Additional port(s) can be employed accordingly. Procedures such as meniscectomy, synovectomy, patellar shaving, or replacement of the anterior cruciate ligament may be performed. Numerous devices have been developed to facilitate these procedures. Examples include a power patellar shaver and other power smoothers. Also available are introducer and vector guides to create tunnels for ligamentous repair. Fixation can be achieved with sutures, staples, interference screws (of metal and bioabsorbable composition) with their assorted screw holders, and so on. Another instrument for intraarticular use is the Caspare suture punch.

A carbon dioxide laser may be employed with some arthroscopes, in which case the knee joint is distended with carbon dioxide and the tourniquet is inflated to prevent dissection by the gas. Nd:YAG and Ho:YAG may utilize the liquid distention medium. See Appendix, pp. 619–624, for laser precautions. Following completion of the procedure(s), the wound is simultaneously copiously irrigated with Ringer's lactate and aspirated. The scope is withdrawn, and the wounds are closed in the usual manner. A soft bandage is applied, held in place by a pressure stocking, for example, a TED hose.

Preparation of the Patient

The patient is supine; arms may be extended on armboards. The patient is placed on the side of the table of the affected leg. Sheet wadding and a tourniquet are applied to the thigh of the operative leg. A leg holder or lateral post is placed on the side of the affected leg (which permits the leg to be angled off the lateral aspect of the table). Apply an electrosurgical dispersive pad.

Skin Preparation and Draping

See Arthrotomy of the Knee, p. 335.

Equipment

Leg holder for skin preparation (optional)
Leg holding post (to help maintain positioning)

Electrosurgical unit
Video monitors (2)
VCR (optional)
Mavigraph (optional)
Arthroscopy cart: Main control unit front panel, fluid pump, cassette, Intellijet suction supply unit (suction level control unit), adjustable IV pole with level-alert sensors (2), waste containers (4), surgical power system for shavers, acromionizer, and so on
Laser unit, for example, Nd:YAG or Ho:YAG

Instrumentation

Shaver handle and motor, scope cannulas and trocars (short, blunt), endoscopic grasping clamps, endoscopic up-biting forceps (assorted), knife handles (2), endoscopic beaver blade handle, small towel clips (2), Kelly clamps (4), Adson forceps (1), toothed forceps (1), straight Mayo scissors, Metzenbaum scissors, Lehey clamp, sharp Senns retractors (2), 1 endoscopic probe, drill key, smoothing device, ligament passer, suction rasp, Key elevator, curette, Weitlaner retractors (small and large), right-angle Kocher clamps (2) 6″, (1) 8″, Pean clamp, needle holder

For patella tendon repair add: Osteotomes, saw with small blade (e.g., Dyonics), rongeurs, bone cutters, ⅛″ drill bit, Gallie needles, Hewson button, Acuflex cruciate ligament instruments (available)

For anterior cruciate ligament add: Vector guides, guide pins, automatic drill, reamer with 6.5 and 10.0 drills, fastlok staple inserter and remover, 1 buckle (2 for allografts), tension device for allografts (Cottony dacron suture with needle for allografts and autografts), ⅛″ drill bit, Gallis needles, Hewson button

Supplies

Basin set
Blade (1) No. 15
Needle 18 gauge spinal
Disposable tubing cassette (attached to main control unit)
Disposable operative cannula and tubing set

PVC tubing (4 lengths; [1] inflow from irrigation bags
to cassette; [2] delivers fluid from cassette through
the arthroscope cannula into the joint space; [3] di-
rects outflow from joint to the cassette; [4] provides
fluid pathway from cassette to waste containers)
Ringer's lactate in 3000 mL bags (2 to 6 extra on hand)
Graft (allograft or autograft, frozen)
Culture tube (anerobic)
Extra graduate
Marking pen
Fastlok staples (for anterior cruciate ligament [ACL])
Skin closure strips
Soft dressing (4 × 4s, ABD pads, TED stockings)
Leg brace for ACL
Antibacterial solution to soak graft
Ziplock baggies (2) for remote controls

Special Notes

Have x-ray films in the room.

The circulator needs to keep Ringer's lactate bag replacements ready at all times.

The circulator turns (Intellijet) control unit on and
gives tubing to scrub nurse.

The scrub nurse removes the cassette and waste and
fluid bag tubing and passes it to the circulator.

The circulator attaches a cassette to the side of the
unit, closes the pinch clamps on the tubing using fluid
bag tubing spikes, connects the waste tubing to the
waste containers, and turns the suction supply switch
on.

The scrub nurse attaches arthroscope cannula and
powered instruments to scrub taking ends.

The circulator then selects pressure range using site
selection key and pushes pump to start. The key on the
control unit display will read "pump running."

White balance the camera.

Position the monitors.

Have on hand assorted abraders and shavers, en-
doblades and acromionizers.

A self-adherent elastic bandage is helpful in holding
an impervious stocking foot protector.

All instruments may be washed and then flash-sterilized except the telescope and camera. Steris 20 solution is recommended for sterilization by soaking.

Remote controls for fluid and monitors may be placed in sterile plastic "baggies" on the field.

For ACL patients the dressing may include a TEMP-PAD which applies cold to the area about the dressing immediately following the surgery.

Thaw grafts in warm normal saline.

Protective goggles may be worn.

EXCISION OF POPLITEAL (BAKER'S) CYST

Definition

Excision of a cyst located in the popliteal space.

Discussion

These cysts are formed by the herniation of synovial membrane or the escape of synovial fluid of the knee joint with the accumulation in one of several bursae in the popliteal space. The cysts also occur in rheumatoid arthritis. Other conditions affecting the knee may be associated (e.g., torn meniscus). Arthrography may be used to delineate the cyst and to distinguish it from other lesions such as tumors and popliteal artery aneurysm.

Procedure

An oblique incision is made over the mass. Deep fascia is incised, exposing the sac that is then dissected free, tracing its attachment to the posterior aspect of the knee joint capsule. The pedicle is ligated and the cyst excised. Tendon bundles may be used to reinforce the closure. The wound is closed. A splint is applied.

Preparation of the Patient

The patient is prone with chest rolls under the thorax and a roll in front of the ankles. The arms are positioned on armboards angled toward the head of the table with the hands pronated. If a tourniquet is used, it is applied on the thigh of the affected leg. A safety strap is secured across the unaffected thigh. Apply electrosurgical dispersive pad.

Skin Preparation

A leg holder may be used. Begin at the back of the knee and include the entire thigh (up to the tourniquet, if used), knee, leg, and foot.

Draping

The leg is abducted, and the foot is held up in a tube (or impervious) stockinette. A large sheet is draped over the end of the table. A folded towel (lengthwise) is wrapped around the top of the thigh and clipped; the stockinette is brought up over the towel. A drape (or split) sheet is draped under the thigh and clipped. A large drape (or split) sheet is draped over the thigh and clipped underneath. The field is covered with additional drape sheets, or the leg is passed through a fenestrated sheet.

Equipment

Leg holder
Electrosurgical unit
Chest rolls, ankle roll, pillows, padding (as necessary for positioning)
Tourniquet and insufflator (available)
Cast cart

Instrumentation

Basic/Minor procedures tray
Basic orthopedic procedures tray
Knee arthrotomy tray (available)

Supplies

Basin set
Blades (2) No. 10, (1) No. 15
Electrosurgical pencil
Needle magnet or counter
Tube (or impervious) stockinette, 6″
Bulb syringe
Esmarch bandage

Special Notes

In the adult patient, a popliteal cyst may be indicative of intra-articular disease; arthrotomy may be necessary.

Adequate padding is required for female breasts and male genitalia.

For tourniquet precautions, see Arthrotomy of the Knee, p. 336.

Protective goggles may be worn.

TOTAL KNEE REPLACEMENT

Definition

Replacement of the articular surfaces of the knee joint by prostheses.

Discussion

The procedure is performed for pain, deformity, and instability secondary to rheumatoid arthritis, osteoarthritis, and posttraumatic conditions. The articular surfaces of the femoral condyles, tibial plateau, anterior trochlear surface of the femur, and articular surface of the patella are trimmed to accept the prostheses. The prostheses are bonded to the bone with methylmethacrylate.

On occasion a single component of the knees articular surface (e.g., medial femoral and tibial condyles) needs to be replaced (unicompartmental). More commonly the entire or total surface requires replacement (tricompartmental).

There are four categories of total knee systems:

1. *Constrained (hinged):* A hinge joint; infrequently used. Examples are Walldius, Guepar, Shiers, and St. Georg prostheses.
2. *Nonhinged constrained:* Spherocentric; allows motion that nearly duplicates that of the normal knee. Examples are Attenborough and Sheehan prostheses.
3. *Non-constrained:* Provides full coverage of the articular surfaces but adds little stability. Examples are Marmor, Savastano, Oxford, Porous Coated

Anatomic (PCA), Bias, Mod II Unicompartmental, TRICON-M, and TRICON-C prostheses.

4. *Partially constrained:* Provides stability as well as full coverage of the articular surface. Examples include Richards Maximum Contact (RMC), Insall-Burstein, Kinematic II, and Freeman-Swanson prostheses.

Procedure

A longitudinal incision extends from over the patella to the tibial tuberosity. The quadriceps tendon is incised superiorly and the knee joint entered. The capsule is incised, the knee is flexed, and the knee joint exposed. The anterior portions of menisci, any osteophytes, and hyperplastic synovium are excised. Soft tissues (if any) are released. Jigs, templates, and spacers of varying sizes for each prosthetic type are employed. Lines may be marked with methylene blue dye and appropriate bone excised (as are the cruciate ligaments and remaining posterior aspect of the menisci). Slots or holes are cut or drilled to accept the prostheses. Methylmethacrylate is used to seat the prosthesis; the excess is removed. The patella may be replaced by prosthesis as well. A check is made of stability, alignment, and range of motion. Realignment of the quadriceps mechanism and patella tendon is carefully performed. Hemostasis is achieved when the tourniquet is released. Suction drains are placed in the joint, and the wound layers are closed in partial flexion (to avoid tension on closure). A bulky dressing is applied. The extremity may be placed in a continuous passive motion (CPM) device when the patient reaches the recovery room, or several days postoperatively. (The CPM device may also be used for other postoperative conditions of the knee, hip, shoulder, and elbow.)

Preparation of the Patient

The patient is supine with the knees over the lower break in the table; arms may be extended on armboards. The patient is secured with a safety strap over the thigh of the unaffected extremity. Sheet wadding and a tourniquet are applied to the top of the thigh of the operative extremity. Apply electrosurgical dispersive pad.

Skin Preparation

A foot holder may be used. Begin at the knee extending from immediately below the tourniquet (on the thigh) to the toes.

Draping

The leg is held up, abducted, and the foot is grasped in a tube (or impervious) stockinette. A large sheet is draped over the end of the table. A drape sheet (cuffed) or a split sheet is draped under the thigh. A folded towel (in thirds, lengthwise) is wrapped around the top of the thigh and clipped; the tube stockinette is brought up over the towel. A drape (or split) sheet is draped over the top of the thigh and clipped underneath. Either a fenestrated sheet or individual drape sheets complete the draping. An additional drape sheet will be needed when the dropped end of the table is returned to normal position.

Equipment

Laminar airflow (if available)
Foot holder
Suction
Electrosurgical unit
Tourniquet and insufflator
Power sources for drill and saw

Instrumentation

Basic orthopedic procedures tray
Knee arthrotomy tray
Osteotomes, gouges
Trial prosthesis, total knee prosthesis, and necessary instrumentation
Power drill and cord
Power oscillating saw with jigs and templates and cord

Supplies

Basin set
Electrosurgical pencil
Suction tubing
Blades (3) No. 10, (1) No. 15
Graduate
Bulb syringes (2)
Tube (or impervious) stockinette, 6″
Esmarch bandage
Needle magnet or counter
Methylmethacrylate kit
Antibiotic irrigation
Closed drainage system (e.g., Hemovac) (optional)
Methylene blue dye (optional)

Special Notes

Laminar airflow may be used.

Have x-ray films in the room.

Have prosthesis and all necessary instrumentation sterile.

Keep conversation and movement in the room to a minimum.

Check levels in the tanks for power equipment.

For tourniquet precautions, see Arthrotomy of the Knee, p. 336.

Protective goggles may be worn.

Follow hospital policy for recording insertion of a prosthesis.

A knee immobilizer may be used following surgery.

OPEN REDUCTION OF THE TIBIAL SHAFT

Definition

Realignment and fixation of the tibia through an operative incision.

Discussion

The type of fixation device is determined by the anatomic considerations of the fracture (i.e., comminuted). Severely comminuted fractures may have to be treated with prolonged traction rather than fixation.

Procedure

The fracture is exposed. Transverse bone screws or plates (including compression plates) are applied to the reduced fracture fragments. When an intramedullary nail is employed (e.g., Lottes, Rush, Enders, Schneider), an incision about the tibial tuberosity is made. A drill reamer penetrates the medullary canal. The measured nail is inserted and aligned to avoid malrotation. It is then driven past the fracture site into the distal portion until the threaded end remains exposed (for later extraction). A counter incision over the fracture site may be needed to effect reduction. Care is taken during the driving of the nail to avoid injury to the shaft. The wound is closed.

Preparation of the Patient

The patient is supine; arms may be extended on armboards. The safety strap is applied to the unaffected thigh. Sheet wadding and a tourniquet are applied to the thigh of the operative leg. Apply electrosurgical dispersive pad.

Skin Preparation

Preparation is best performed by two people to prevent further injury to the bone. Begin at the fracture site; cleanse the leg, thigh (up to the tourniquet), and foot (including interdigital spaces and nails).

Draping

The leg is abducted, and the foot is held up in a tube (or impervious) stockinette. A large sheet is draped over the end of the table. A folded towel (in thirds, lengthwise) is wrapped around the top of the thigh and clipped; the stockinette is brought up over the towel. A drape (or split) sheet is draped under the leg. A large drape (or split) sheet is draped over the thigh and clipped underneath. The leg is passed through a fenestrated sheet, or additional drape sheets complete the draping.

Equipment

Suction
Electrosurgical unit
Tourniquet and insufflator
Power source for drill

Instrumentation

Basic orthopedic procedures tray
Bone holding instruments tray
Fixation device (and necessary instrumentation)
Power drill, cord, and drill bits

Supplies

Basin set
Sheet wadding
Blades (2) No. 10
Tube (or impervious) stockinette
Esmarch bandage
Needle magnet or counter
Graduate
Bulb syringe
Suction tubing
Electrosurgical pencil
Antibiotic irrigation (optional)

Special Notes

Have x-ray films in the room.
  Check pressure level in the tank for the power drill.
  For tourniquet precautions, see Arthrotomy of the Knee, p. 336.
  Protective goggles may be worn.

OPEN REDUCTION OF THE ANKLE

Definition

Realignment and fixation of fractures of the medial malleolus (tibia), lateral malleolus (fibula), and/or posterior malleolus (posterior aspect of distal tibia).

Discussion

This procedure is performed for acute fractures or nonunion of fractures. Many anatomic variations of ankle fractures and dislocations occur.

Procedure

For fracture of the lateral malleolus, an anterolateral incision is made over the fracture site avoiding the sural nerve. The malleolus is exposed. and the fracture is fixed with screws that engage the opposite cortex. Care is taken not to compromise the tendon sheaths. After the incision is closed, a short leg cast is applied.

Preparation of the Patient

The patient is supine; arms may be extended on armboards, and the safety belt is secured over the unaffected extremity. Apply sheet wadding and a tourniquet to the thigh of the operative leg. Apply electrosurgical dispersive pad.

Skin Preparation

The preparation is performed by two people, or a knee holder may be employed. Begin at the ankles and continue to foot (including interdigital spaces, nails). Next prepare the leg (including the knee).

Draping

The leg is abducted, and the foot is held up in a tube (or impervious) stockinette. A large sheet is draped over the end of the table. A folded towel (in thirds, lengthwise) is wrapped around the top of the thigh and clipped; the tube stockinette is brought up over the towel. A drape (or split sheet) is draped under the leg. A large drape (or split) sheet is draped over the thigh and clipped underneath. The extremity is passed through a fenestrated sheet, or additional drape sheets cover the field.

Equipment

Leg holder (optional)
Suction
Electrosurgical unit
Tourniquet and insufflator
Power source for drill
Cast cart

Instrumentation

Basic orthopedic procedures tray
Power drill, cord, and drill bits
Kirschner wires and Steinmann pins
Fixation device with instrumentation (e.g., Rush rods
  or compression plate and screw sets)

Supplies

Sheet wadding
Basin set
Blades (2) No. 10, (1) No. 15
Needle magnet or counter
Suction tubing
Tube (or impervious) stockinette
Esmarch bandage
Bulb syringe
Graduate
Electrosurgical pencil
Antibiotic irrigation (optional)

Special Notes

Have x-ray films in the room.
  For tourniquet precautions, see Arthrotomy of the
Knee, p. 336.
  Protective goggles may be worn.
  Be prepared for the application of a cast.

ARTHROSCOPY OF THE ANKLE AND FOOT

Definition

Endoscopic visualization of the ankle joint and joints of
the foot.

Discussion

Arthroscopy is indicated when other diagnostic modalities such as arthrography or MRI scan do not reveal
the etiology of various ankle and foot problems such as
pain, swelling, instability, or locking. Therapeutic indications include treatment of injuries to cartilage and
soft tissue, loose bodies, synovitis, osteophytes, osteochondral defects, and arthrofibrosis. On occasion an

additional, but as yet controversial, application is arthrodesis of the ankle.

Contraindications to this approach include soft tissue (but not intra-articular) infection and severe degenerative joint disease.

Procedure

According to the pathology and being cognizant of neuromuscular and tendinous structures, three anterior portals (anterolateral, anterocentral, and anteromedial) and three posterior portals (posterolateral, transachilles tendon, and posterior medial) may be made. Most commonly the anteriomedial, anterolateral, and posterolateral portals are employed. Transmalleolar portals are employed. Transmalleolar portals may be used for drilling osteochondrial lesions of the talus. An external (noninvasive) sterile strap is applied. When the ankle joint is tight, invasive pins (e.g., Steinman) may be placed in the distal tibia and calcaneus or talus, penetrating only the lateral cortex of the bone. Care is taken to avoid injuring underlying structures with excessive distraction (greater than 7 or 8 mm is avoided). Lactated Ringer's solution (10 mL) is infused through an 18-gauge needle to assist in the establishment of the anteromedial portal. After a skin incision is made with a No. 11 Bard Parker blade, a clamp is used to spread the soft tissue to the joint capsule, after which a 2.7 mm or 4.0 mm cannula is carefully inserted into the joint, infusing more fluid as necessary. Under direct visualization the additional portals are similarly established. It is important to infuse adequate fluid to maintain distention.

The joint is thoroughly examined in systematic fashion.

According to the pathology a definitive procedure is performed (e.g., loose body removal, debridement, synovectomy, shaving of osteochondral lesions, insertion of pins, or placement of fixation devices).

Preparation of the Patient

The patient is in the supine position with the arms extended on armboards and the safety belt secured over the unaffected extremity. The hip on the affected side is flexed 45 to 50° using a nonsterile thigh holder. (The holder should support the proximal thigh to the region of the popliteal fossa.) Additional foam padding is used with the thigh holder to avoid injury to the sciatic nerve. A sterile foot holder is used to support the foot and ankle in the desired position when invasive distraction is employed. The sterile strap that is used with the noninvasive ankle distractor is sufficient when noninvasive distraction is adequate. A tourniquet and sheet wadding are applied to the proximal thigh. Apply an electrosurgical dispersive pad.

Skin Preparation

Begin at the ankle and continue to the foot (including the interdigital spaces and nails). Next prepare the leg including the knee.

Draping

See Open Reduction of the Ankle, p. 349.

Equipment

Tourniquet and insufflator
Leg holder
Suction
Electrosurgical unit
Video monitor
VCR (optional)
Mavigraph (optional)
Camera control unit
Xenon light source

Instrumentation

Similar as for Arthroscopy of the Knee, p. 339, except
    perhaps smaller scopes and trocars, for example, 4.0
    mm and 2.7 mm
Steinman pins (optional)

Supplies

Sterile foot holder
Sheet wadding

Foam padding
Pillows, as needed for positioning
Basin set
Blades (1) No. 15, (1) No. 11
18-gauge needle
Syringe, 10 or 20 mL
Graduate or small basin
Electrosurgical pencil

Special Notes

The scrub nurse attaches arthroscope cannula and powered instruments to power tubing ends.

White balance the camera.

Position the monitors.

Have Hand and Foot tray available.

All instruments should be meticulously washed and then flash-sterilized, except the telescope and camera. Steris 20 solution is recommended to sterilize these instruments by soaking.

Remote control for video monitor may be placed in sterile plastic bag for use on the field.

Splint material should be available, as desired.

TRIPLE ARTHRODESIS OF THE ANKLE

Definition

Fusion of the talocalcaneal (subtalar), talonavicular, and calcaneocuboid joints.

Discussion

Arthrodesis is performed to relieve pain, provide stability, and arrest a joint-destroying disease process. Multiple combinations of ankle joint arthrodeses and techniques may be employed, which are classified as intraarticular, extra-articular, or a combination of the two.

Procedure

An incision is made from the dorsal prominence of the lateral aspect of the foot to the midportion of the calcaneus. Tendons are retracted exposing the floor of the sinus tarsi. The periosteum of the calcaneus is exposed, and the calcaneocuboid joint capsule is incised. The articular surfaces are excised; the bone fragments are saved. The talonavicular joint capsule is incised, and the head of the talus is excised. The proximal articular surface of the navicular is removed. The subtalar joint is incised, and the articular surface removed with that of the sustenaculum tali and anterior facet of the talus. Bony surfaces are trimmed to correct deformity and to provide for maximum contact. An accessory medial incision may be required. Bone chips are packed into the defect. Soft tissues are sutured to fill the sinus tarsi obliterating dead space. Kirschner wires may be used to maintain alignment. A long leg cast is carefully applied, molding the foot to correct shape and aligning the malleoli. Ten to fourteen days postoperatively, remanipulation of the foot under anesthesia may be necessary.

Preparation of the Patient, Skin Preparation, Draping, Equipment, and Supplies

See Open Reduction of the Ankle, pp. 349–350.

Instrumentation

Basic orthopedic procedures tray
Power drill, cord, drill bits
Osteotomes, curettes, gouges
Steinmann pins, Kirschner wires
Fixation device and instrumentation (e.g., screws, staples)
Vertebral spreader (small)

Special Notes

See Open Reduction of the Ankle, p. 350.

TOTAL ANKLE JOINT REPLACEMENT

Definition

Substitution of the articular surfaces of the distal tibia and the talus with high density polyethylene and metal components, which are fixed with methylmethacrylate.

Discussion

Indications for this procedure include traumatic, degenerative, and rheumatoid arthritis. In general, younger, more active patients will have better ankle function with fusion (arthrodesis). Elderly, less active patients are usually better candidates for joint replacement. The prostheses are classified as: constrained (restricted motion), semiconstrained (semirestricted motion), or nonconstrained (unrestricted motion).

Procedure

An anterolateral incision is made. Tendons and neurovascular structures are retracted. The tibiotalar joint and dome of the talus are exposed. Using special templates, osteotomy incisions for the tibia and talus are outlined and made with an oscillating saw. Care is taken to avoid injury to posteromedial neurovascular bundle and the anterior talofibular ligament. A template is used to cut a section of tibia to accept the stem of the prosthesis. Holes are made in the talus with a curette to provide fixation points for the cement. Trial insertion of the prosthesis is made, and range of motion is determined. The metallic tibial prosthesis is permanently seated after prepared methylmethacrylate is applied. Similarly, the polyethylene talarprosthesis is seated; excess methylmethacrylate is trimmed. The wound is irrigated. The incision is closed over suction drains. A splint is applied over a bulky dressing.

Preparation of the Patient, Skin Preparation, and Draping

See Open Reduction of the Ankle, p. 349.

Equipment

Laminar airflow (if available)
Suction
Electrosurgical unit
Tourniquet and insufflator
Cast cart

Instrumentation

Basic orthopedic procedures tray
Osteotomes, curettes
Power oscillating saw with jigs, templates, and cord
Trial prosthesis, total ankle prosthesis, and specific instrumentation
Power burr set (available)

Supplies

Basin set
Tube (or impervious) stockinette
Esmarch bandage
Needle magnet or counter
Blades (2) No. 10, (1) No. 15
Suction tubing
Electrosurgical pencil
Bulb syringes
Graduate
Methylmethacrylate kit
Antibiotic irrigation (optional)
Closed drainage system (e.g., Hemovac)

Special Notes

Laminar air flow may be used.

Keep conversation and movement in the room to a minimum.

Have x-ray films in the room.

Check pressure level in the tanks for the power equipment.

For tourniquet precautions, see Arthrotomy of the Knee, p. 336.

Have prosthesis and all necessary instrumentation sterile.

Protective goggles may be worn.

Follow hospital policy recording insertion of a prosthesis.

BUNIONECTOMY

Definition

Excision of a soft tissue and/or bony mass at the medial site of the first metatarsal head.

Discussion

Correction may be achieved by a variety of procedures. Excision of exostosis, realignment of the great toe, or transfer of tendons and/or osteotomy of the first metatarsal shaft may be performed. The most frequently performed procedures are the Keller and the Chevron; others include the McBride and Silvers.

Procedure

Keller Procedure. A curved incision is made dorsally along the medial aspect of the first metatarsophalangeal joint. Care is taken to preserve the cutaneous nerves.The capsule and periosteum at the base of the proximal phalanx are incised and retracted. The metatarsal head is dislocated. The proximal half of the phalanyx is resected. Exostosis and osteophytes are excised. The sesamoids are excised if they are enlarged, deformed, or arthritic. A Kirschner wire is inserted, aligning the toe and the metatarsal head. or the resected joint surfaces may be replaced by Silastic prosthesis. A figure-of-eight suture is placed in the capsule and periosteum to cover the end of the phalanx. The wound is closed.

Chevron Procedure. The Chevron procedure utilizes an osteotomy in which the method of fixation involves divergent absorbable pins.

Preparation of the Patient

The patient is supine; arms may be extended on armboards, and the safety belt is secured over the unaffected extremity. Sheet wadding and a tourniquet are applied to the thigh of the operative leg. Apply electrosurgical dispersive pad.

Skin Preparation

A leg holder may be used. Begin with the great toe, and prepare all nails and interdigital spaces. Cleanse foot and leg extending up to the knee.

Draping

The leg is abducted and the foot is grasped in a tube (or impervious) stockinette. A large sheet is draped over the end of the table. A folded towel (in thirds, length-wise) is wrapped around the top of the leg and clipped; the tube stockinette is brought up over the towel. A drape (or split) sheet is draped under the leg and clipped. A large drape (or split) sheet is draped over the thigh and clipped underneath. The extremity is passed through a fenestrated sheet, or additional drape sheets cover the field.

Equipment

Leg holder (optional)
Electrosurgical unit
Tourniquet and insufflator
Power sources for drill and saw

Instrumentation

Minor orthopedic tray
Osteotomes
Kirschner wires
Power saw and cord
Small power drill, cord, and drill bits

Supplies

Basin set
Sheet wadding
Tube (or impervious) stockinette, 6″
Blades (2) No. 10, (1) No. 15
Needle magnet or counter
Esmarch bandage
Bulb syringe
Graduate
Electrosurgical pencil
Antibiotic solution (optional)

Special Notes

Have x-ray films in the room.

Check pressure levels of the tanks for the drill and saw.

For tourniquet precautions, see Arthrotomy of the Knee, p. 336.

Protective goggles may be worn.

CORRECTION OF HAMMER TOE DEFORMITY WITH INTERPHALANGEAL FUSION

Definition

Resection and fixation of the proximal interphalangeal joint.

Discussion

The procedure corrects the deformity and prevents its recurrence. Corns are not disturbed because they disappear following the procedure.

Procedure

A longitudinal incision is made over the dorsum of the proximal interphalangeal joint. The extensor tendon is split and retracted, exposing the joint. The base of the middle phalanx and the head of the proximal phalanx are excised. The remaining parts of the proximal and middle phalanges are fixed with a Kirschner wire drilled through the distal phalanx and out through the skin. A dorsal capsulotomy may be performed through a second incision to release a contracture. The wounds are closed. The wires may be capped.

Preparation of the Patient, Skin Preparation, Draping, Equipment, Instrumentation, Supplies, and Special Notes

See Bunionectomy, pp. 357–358.

METATARSAL HEAD RESECTION

Definition

Excision of the metatarsal head(s).

Discussion

The procedure is indicated in patients with pain related to the prominence of the metatarsal heads; it is often performed on patients with rheumatoid arthritis and dorsally dislocated toes.

Procedure

A longitudinal incision is made in the interspace adjacent to the particular metatarsal head to be excised. The metatarsal head and neck, as well as the articular surface of the phalanges, are freed of soft tissue and resected. Contracted soft tissue is released. The end of the metatarsal is smoothed with a bone rasp. A Kirschner wire is inserted through the medullary canal of the metatarsal stump, aligning it in proper relation to the appropriate toe. The wound is closed. A bulky pressure dressing is applied. The wire may be capped.

Preparation of Patient, Skin Preparation, Draping, Equipment, Instrumention, Supplies, and Special Notes

See Bunionectomy, pp. 357–358.

PROCEDURE FOR CORRECTION OF SCOLIOSIS

Definition

The insertion of various rods, frames, and other fixation devices that act as internal splints until the vertebrae involved in the curvature fuse in an improved position.

Discussion

Surgical treatment of scoliosis is performed when musculoskeletal and respiratory functions become compromised or for cosmetic purposes. A variety of systems (each requiring its own instrumentation) employing compression and distraction rods, hooks, spring hooks, buttons, wires, and so on is in use. The need for a plaster cast or jacket postoperatively varies with the procedure and individual patient requirements. Younger patients are more amenable to corrections. In the Harrington rod procedure a longitudinal compression rod is placed along the convex aspect of the curvature, and a distraction rod is placed on the concave side. Appropriate hooks are attached to the rods that when tightened, diminish the curvature.

A variation of this technique using the Cotrel-DuBousset system employs transverse rods (in addition to the longitudinal rods), which apply corrective forces to segmental areas of the curvature, as well as the full length of the curvature.

Correction can also be accomplished with the Luque system of L-shaped rods and wires, which distributes the corrective forces to vertebral levels rather than the entire length of the deformity.

In the Wisconsin compression rod system, Keene hooks are applied to multiple transverse processes or laminae.

An alternative anterior approach (by anterolateral thoracotomy) for a thoracolumbar deformity utilizes the Dwyer system. A cable is placed through special screws that also anchor special staples placed in the vertebral bodies on the convex side of the curvature. The involved invertebral discs are removed and the cable tightened. Bone grafts (from a rib) are utilized.

Procedure

Harrington Rod. Incision is made over spinous processes of involved segments; by staying in the midline, blood loss is minimized. The vertebral levels are identified using radiography as necessary. Muscular and ligamentous structures are reflected using elevators (Cobb) and curettes about the area to be fused. Bleeding is controlled with cautery and bone wax. Distraction hooks are placed on the concave side of the curvature avoiding penetration into the medullary cavity. Bone slots may be cut to accept the hooks. The distraction rod is then placed. Hooks for the compression rod are placed. Bone grafts from the posterior iliac crests are obtained and kept moist; the iliac wound is closed. The concave vertebral facets are obliterated and decortication of the laminae and transverse processes are performed. Spinal fusion is achieved with bone grafts packed in predominantly on the concave side. Suction drains are placed and the wound closed. Casting or replacement of preoperative bivalved cast may be employed but usually not until several days postoperatively.

Preparation of the Patient

The patient is prone on the Andrews or Wilson frame or on the operating room table with arms on armboards angled toward the head of the table and the hands pronated. Chest rolls are placed under the thorax and abdomen, and a roll is placed in front of the ankles. All pressure points, for example, elbows and knees, require adequate padding. A sterile, plastic adhesive drape may be used to drape buttocks out of the field before skin preparation. Apply electrosurgical dispersive pad.

Skin Preparation

Begin at the midline of the back extending from the base of the skull to the midthighs and down to the table at the sides. (Particular attention is paid to the area above the iliac crests.)

Draping

Folded towels are placed around the site of the incision and the iliac crests. A sterile, plastic adhesive drape may be used. Four drape sheets may be used to drape the head, foot, and sides of the table. A laparotomy sheet that is cut out over the iliac crest(s) completes the draping.

Equipment

Special frame (e.g., Andrews or Wilson) (optional)
Chest rolls, ankle roll, pillows, padding (for positioning)
Suctions (2)
Scales (for weighing sponges)
Electrosurgical unit
Fiberoptic headlight and light source (available)
Cell Saver (available)
Cast cart

Instrumentation

Laminectomy tray
Kerrison rongeurs and Pituitary forceps tray
Spinal fixation device and specific instrumentation (e.g., Harrington rod: distraction and compression rods and hooks, hook clamps, rod clamps, spreader,

drivers, wrench, outrigger distraction unit, Harrington elevator, sacral rod, nut and eyelet)
Self-retaining retractors (e.g., Weitlaners, Beckman)
Large bone cutter, large pin cutter, Steinmann pins,
and protractor

Supplies

Basin set
Blades (2) No. 10, (1) No. 15
Suction tubings (2)
Electrosurgical pencil
Needle magnet or counter
Bone wax
Cottonoids (assorted sizes)
Gelfoam (usually soaked in thrombin 1000 units in 10
mL of saline)
Sterile, plastic adhesive drapes (2) (buttocks and oper-
ative site)
Stainless steel wire, 16 or 18 gauge (for Wisconsin,
Luque)
Graduate
Bulb syringes (2)
Antibiotic irrigation (optional)
Closed drainage system (e.g., Hemovac)

Special Notes

Have x-ray films in the room.
Check with the blood bank that all blood ordered is
available.
Weigh sponges.
Measure blood loss accurately.
Skin and subcutaneous tissues may be injected with
vasoconstricting agent such as epinephrine (advise
anesthetist accordingly).
Have additional suction collection devices ready.
Protective goggles may be worn.

AMPUTATION OF LOWER EXTREMITY

Definition

Severance of a thigh, leg, foot, digit(s), or portions
thereof.

Discussion

Amputation may be necessitated by, among others, gangrene secondary to diabetes, vascular insufficiency, malignancy, or severe trauma. Commonly performed amputations include above the knee (AK), below the knee (BK), and transmetatarsal (TM).

Procedure

For an above the knee amputation the incision is made creating musculocutaneous flaps for better coverage of the femoral stump. The distal adductor canal is entered, and the neurovascular bundle (superficial femoral artery and vein and saphenous nerve) is ligated and divided. Muscles are further transsected circumferentially. The sciatic nerve is ligated and divided. The femoral periosteum is incised and the bone transsected with a saw. Bone edges are smoothed with a rasp. Hemostasis is achieved, and the wound is closed. A closed suction unit may be employed. A bulky dressing can be applied, but preferably a plaster cast or temporary prosthesis is used to minimize postoperative edema and to prepare the stump for a permanent prosthesis later on.

Preparation of the Patient

The patient is supine; arms may be extended on armboards, and the safety belt is secured over the unaffected extremity. Apply electrosurgical dispersive pad.

Skin Preparation

At the surgeon's discretion, a grossly septic distal part need not be prepared. The extremity may be isolated by covering it with a Mayo stand cover or a sterile, plastic adhesive drape.

Transmetatarsal. Begin at the ankle, extending up to the knee and down to the foot and toes (as directed).

Below the Knee. Begin below the knee, include the thigh and extend distally to include leg, foot, and toes (as directed).

Above the Knee. Begin at the thigh, extending distally to include the knee, leg, foot, and toes (as directed).

Draping

The distal portion of the extremity may be wrapped in a Mayo stand cover or a sterile, plastic adhesive drape before the preparation or immediately following the preparation. The extremity is abducted, and the foot is grasped in a tube (or impervious) stockinette. A large sheet is draped over the end of the table. A drape (or split) sheet is draped under the thigh and clipped. A folded towel (in thirds, lengthwise) is wrapped around the thigh and clipped. A sheet is draped proximal to the thigh and clipped underneath. The extremity is passed through a fenestrated sheet, which covers the field. During surgery an extra Mayo cover may be used to hold the amputated part.

Equipment

Electrosurgical unit
Power source for power saw (optional)
Cast cart (optional)

Instrumentation

Basic orthopedic procedures tray
Amputation saw and knife, bone hook
Oscillating power saw and cord (optional)

Supplies

Basin set
Tube (or impervious) stockinette, 6″
Blades (2 to 4) No. 10
Needle magnet or counter
Bulb syringe
Graduate
Electrosurgical pencil
Culture tubes, aerobic and anaerobic
Antibiotic irrigation (optional)
Closed suction unit (e.g., Hemovac)

Special Notes

When preparing, begin with the cleanest area and work toward the dirtiest area (gangrenous part). Do not use sponges from a "dirty" area on a "clean" area.

Dispatch aerobic and anaerobic cultures promptly.

Protective goggles may be worn.

Ask the surgeon if a bulky dressing, plaster cast, or temporary prosthesis will be applied at the conclusion of the procedure.

Determine where amputated part is to be sent (e.g., laboratory, morgue). Be certain it is well wrapped and labeled correctly.

Chapter 16

Neurosurgical Surgery

CRANIOTOMY

Definition

Opening of the skull.

Discussion

The most basic form of craniotomy is the burr hole, a
limited opening through which blood or fluid may be
evacuated, or instruments inserted, to divide neural
tracts (as in prefrontal lobotomy).

Burr holes also may be employed as a preliminary to
other procedures, serving as points that are connected,
for example, when a bone flap is raised. When bone is
excised to permit better exposure or because it is involved in a disease process, it is referred to as a *craniectomy*. *Trephination* may refer to larger burr holes.

Additional uses of the burr hole include biopsy of an
intracranial mass and aspiration of the contents of an
abscess. This stereotactic guided procedure may often
be performed through a limited twist drill opening.
After any of several guidance (e.g., Brown-Roberts-
Wells) devices are affixed to the skull, CT, MRI, or ul
trasound scans localize the lesion. Appropriate instruments are inserted and the procedure performed. In
some institutions this may be done in a specialized x-
ray unit or after the imaging localization is complete

the patient is returned to the operating room for the definitive procedure.

Numerous neurosurgical conditions are treated by craniotomy. Some of those commonly encountered and their treatments include:

Intracranial Aneurysm. An arterial dilation secondary to muscular weakness in a vessel wall prone to rupture (hemorrhage). The patient's blood pressure is controlled and the aneurysm isolated by the application of clips, or the aneurysm can be coated with methylmethacrylate or a cyanoacrylate used to strengthen the aneurysm wall or provide external support.

Arteriovenous Malformation. The capillary bed is bypassed, thus making the veins more prone to rupture. The feeding vessels may be clipped, coagulated, or treated by laser.

Occluded Intracranial Vessel. The superficial temporal artery may be microsurgically anastomosed to the middle cerebral artery distal to the occlusion. The superficial temporal artery is dissected free for an appropriate distance and then passed intracranially through a frontotemporal burr hole preparatory to anastomosis.

Tumors near the Pituitary. The tumor (e.g., optic glioma, craniopharyngioma, suprasellar, and parasellar) is resected; sometimes complete resection is not possible. These tumors are resected by a frontal or frontotemporal approach.

Cerebrospinal Fluid Otorrhea or Rhinorrhea. A skull fracture with a tear in the dura mater and the leakage of cerebrospinal fluid from the ear (otorrhea) or the nose (rhinorrhea). The approach for repair of a dural tear with cerebrospinal otorrhea is temporal or suboccipital. Frontal craniotomy may be performed for cerebrospinal rhinorrhea.

Subdural or Epidural Hematoma (Acute, Subacute, or Chronic). The evacuation of blood, clots, and membranes; the elevation and debridement of associated depressed fractures; and the excision of devitalized brain.

Acoustic Neuroma. Excision of the tumor (without damaging the facial nerve) by a posterior fossa approach. Removal of the bony superior wall of the auditory canal may be necessary to expose the tumor. Some small tumors may be removed by drilling directly through the temporal bone. A nerve stimulator, microscope, and a high-speed power drill may be used.

Neurological Disorders. Examples are trigeminal neuralgia for which rhizotomy is performed or absolute alcohol injected. For Parkinson's disease, a cryoprobe is inserted under stereotaxic control into the globus palidus through a burr hole, producing a destructive lesion.

Hydrocephalus. Treated by insertion of a ventriculoperitoneal or ventriculoatrial shunt (see Ventricular Shunts, p. 381).

Congenital Abnormalities. Premature closure of the sutures is an example. These sutures are resected and the edges covered with Silastic sheeting to prevent healing of the suture lines.

Media attention has been given to the use of the gamma knife. This radiotherapeutic modality is a nonsurgical procedure that can be used to treat many of the conditions above, particularly when the lesion is small, (relatively) inaccessible to surgery techniques, or in poor-operative-risk patients. After a brain lesion is defined by various imaging techniques, the stereotactic gamma knife head form is fixed to the cranium and then emits an appropriate dosage of ionizing radiation by simultaneously focusing a number (e.g., 201) of cobalt 60 source beams at the localized target lesion, relatively sparing adjacent normal tissue. Local anesthesia with sedation or general anesthesia may be employed; the procedure is performed in a special suite of the radiotherapy department. This modality of radiotherapy is not "new," but the gamma knife modification involves less manipulation of the patient and radiation source as compared with prior established similar methods.

Procedure

The incision may be marked. The layers of the scalp are incised, and scalp clips are applied. The scalp is covered with a moist sponge and reflected. Burr holes are made, and the dura mater is carefully separated from the skull. A craniotome may be used to remove the bone, or a bone flap that is hinged on the adjacent periosteum and musculature is made. Bleeding is controlled with electrosurgical forceps, gelatin sponge, and bone wax. If the bone flap is to be replaced at the end of the operation, drill holes are made in the periphery of the skull; the dura and brain are protected. Matching holes are drilled in the bone flap. The dura mater is incised, vessels in the dural margins are coagulated or ligated with hemoclips, and the dura mater may be tacked up to the pericranium. Moist cottonoids are placed as necessary; the brain is continually moistened by saline irrigation or moist cottonoids to prevent cortical injury caused by drying. Lumbar drainage of cerebrospinal fluid and intravenous administration of mannitol or urea and steroids may be done to decrease cerebral edema before any cortical incision is made. A subcortical mass is approached by the most direct route except when this is through a vital region such as a motor or speech area. In these cases, the incision is made in a less important area and continued obliquely. An ultrasonic probe can be employed intraoperatively to facilitate in defining such subcortical mass. Care is taken to cover areas adjacent to the incision with moist cottonoids. Blood vessels are electrocoagulated or clipped. The pia mater and gray matter are usually incised with a knife. The white matter is divided by a dissector or suction tip. Moist cottonoids and cotton balls are employed to restrict capillary oozing or to tamponade blood vessels. During the resection of a brain tumor, the center of the neoplasm may be evacuated or a neoplastic cyst aspirated to facilitate dissection and exposure. Tumor removal may be completed with curettes, pituitary forceps, and a brain spoon. When cerebral resection is completed, the wound is irrigated, and hemostasis is ensured. The dural flap is closed, making the suture line watertight. If the dural defect is too large to be closed, a dural graft may be inserted (using temporalis fascia, periosteum, fascia lata, or an artificial dural substitute). The dura mater may be left open after operations in the posterior fossa (if there is adequate closure of the nuchal muscles), beneath simple burr holes, and following subtemporal cranicctomy for subdural hematoma. The bone flap is wired back. Burr holes may be covered with silicone rubber buttons, methyl-methacrylate, or autogenous bone chips. As the scalp is closed, skin clips are removed. The wound is dressed and the head is wrapped in a turbanlike gauze bandage.

Preparation of the Patient

The patient's hair may be partially or completely removed following the patient's arrival in the surgery department. A cubicle in the preoperative area or the recovery room can be screened off to maintain the patient's privacy. The hair is cut with electrical clippers and the scalp is carefully shaved with disposable razors and warm soapy water. The patient's hair is saved in a bag labeled with the patient's identification and returned to him or her postoperatively. A hypothermia mattress may be put on the table. The patient's temperature is monitored. A Foley catheter is often inserted in the bladder. Elastic bandages or antiembolic hose may be applied from the toes to the groin to prevent venous stasis and to help maintain blood pressure. A right atrial or central venous pressure line may be inserted. Hypotension may be induced by drugs injected intravenously. The surgeon may mark the site of the incision with an indelible marking pen. The position of the patient depends upon the location of the lesion and the preference of the surgeon. After the patient is positioned, apply electrosurgical dispersive pad.

Supine. The patient is supine with arms extended on armboards or tucked in at the patient's sides; the head may be stablized by the insertion of the sterile pins from a headrest attachment to the table, or it may simply be positioned on a doughnut headrest.

Sitting. The patient is supine with the knees over the lower break, the table is raised from the middle break, and the foot of the table is lowered. A padded footboard supports the feet. The arms are placed in the patient's lap on a pillow and secured with padded restraints. The safety strap is secured across the thighs. The head may be stabilized by the insertion of the sterile pins of a headrest attachment to the table.

Prone. The patient is intubated on the gurney and carefully rolled over to the prone position onto the table. The arms are extended on armboards (angled toward the head of the table) with the hands pronated. Chest rolls are placed under the patient from the acromioclavicular joints to the iliac crests to facilitate breathing. A pillow or roll is placed in front of the ankles. Padding is placed under the elbows and knees. Female breasts and male genitalia are protected from pressure. The safety strap is secured across the patient's thighs.

Skin Preparation

Check with the surgeon regarding the type of solution to be used and the area to be prepared. Care is taken to avoid getting preparation solution in the eyes. Antibiotic ointment may be put in the eyes and nonirritating tape may be used to tape lids shut. Small cotton pledgets are helpful in preventing solution from pooling in the ears.

Draping

The surgeon usually prefers to do the draping. Folded towels are placed around the operative site and secured by towel clips or sutures. To suture towels in place, heavy silk suture on a cutting needle, a needle holder, toothed forceps, and suture scissors are needed. A sterile, plastic adhesive drape may be used; the prepared area must be dry or the adhesive drape will not stick. If an overhead table (e.g., Mayfield) is used, a large drape sheet, fanfolded at the front edge of the table, is used. The fanfolded sheet is brought down toward the operative site and secured; this covers the space between the unsterile area under the table and the operative field. A disposable craniotomy sheet eliminates the need for multiple drape sheets; otherwise, individual drape sheets cover the field.

Equipment

Headrest clamp (e.g., Mayfield, Crutchfield, Gardner)
Overhead table (e.g., Mayfield)

Hypothermia/hyperthermia mattress (optional)
Pillows, chest rolls, and padded restraints, as needed
for positioning
Suction (2)
Electrosurgical unit (monopolar)
Electrosurgical unit (bipolar)
Temperature monitoring device
Fiberoptic light source for retractors (optional)
Power sources for power drill and saw
Loupes and/or microscope (e.g., Zeiss)
Blood warming units
Blood pumps (for infusion of blood)
Footstools (6 to 8)
Scales
Cell Saver (available)
Carbon dioxide laser (available, depending on proce-
dure): see Appendix, pp. 619–624, for precautions

Instrumentation

Craniotomy tray
Microsurgical instruments (optional) (e.g., microfor-
ceps, scissors, needle holders, curettes, suction tips,
bayonet bipolar electrosurgical forceps, dissectors,
elevators)
Power saw and/or drill (optional)
Aneurysm clips and appliers (assorted) (e.g., Heifetz,
Yasargil, Sundt-Kees, Mayfield, Keer, Olivecrona)
for aneurysm, arteriovenous malformation, pituitary
tumors

Supplies

Basin set
Blades (2) No. 10, (1) No. 15, (1) No. 11
Needle magnet or counter
Suction tubing
Needle and local anesthesia with epinephrine (to inject
site of incision for hemostasis)
Nerve stimulator (locator)
Bulb syringes (2)
Graduate
Electrosurgical pencil

Telfa (for specimens)
Cottonoids, assorted (e.g., ½″ × ½″, 1″ × 1″, 1″ × 3″, ½″ × 3″)
Bone wax, 2 packages
Hemostatic agents (e.g., Surgicel, Gelfoam and thrombin, Avitene)
Cotton balls
Hemoclips (small, medium)
Scalp clips (e.g., Raney, Michel)
Drain (e.g., Hemovac) (optional)
Antibiotic irrigation (optional)
Medications
Sodium nitroprusside (Nipride) to induce hypotension.
   Note: Nipride when mixed in solution for intravenous use is unstable in light. Cover bottle and tubing with aluminum foil.
Dexamethasone (Decadron), a synthetic steroid, to decrease inflammation
Mannitol, 20% with filter, to reduce intracranial pressure
Methylmethacrylate kit (optional)

Special Notes

Planning prior to bringing the patient to the operating room is essential. Consider equipment, special physical needs of the patient, surgical approach, position, instrumentation, supplies, and medications.

Headrest clamps attached to the table headrest attachment (e.g., Mayfield, Crutchfield, or Gardner) secure the skull by two or three sterile fixation pins. Insertion sites for the pins are prepared with preparation solution.

Have x-rays and CT scan films in the room.

Check with the blood bank that blood is available as ordered.

Extra care is taken to be certain that all bony prominences are padded (these procedures can be lengthy) to avoid damage to skin and nerves.

An electrosurgical dispersive pad is necessary if the monopolar electrosurgical unit is used.

Have a second suction unit available.

Have all equipment (electrosurgical unit, suction, microscope, drills, etc.) connected and ready before the skin incision is made.

A kickbucket may be used to catch irrigation and blood below the head of the table (gather drapes to form a funnel) if a special craniotomy sheet is unavailable.

Towels around the operative site may be secured with suture; have heavy suture, cutting needle, needle holder, and forceps with teeth ready.

If the lines of the incision are marked, methylene blue is *never* used because it produces an inflammatory reaction in nervous tissue.

Keep both (bulb or Asepto) syringes filled at all times. Measure irrigation used accurately.

Place moistened cottonoids, cotton balls, and bone wax within the surgeon's view on a neurosurgical sponge (pattie) plate.

Record the number of cotton balls used, in addition to sponges and cottonoids. Saline or Ringer's lactate is used during bipolar coagulation to minimize tissue heating.

Drill sites or saw incisions into the cranium are irrigated with saline to minimize the heat (produced by friction).

Aneurysm clips are applied with clip appliers only and should be discarded after being compressed.

If methylmethacrylate is used to coat a blood vessel, all surrounding tissues are protected with moistened cottonoids.

Protective goggles may be worn.

CRANIOPLASTY

Definition

Repair of a cranial defect.

Discussion

Cranial defects may result from fractures, infections, surgical procedures (e.g., cranial bone biopsy, craniectomy), or a congenital deformity. Indications for the procedure include protection from external trauma, alleviation of pain or seizures, and cosmesis. The artificial cranium may be fashioned from autogenous bone grafts, metal (e.g., tantalum), or acrylic material (e.g., methylmethacrylate). Methylmethacrylate is the pre-

ferred material for cranioplasty, except in cases of wound infection, in which autogenous grafts are better accepted.

Procedure

The scalp is incised over the defect. The defect may be trimmed as necessary. Methylmethacrylate is mixed according to manufacturer's directions (i.e., until dough-like, put in a polyethylene bag, and rolled flat). The surgeon then molds the material to fit the defect. Acrylic is removed from the polyethylene bag and allowed to harden. Excess material may be trimmed with rongeurs or a power saw. A craniotome may be used to smooth rough spots. Holes are drilled in the periphery of the acrylic plate and the cranial defect. The plate is placed over the defect and secured by stainless steel wire passed through the holes. The wound is irrigated and closed.

Preparation of the Patient

The hair over the area of the defect must be removed. Complete hair removal may be indicated; check with the surgeon. The patient's hair is removed, saved in a bag, and labeled with patient's identification prior to entering the operating room and returned to him or her postoperatively. See Craniotomy Preparation of the Patient, pp. 371–372. The position of the patient depends on the area of the defect. Apply electrosurgical dispersive pad.

Skin Preparation

Check with the surgeon regarding the type of solution to be used and the area to be prepared. Care is taken to avoid getting preparation solution in the eyes. Antibiotic ointment may be instilled in the eyes and a nonirritating tape may be used to tape the lids shut. Small cotton pledgets may be used to prevent solution from pooling in the ears.

Draping

The surgeon usually prefers to do the draping. Folded towels are placed around the operative site and secured

by towel clips or sutures. A sterile, plastic adhesive drape may be used; the prepared area must be dry or the adhesive drape will not stick. The patient is covered with a craniotomy sheet, or individual drape sheets may be used.

Equipment

Suctions (2)
Electrosurgical unit
Power sources for power saw and power drill

Instrumentation

Craniotomy tray
Power saw or craniotome and cord
Power drill, burrs, and cord

Supplies

Basin set
Blades (2) No. 10
Needle magnet or counter
Sterile, plastic adhesive drape
Suction tubing
Asepto or bulb syringes (2)
Graduate
Electrosurgical pencil
Bone wax
Scalp clips (e.g., Raney, Michel)
Cranioplasty kit (methylmethacrylate, polyethelene bag, roller, mixing bowl, and spoon)
Stainless steel wire
Cottonoids, large (e.g., 1″ × 3″)
Antibiotic irrigation (optional)

Special Notes

If suture is used to secure the towels, have ready heavy silk suture on a cutting needle, needle holder, toothed forceps, and suture scissors.

Methylmethacrylate is mixed by adding one volume of liquid monomer to one volume of powered polymer. When mass is doughy, put in plastic bag and roll flat.

The surgeon will then mold the plate. When cool, excess material will be sawed or cut off with rongeurs. The process from mixing to hardening takes 7 minutes.

TRANSSPHENOIDAL HYPOPHYSECTOMY

Definition

Excision or destruction of all or a portion of the pituitary gland.

Discussion

Hypophysectomy is performed for endocrine disorders, primary tumors of the pituitary, some presentations of diabetic retinopathy, and hormonally dependent metastatic breast and prostatic carcinoma. Its use in control of other malignancies is controversial (e.g., malignant melanoma, hypernephroma, thyroid cancer). A side effect of hypophysectomy is the production of diabetes insipidus which can be controlled by vasopressin (Pitressin) replacement. More than 90 percent removal of the gland is usually necessary to effect the desired results. Radiotherapy to ablate the pituitary by either interstitial radiation (placed by stereotaxic approaches) or external beam radiation give less than favorable results. Open craniotomy presents greater stress and risk to these often frail patients.

Stereotaxic hypophysectomy, a modality that can be performed under local anesthesia, employs an integrated system controlled by computer. The patient's head is secured in a stereotaxic frame. Preoperatively the patient undergoes computerized axial tomography, tomographic pneumoencephalography, and vascular angiography. Using coordinates thus established, the surgeon places the patient in the same frame in surgery, the patient is anesthetized and, under computerized control, checked by fluoroscopy. After a drill is used to perforate the sphenoid sinus and the floor of the sella turcica, a cryoprobe is placed in the sella turcica (position predetermined) via cannula. Cryodestruction is then performed. On removal of the probe, a silicone plug is placed in the sellar opening to prevent cerebrospinal fluid leakage. This procedure is usually performed in a specially designed radiology suite.

Procedure

General anesthesia is administered by endotracheal tube. The nasal cavity and gums are infiltrated with a local anesthetic containing epinephrine to minimize blood loss and aid in elevation of the mucosa. A horizontal incision is made under the upper lip and extended over the maxilla into the nasal cavity. The mucosa is elevated, and a portion of the cartilaginous septum is excised and saved in a saline soaked sponge. Using a bivalve nasal speculum, the floor of the sphenoidal sinus is exposed and incised by rongeur. The boundaries of the sella are determined by direct vision with microscope and by fluoroscopy. The sella is entered in the midline; a sphenoidal punch is used to enlarge the opening, exposing the dura of the pituitary fossa. The dura is incised avoiding entry into the pituitary capsule. The gland is dissected extracapsularly, and the stalk is identified. Care is taken not to penetrate the posterior wall of the sella. Again, fluoroscopy confirms the position of the instruments. A sickle knife or scissors may be used to sever the stalk. Further dissection, with a specifically designed blunt dissector, frees the remainder of the gland from its dural attachments, and the gland is delivered intact. Gelfoam soaked in thrombin can be used to control oozing.

A patch of fascia lata and muscle is excised from the previously prepared thigh and packed into the empty sella. A segment of previously excised cartilaginous nasal septum is used to seal the muscle plug to the floor of the sella, "snapping" it into place. Antibiotics may be instilled. Nasal packing reapproximates the nasal mucosa. The gingival incision is closed with absorbable suture. The thigh incision (donor site) is closed.

Preparation of the Patient

The patient may be supine with arms tucked in at the sides; the head may be supported by a headrest. One leg (usually the right) is not restrained by the safety belt to provide access for the muscle tissue graft.

The procedure is usually performed under general anesthesia with endotracheal intubation. The nasal cavity and gums are infiltrated with local anesthesia containing epinephrine. Apply electrosurgical dispersive pad.

Skin Preparation

The thigh is prepared from the knee to the groin, and down to the table at the sides. Check with the surgeon for the type of solution to be used and the area to be prepared; the area may include the face and oral and nasal cavities (the surgeon may do this preparation). In addition to the standard preparation tray, include bayonet forceps, nasal speculum, long cotton-tipped applicators, and hemostat.

Draping

The patient's face is draped with folded towels, as is the prepared thigh. The patient may be covered with a disposable fenestrated sheet (an opening can be cut for access to the thigh). A drape is necessary for the image intensifier and the microscope.

Equipment

Headrest (e.g., Richards, doughnut, Shea)
Suction
Electrosurgical unit (bipolar)
Microscope
Image intensifier (with C-arm) and TV monitor
Fiberoptic headlight and light source (available)

Instrumentation

Craniotomy tray
Limited procedure tray (muscle tissue graft)
Bayonet bipolar electrocoagulating forceps, microtip
Bivalve nasal speculum (long blades), punch forceps, small ring curettes (angled), Hardy's enucleator (angled), pituitary spoon (angled), microscissors

(straight, curved, angled), microdissectors (angled), sickle knife (angled)

Supplies

Basin set
Blades (1) No. 10, (2) No. 15, (1) No. 12
Needle magnet or counter
Electrosurgical pencil
Suction tubing
Bulb syringes (2)
Cottonoids (e.g., ½″ × ½″, ½″ × 1″ frequently used)
Syringe (e.g., 10 mL Luer-lock, control) long needle; local anesthesia with epinephrine
Bone wax
Nasal packing (e.g., ½″ petrolatum-impregnated gauze)
Hemostatic agents (e.g., Gelfoam and thrombin, Surgicel, Avitene)
Antibiotic irrigation (optional)

Special Notes

Lead aprons are worn during fluoroscopy.

A second Mayo stand may be used for taking the muscle tissue graft.

Have materials available for aerobic and anaerobic cultures.

VENTRICULAR SHUNTS

Definition

Refers to the insertion of a valve system to divert the flow of cerebrospinal fluid from the ventricular system.

Discussion

Shunting the ventricular fluid to a body cavity outside the cranium is performed to treat hydrocephalus (congenital, neoplastic, traumatic, and infectious). The distal end of the shunt is placed in the peritoneal cavity unless contraindicated by intraperitoneal disease. If peritoneal placement cannot be performed, the shunt may be indirectly placed in the right atrium by way of the internal jugular vein, or directly placed in the atrium by thoracotomy. The advantages of peritoneal over atrial placement of the distal catheter are avoidance of vascular and cardiopulmonary complications, faster, simpler placement of the distal catheter, space to place a longer distal catheter (prolonging the interval before revision), and easier replacement of the distal catheter.

Procedure

Ventriculoperitoneal Shunt for Hydrocephalus. Lines are marked for a right-sided shunt incision (several centimeters above and posterior to the ear), and a transverse right-upper-quadrant incision of the abdomen. The scalp is incised and reflected on its base. Bleeding is controlled by electrocoagulation. The burr hole site in the periosteum is electrocoagulated and a self-retaining retractor is placed. The periosteum is incised, and a burr hole is made and enlarged as necessary to accommodate the reservoir. The dura is electrocoagulated, and the outer layer incised. Bipolar electrocautery is used to seal the dura to the pia and cortex. A straight ventricular catheter is passed into the posterior aspect of the lateral ventricle, the stylet is removed, and the opening pressure recorded. A premeasured length of catheter is advanced anterior to the foramen of Munro. Air (5 to 10 mL) is injected, and an x-ray film is taken to confirm the position of catheter placement.

The transverse abdominal incision is carried down to the anterior rectus sheath. A distal catheter is passed from the scalp incision to the abdominal incision subcutaneously. The reservoir is attached to the proximal end of the valve with a connector and suture. The reservoir is attached to the ventricular catheter with suture. The valve mechanism is placed in the subgaleal space behind the ear. A longitudinal incision is made in the anterior rectus sheath. The rectus abdominus muscle is split. An incision is made in the posterior rectus sheath and transversalis fascia. The peritoneum is grasped and incised (1 mm). The peritoneal catheter, passed intraperitoneally, is attached to the reservoir. Wounds may be irrigated with antibiotic solution. The abdominal wound is closed. An antibiotic may be injected into the ventricle through the reservoir after compression of the valve. The scalp incision is closed.

Preparation of the Patient

The patient is supine with the right arm tucked in at the patient's side and the left arm extended on an armboard. The patient's head is slightly elevated and turned to the left; a headrest may be used. See Pediatric General Information, pp. 518–520, for measures to maintain pediatric patient's body temperature, to restrain the extremities, and so on. Fluoroscopy or x-rays may be employed to determine the correct placement of the catheter.

Skin Preparation

Check with the surgeon regarding preparation and the solution to be used. In pediatric patients, hair is shaved in the operating room prior to the skin preparation. The area to be prepared may include the exposed scalp and the right side of the face extending from the forehead to the shoulder (including the lateral aspect of the face to the orbital rim and the neck), and down to the table at the sides.

Draping

The surgeon usually does the draping. Folded towels are placed around the operative site. The superior tip of the ear may be sutured forward to the skin (to keep it out of the field). A sterile, plastic adhesive drape may be used. A fenestrated sheet may be used to cover the field.

Equipment

Suction
Electrosurgical unit (biopolar)
Headrest (e.g., doughnut) (optional)
Restraints, softpadded (pediatric)
Power source for power drill

Scale (optional)
Body heat maintenance equipment (e.g., heating lamps, warming mattress)

Instrumentation

Craniotomy tray
Power drill (e.g., micro Stryker) and cord
Shunt, ventricular catheter, peritoneal catheter
Small bulldog clamp
Uterine packing forceps or a long passing instrument

Supplies

Basin set
Blades (2) No. 15
Needle magnet or counter
Sterile, plastic adhesive drape (optional)
Suction tubing
Plastic syringe (3 mL) and blunt needle (e.g., 18 gauge) to pump through shunt reservoir and tubing
Shunt (e.g., Rickham reservoir, Holter valve, and catheter)
Cottonoids (e.g., $\frac{1}{2}'' \times \frac{1}{2}''$)
Gelfoam and thrombin
Bulb syringe
Graduate
Antibiotic irrigation (optional)

Special Notes

Take extra precautions to correctly identify the pediatric patient.

Check with the surgeon and anesthetist regarding measures to be employed to prevent loss of body heat, such as heating lamps, warming mattress, and wrapping extremities. Use warmed solutions.

Determine the area to be prepared. Do not allow solution to pool under the patient. Do not allow solution to run into eyes or pool in the ear. Ask if the patient's head is to be shaved partially or completely.

Employ measures to protect the eyes, for example, eye ointment and hypoallergenic tape (to tape eyes shut).

Notify the x-ray department before the surgery

starts regarding the necessity for equipment such as a portable x-ray machine or fluoroscopy unit.

Ask if sponges are to be weighed.

Follow hospital policy for recording insertion of an implant.

Regarding the Implant. A reservoir such as the Rickham reservoir may be inserted into the system between the valve and the catheter.

Check valve patency and pressure with normal saline before use.

Flush unit with saline or Ringer's solution (surgeon's preference); do *not* allow air into the unit.

Observe x-ray precautions, see p. 21.

Regarding the Shunt Unit. Handle the unit only as much as absolutely necessary. Avoid contact with lint or other foreign materials; do not place on gauze sponges. Always place the unit in a basin.

The valve must be properly oriented to allow a one-way passage of fluid only.

Antibiotic solution may be used for irrigation.

LAMINECTOMY

Definition

Laminectomy is the removal of one or more vertebral laminae.

Discussion

Indications for laminectomy, hemilaminectomy, and an interlaminar procedure include herniated disc, compression fracture, dislocation, and spinal cord tumor. Other procedures may be performed in conjunction with laminectomy such as *cordotomy,* that is, the division of the anterolateral tracts of the spinal column for intractable pain, and *rhizotomy,* that is, the interruption of spinal (sensory) nerve roots for relief of spasm or intractable pain.

Procedure

Laminectomy for Herniated Intervertebral Disc. A midline vertical incision may be used. The wound is deepened with a knife or, more frequently, with an electrosurgical pencil. Self-retaining retractors are placed, and the fascia is incised. The paraspinous muscles and periosteum are reflected (this may be done unilaterally on the side of the involved disc). Sponges are packed along the vertebrae with a periosteal elevator to aid in blunt dissection and effect hemostasis. A larger retractor (e.g., Beckman, Taylor, or Scoville) is placed for exposure. Small portions of the laminae overlying the herniated disc are removed with a Kerrison rongeur; portions of vertebral spines and intervertebral facets may also be excised. Hemostasis is achieved with bone wax. The ligamenta flava are incised; care is taken to avoid injury to the epidural veins. If the electrosurgical pencil is used, the vein is held away from the dura to prevent thermal injury to neural tissues. Moistened cottonoids are placed to protect the dura. Additional ligament or bone may be removed to provide adequate exposure. Nerve roots are cautiously retracted exposing the herniated disc, which is removed with a pituitary rongeur and curettes; care is exercised anteriorly to avoid the aorta and vena cava. The wound is irrigated. The area is examined to ensure that all protruding disc has been removed. Hemostasis is achieved. The wound is closed in layers.

Preparation of the Patient

Check with the surgeon regarding removal of the patient's hair. The position of the patient depends on the type of laminectomy to be performed and the surgeon's preference. Cervical laminectomy is most frequently performed in the sitting position. Thoracic and lumbar laminectomies are most frequently performed in the prone or a modified knee-chest position. Occasionally, the lateral position is used for thoracic or lumbar laminectomy. Antiembolic hose or woven elastic bandages (e.g., Ace) may be applied to the legs to prevent venous stasis and to help maintain blood pressure.

Sitting. The patient is supine with knees over the lower break of the table. The head of the table is raised from the middle break. The foot of the table is lowered; a padded footboard supports the feet. The arms are placed in the patient's lap on a pillow and secured with padded restraints. The safety strap is secured above the knees. The Mayfield (skull) clamp is attached to a headrest table attachment. Preparation solution is applied to the insertion sites of the pins; some hair will need to be shaved.

Prone. Following placement of an intravenous line, the administration of general anesthesia, and the insertion of an endotracheal tube (while the patient is on the gurney or the hospital bed), the patient is carefully rolled over to the prone position onto the table. The arms are extended on armboards angled toward the head of the table with the hands pronated. Chest rolls are placed under the patient from the acromioclavicular joint to the level of the iliac crests to facilitate breathing. A pillow or roll is placed in front of the ankles. Pads are placed under the elbows and knees. Female breasts and male genitalia are protected from pressure. The safety strap is secured across the patient's thighs. A sterile, plastic adhesive drape may be put on the buttocks at this time to seal the rectal area out of the field.

Modified Knee-Chest. Following placement of an intravenous line, the administration of general anesthesia, and the insertion of an endotracheal tube (while the patient is on the gurney), the patient is carefully rolled over to the prone position onto the table. Adjust the patient's position so the hips are over the middle break in the table. The foot of the table is lowered, and a padded extension is added on perpendicular to the table. The arms are extended on armboards angled toward the head of the table with the hands pronated. Chest rolls are placed under the patient from the acromioclavicular joint to the level of the iliac crests to facilitate breathing. Pads are placed under the elbows and knees. Female breasts and male genitalia are protected from pressure. Pillows are placed in front of the ankles and under the feet. The patient's position is secured with the safety strap or 7.5 cm (or 3 inch) wide adhesive tape across the thighs. A sterile, plastic adhesive drape may be put on the buttocks at this time to seal the rectal area out of the field. After the patient is positioned, apply electrosurgical dispersive pad.

For *cervical laminectomy,* hair on the lower portion of the scalp (supra-auricular border) and the neck is removed after the patient has arrived in the surgery department, but before entering the operating room. Hair on the top of the head need not be removed. Long hair is secured at the top of the head. The hair to be removed is clipped with electric clippers. The area is then shaved with warm soapy water and disposable razors.

For *thoracic* or *lumbar laminectomy,* hair present on the dorsal thorax is shaved in the operating room.

Skin Preparation

Check with the surgeon regarding the area to be prepared.

Cervical. Begin cleansing at the midline, extending from the supra-auricular border to the level of the axillae, and down to the table at the neck and shoulders.

Thoracic. Begin cleansing at the midline, extending from the base of the skull to the level of the waist, and down to the table at the neck and sides.

Lumbar. Begin cleansing at the midline, extending from the shoulders to the coccyx (or the adhesive drape), and down to the table at the sides.

Draping

The surgeon usually prefers to do the draping. Folded towels are placed around the operative site and secured with towel clips or sutures. To suture towels, heavy silk sutures on a cutting needle, needle holder, toothed forceps, and suture scissors are needed. A sterile, plastic adhesive drape may be used. The field is covered with a craniotomy sheet or a sheet with a moderate-sized fenestration for a cervical procedure. For a thoracic or lumbar procedure, the field may be covered with a laparotomy sheet.

Equipment

Suction
Electrosurgical unit (monopolar)
Electrosurgical unit (bipolar)
Power source for power drill (optional)

Fiberoptic headlight and light source
Pillows and pads for elbows and knees, chest rolls (for prone or modified knee-chest position)
Pillows and padded arm restraints (for sitting position)
Headrest, for example, Mayfield (for cervical approach)
Scales (to weigh sponges)

Instrumentation

Laminectomy tray
Kerrison rongeurs and pituitary forceps tray
Power drill (e.g., micro Stryker), drill bits, cord (optional)

Supplies

Basin set
Suction tubing
Blade (3 or 4) No. 10, (1) No. 15
Sterile, plastic adhesive drapes (2)
Needle magnet or counter
Bone wax
Bulb or Asepto syringes (2)
Electrosurgical pencil
Gelfoam and thrombin (e.g., 5000 units)
Roller gauze, 2″ (to hold retractor)
Cottonoids (e.g., ½″ × ½″, 1″ × 1″)
Antibiotic irrigation (optional)

Special Notes

Have x-ray films in the room.

Check with the blood bank that blood is available as ordered.

Save the patient's hair in a bag labeled with the patient's identification.

Utmost care must be taken when moving the patient from the gurney to the table. Have adequate assistance.

In positioning, protect bony prominences from pressure to prevent skin and nerve damage.

Protect the eyes from injury (e.g., by using eye ointment and taping lids shut).

Have all equipment (e.g., suction, electrosurgical unit) ready before the incision is made.

Keep both bulb or Asepto syringes filled at all times. Irrigation temperature should be tepid.

Place moistened cottonoids and bone wax within the surgeon's view on a neurosurgical sponge ("pattie") plate.

Saline or Ringer's lactate is used during bipolar coagulation to minimize tissue heating.

When a Taylor retractor is used, after it has been appropriately placed, the surgeon wraps the roller gauze around the tail of the retractor, and drops the roll to the circulator, who secures it to the table.

EXCISION OF CERVICAL INTERVERTEBRAL DISC WITH FUSION, ANTERIOR APPROACH

Definition

Excision of a herniated intervertebral disc with the stabilization of the cervical spine.

Discussion

The procedure is indicated when nerve deficits and pain caused by spondylosis or herniated disc persists, despite conservative treatment of bedrest and traction. The anterior approach is preferred when spondylotic bars compromise the cord or the nerve root; the posterior approach is employed when multiple nerve roots must be decompressed. Fusion is accomplished with a bone graft, usually obtained from the iliac crest.

Procedure

A transverse incision is made at the level of the cricoid cartilage. The incision is deepened, usually to the right of the midline, retracting the carotid sheath and prevertebral muscles laterally, and the trachea and esophagus medially to expose the spine. Care is taken to avoid injury to the carotid sheath contents, vertebral vessels, and recurrent laryngeal nerve. The anterior longitudinal ligament is incised exposing the intervertebral disc. The disc level may be confirmed by x-ray (using a needle as a marker). A bone graft may be taken from the iliac crest using either an osteotome (after the periosteum has been reflected) or a dowel cutter. All bone chips are kept moist and saved for later packing of the fusion site. The iliac crest wound is closed after hemostasis is achieved. The diseased disc is incised and removed piecemeal with rongeurs. Bony spurs compressing the nerve roots or dura are excised with small rongeurs and/or burrs. The intervertebral space is packed with the bone graft (and chips). A depth gauge may be used to determine the size to use for the bone plug. After hemostasis is achieved, the cervical wound is closed in layers.

Preparation of the Patient

The patient is supine with the head turned to the left and the right hip elevated (e.g., with a folded sheet).

Skin Preparation

For *cervical incision:* Begin at the neck extending from the infra-auricular border to the nipples, and down to the table at the sides of the neck and shoulders.

For *donor site incision* (e.g., iliac crest): Begin cleansing the iliac crest area extending from the midthorax to the upper thigh, down to the table on the right side, and well beyond the midline on the left side.

Draping

The patient is draped with four folded towels at the neck and four folded towels at the hip; towel clips or suture may be used to secure the towels. A sterile, plastic adhesive drape may be used. A sheet with a small fenestration is used for the cervical incision; a laparotomy sheet is used for the donor graft incision.

Equipment

Suction
Electosurgical unit (bipolar)
Fiberoptic headlight and power source

Power source for power drill (optional)
Loupes or microscope (optional)

Instrumentation

Laminectomy tray
Kerrison rongeurs and pituitary forceps tray
Cervical fusion instruments (e.g., Cloward self-retaining retractors, drill guards, drills, dowel cutters, bone graft holder, impactor, vertebral spreaders)
Hudson brace, mallet, depth gauge
Power drill (e.g., Stryker), small burrs, and cord (optional)
Hemoclip appliers (short, medium)

Supplies

Basin set
Suction tubing
Blades (2) No. 10, (1) No. 15, (1) No. 11
Bayonet bipolar electrocoagulating forceps
Needle (inserted into disc space to determine level)
Cassette drape
Gelfoam
Thrombin (e.g., 5000 units)
Cottonoids (e.g., ½″ × ½″)
Graduate
Bulb syringes (2)
Hemoclips (small, medium)
Microscope drape (optional)
Sterile, plastic adhesive drape (optional)

Special Notes

Have x-ray films in the room.

Notify the x-ray department regarding portable films to be taken.

Observe x-ray precautions, see p. 21.

The site of the donor graft is covered with a towel until the surgeon is ready to take the graft.

A Stryker drill with a small burr may be used on the vertebrae to facilitate access to the disc.

The cervical incision is covered with a towel while the graft is taken from the donor site (e.g., iliac crest).

Chapter 17

Plastic Surgery

CLEFT LIP REPAIR

Definition

Correction of a congenital deformity of the lips and face.

Discussion

Cleft lip results from a fusion failure during the embryonic processes. Each cleft lip deformity varies. There are four categories:

1. Unilateral incomplete cleft with nasal deformity
2. Unilateral complete cleft with nasal deformity
3. Bilateral incomplete cleft with or without adequate columella
4. Bilateral complete cleft on one side and incomplete on the other side

The cleft lip can be closed in the neonate, but repair at 3 months of age is preferable, as growth of the tissues facilitates the initial detailed surgery. Palatal and alveolar deformities may also be present.

Procedure

General anesthesia is administered, and an endotracheal tube is inserted. In addition, a local anesthetic containing epinephrine is infiltrated locally to aid in hemostasis. Simple closure does not usually suffice but may render subsequent stages easier. More often, any of several flaps are isolated and advanced. Proper restoration of the philtrum and shape of the bow of the lip is sought. Secondary repairs are performed according to individual situations even months or years later. Similarly, palatal and alveolar deformities are repaired in due time to commensurate with the patient's feeding requirements and tissue growth. Postoperatively, the child's arms are restrained. The incision is protected with antibiotic ointment, and the cheeks are splinted with a Logan's bow (to counter the effects of crying).

Preparation of the Patient

The patient is supine. The head should be at the top edge of the table; a headrest or support may be used. Following induction of general anesthesia, the table is usually turned so that the surgeon may stand or sit at the head of the table and the anesthetist is at the patient's side. For the pediatric patient special measures must be taken to prepare the room, restrain the patient, and maintain the patient's body temperature. Refer to Pediatric General Information, pp. 518–520.

Skin Preparation

Check with the surgeon regarding choice of preparation solution. Begin at the upper lip, cleanse the face extending from the hairline to the shoulders, and down to the table at the sides of the neck.

Draping

The patient is usually draped with a head drape (drape sheet and two towels under the head with the uppermost towel wrapped around the head and clipped). A split (or drape) sheet covers the patient's body.

Equipment

Padded restraints
Headrest (e.g. doughnut) (optional)
Warming mattress or heat lamps (optional)
Suction

Electrosurgical unit (bipolar)
Sitting stools (optional)

Instrumentation

Basic plastic procedures tray
Lip clamp
Beaver knife handle

Supplies

Basin set
Bayonet bipolar electrocoagulating forceps
Blades (1) No. 15, (1) No. 11
Beaver blades (1) No. 64, (1) No. 65
Marking pen or methylene blue
Needle magnet or counter
Syringes (2) Luer-lock control, and needles (2) 25 or 27
    gauge
Local anesthetic with epinephrine
Suction tubing
Antibiotic ointment
Logan's bow

Special Notes

Do not allow preparation solution to pool in or around
the eyes.

CLEFT PALATE REPAIR

Definition

Correction of congenital defects in the palate.

Discussion

The defects result from lack of embryonic development
of elements of the prepalate (face, lips, premaxilla, and
incisors) and the palate (hard and soft palate, uvula,
and additional maxillary teeth). Multiple combinations
and defects exist. In severe defects, nursing and respiratory problems may be present. To minimize speech
difficulties, repair is desirable prior to age 2 years. Mobilization of lateral tissue (by undermining it) allows

for midline closure. Anterior detachment of the hard and soft palate allows "push back" of the whole palate. Secondary repairs are performed to correct residual fistula, to correct speech problems, and to facilitate dental restoration.

Procedure

General anesthesia is administered, and an endotracheal tube is inserted. In addition, a local anesthetic containing epinephrine is infiltrated locally to aid hemostasis. For repair of a complete unilateral (prepalatal and palatal) defect, soft palate margins are incised. Layers for oral mucosa, muscle, and nasal mucosa are developed. The pterygoid hamulus is fractured, and mucoperiosteal flaps are elevated. Nasal mucosal flaps are freed and sutured. The nasal mucosa of the soft palate is sutured. The greater palatine vessels are preserved. Holes may be drilled in the hard palate for suture placement. Bone grafts may be employed. Muscle layers, and the oral mucosa are sutured.

Preparation of the Patient

The patient is supine with the head at the foot of the table. The table may be in slight reverse Trendelenburg position. For the pediatric patient special measures must be taken to prepare the room, restrain the patient, and maintain the patient's body temperature. Refer to Pediatric General Information, pp. 518–520.

Skin Preparation

Check with the surgeon regarding choice of preparation solution. Begin at the upper lip, cleanse the face extending from the hairline to the shoulders, and down to the table at the sides of the neck.

Draping

See Cleft Lip Repair, p. 394.

Equipment

Padded restraints
Warming mattress or heating lamps (optional)

Suction
Electrosurgical unit (bipolar)
Sitting stools (optional)
Power source for power drill

Instrumentation

Basic plastic procedures tray
Power drill (small), cord, and drill bits (fine)

Supplies

Basin set
Bayonet bipolar electrocoagulating forceps
Blades (1) No. 15, (1) No. 11, (1) No. 12
Syringes (2) Luer-lock control, and needles (2) 25 or 27
    gauge
Local anesthetic with epinephrine
Suction tubing
Needle magnet or counter

Special Notes

Some surgeons may allow the patient's head to extend
over the edge of the table, supporting it in the surgeon's
lap. The surgeon's lap is covered with a drape sheet
clipped to the table.

The table may be turned to facilitate access.

REDUCTION OF A NASAL FRACTURE

Definition

Molding and realignment of the nasal bones and septum.

Discussion

Fractures of the nasal bones, cartilage, septum, and
frontal processes of the maxilla occur in multiple combinations. Most often reduction is accomplished by the
closed method.

Procedure

A forceps (e.g., Asch) is placed to provide traction under
the nasal bones. External digital manipulation reduces
the fracture. Nasal packing is inserted, and a nasal

splint is applied. If the results of closed reduction are unsatisfactory, open reduction exposing the septum and portions of the nasal bones may be required. Modified rhinoplastic techniques are necessary to realign malpositioned bony and cartilaginous fragments, which may be stabilized by intranasal sutures. Nasal packing is inserted, and an external nasal splint is applied.

Preparation of the Patient

The patient is supine; arms may be tucked in at the patient's side and secured with padded restraints. The procedure may be performed under local anesthesia. The surgeon usually does a preliminary nasal preparation. If an anesthetist is not in attendance, see circulator responsibilities, pp. 34–35.

Preliminary Nasal Preparation (on a "Clean" Tray)

Packing (e.g., ½" plain gauze or cotton)
Cotton-tipped applicators (long; wood or metal)
Medicine cups (2)
Topical anesthetic (e.g., cocaine 4% or 5%)
Local anesthetic with epinephrine
Syringes (2) Luer-lock control, and needles (2) 25 or 27 gauge
Atomizer
Scissors (e.g., straight Mayo)
Bayonet forceps

Skin Preparation

Closed Reduction. None is required for closed reduction.
Open Reduction. Check with the surgeon regarding the type of preparation solution. Begin at the nose, cleanse the face and neck extending from the hairline to the shoulders, and down to the table at the sides of the neck.

Draping

Closed Reduction. None is required for closed reduction; the patient's body may be covered with a drape sheet. The Mayo stand is draped. Gloves are worn.
Open Reduction. See Cleft Lip Repair, p. 394.

Equipment

Restraints, padded
Suction
Fiberoptic headlight and light source

Instrumentation

Closed. Frazier suction tip, bayonet forceps, Asch forceps (or rubber shod Crile forceps, straight)
Open. Nasal procedures tray

Supplies

Closed
Suction tubing
Small basin
Nasal splint
Nasal packing

Open
Basin set
Blades (2) No. 15
Suction tubing
Needle magnet or counter
Antibiotic ointment (optional)
Nasal packing
Nasal splint

Special Notes

Do not allow preparation solution to pool in or around the eyes.
    The table may be turned for easier access.
    The table may be flexed for patient's comfort.

REDUCTION OF A MANDIBULAR FRACTURE

Definition

Correction of malocclusion resulting from a fracture of the lower jaw.

Discussion

Numerous presentations occur; all should be reduced and fixed as soon as possible after the injury. When the fracture is anterior (so that teeth are on either side of the fracture), intermaxillary fixation may suffice. For fractures posterior to the teeth, intermaxillary fixation and open reduction are necessary.

Procedure

Closed Reduction. For closed reduction, an arch bar is bent to conform to the teeth and the dental arch. Fine wire encircles the necks of the teeth, attaching the teeth to the bars. The maxillary and mandibular bars may be placed in occlusion, or multiple small latex bands may be attached to the bars, which also produce occlusion.

Open Reduction. In open reduction, an incision (one or more) is made below the inferior border of the mandible. The fracture site(s) is(are) exposed, and the periosteum reflected. The fracture is reduced. Holes may be drilled into the mandible on both sides of the fracture. Wires passed through the holes maintain alignment. The fracture site may be stabilized with bone fragments. The wound(s) is(are) closed in layers. A small drain may be placed. Arch bars may be applied prior to or following the open reduction.

Preparation of the Patient

The patient is supine; arms may be tucked in at the patient's sides and secured with padded restraints. The head may be positioned on a headrest. Apply electrosurgical dispersive pad for open reduction.

Skin Preparation

Closed Reduction. None is required.
Open Reduction. Check with the surgeon regarding choice of preparation solution. Cleanse face, ears, and neck (including the sides and back of the neck) extending from hairline to shoulders. Some surgeons prepare the inside of the mouth with swabs saturated in preparation solution.

Draping

Closed Reduction. None is required; however, a Mayo stand cover and a drape sheet (for back table) are

necessary. A sheet may be draped over the patient's
body and a towel placed over the eyes. This procedure
is "clean," not sterile. Gloves (only) are required.

Open Reduction. See Open Reduction of a Carpal
Bone Fracture, p. 297.

Equipment

Headrest (e.g., Richards, Shea, doughnut)
Restraints, padded
Suction
Electrosurgical unit
Power source for power drill
Fiberoptic headlight and light source

Instrumentation

**Closed Reduction and Application of
Intermaxillary Wiring**
Suction tip (e.g., Yankauer)
Arch bars and latex bands (or other intermaxillary
wiring device)
Wire cutters, Freer septal elevator, Weider tongue
depressors (large and small), Heaney needle holders
Minor orthopedic procedures tray (available)

Open Reduction
Minor orthopedic procedures tray
Weider tongue depressors (large and small)
Power drill (e.g., Mini Stryker or Hall II, cord, drill
bits)

Supplies

Closed Reduction
Small basin
Suction tubing
Stainless steel wire (25 or 26 gauge)

Open Reduction
Basin set
Suction tubing
Stainless steel wire (25, 26, or 28 gauge)
Blades (2) No. 15
Marking pen

Electrosurgical pencil
Bulb syringe
Drain (e.g., Penrose ¼", optional)
Local anesthetic with epinephrine (hemostasis),
syringes (2) Luer-lock control, and needles (2) 25 or
27 gauge (optional)
Nerve stimulator (locator) (e.g., Concept) (op-
tional)

Special Notes

The table may be turned to facilitate access.

Do not allow preparation solution to pool in or around
eyes or ears.

If arch bars (or other intermaxillary wiring devices)
are applied first, a separate setup is required for the
open reduction.

The surgeon may request the scrub person to irrigate
(slow trickle of saline) over the drill point to prevent
buildup of heat from the friction of the power drill.

Protective goggles may be worn.

Always have (disposable) wire cutters accompany
patient on leaving the operating room.

REDUCTION OF A ZYGOMATIC FRACTURE

Definition

Correction of fracture(s) of the cheek (zygoma or malar
bone).

Discussion

The two most common zygomatic fractures are depressed fractures of the arch and trimalar fractures.
Closed reduction is the treatment for zygomatic arch
fractures. Trimalar fractures are treated by open reduction and internal fixation.

Procedure

Small, access incisions to the fracture fragments are
made in the lateral third of the eyebrow and in the infraorbital region. Holes are drilled in the fragments,
through which stainless steel wires are passed. The

fragments are realigned, and the position is maintained by the wires. The incisions are closed.

Preparation of the Patient

The patient is supine; arms may be tucked in at the patient's sides and secured with padded restraints. The head may be positioned on a headrest. Apply electrosurgical dispersive pad if monopolar electrosurgical unit is used.

Skin Preparation

Closed Reduction. None is usually required. Check with the surgeon.

Open Reduction. Check with the surgeon regarding the type of preparation solution. Begin cleansing the affected cheek. Cleanse the face and neck from the hairline to the shoulders; include the ear on the affected side.

Draping

None is usually required for *closed reduction;* the patient's body may be covered with a drape sheet. If instrumentation is used, the Mayo stand and back table are draped.

For *open reduction,* see Cleft Lip Repair, p. 394.

Equipment

Restraints, padded

Open Reduction
Headrest (e.g., Richards, Shea, doughnut)
Suction
Power source for power drill
Electrosurgical unit, monopolar or bipolar

Instrumentation

Closed Reduction. Check with the surgeon.

Open Reduction
Limited procedure tray
Minor orthopedic procedures tray (available)

Kerrison rongeurs, bone hook
Power drill, cord, and drill bits
Wire cutter

Supplies (Open Reduction)

Basin set
Blades (2) No. 15
Marking pen
Electrosurgical pencil or bayonet bipolar electrocoagu-
    lating forceps
Suction tubing
Bulb syringe
Stainless steel wire (e.g., 25, 26, or 28 gauge)
Local anesthetic with epinephrine (hemostasis), sy-
    ringes (2) Luer-lock control, and needles (2) 25 or 27
    gauge

Special Notes

Do not allow preparation solution to pool in or around
eyes and ears.
    The table may be turned to facilitate access.
    The table may be flexed for the patient's comfort.

OPEN REDUCTION OF AN ORBITAL
FLOOR FRACTURE

Definition

Elevation and restoration of the integrity of the thin
bone that supports the eye and intraorbital tissues.

Discussion

Orbital floor fractures often occur in combination with
other facial fractures (maxillary and zygomatic).
Blowout fracture refers to an isolated depressed fracture of the orbital floor (with the infraorbital rim intact), often with the orbital contents protruding into
the maxillary sinus. Various structures including the
infraorbital nerve and extraoccular muscles must be
recognized and protected. Repair should be done
promptly.

Procedure

An incision is made over the infraorbital rim (avoiding injury medially to the orbicularis oculi muscle) and continued down to the periosteum. The periosteum is incised and reflected over the fracture site. Debris is removed from the fracture site. The defect may be covered with a synthetic material (e.g., a Teflon or Silastic sheet), autogenous cartilage, or bone. The globe is rotated to test the security of the implant and to make certain the inferior rectus muscle is not trapped. The periosteum is sutured back to its site of origin, as are the orbicularis oculi muscle and skin. An ice pack may be applied following the application of an antibiotic eye ointment and an eye patch.

Preparation of the Patient

The patient is supine; arms may be tucked in at the patient's sides. The head may be positioned on a headrest. Apply electrosurgical dispersive pad if monopolar electrosurgical unit is used.

Skin Preparation

Check with the surgeon regarding the type of preparation solution to be used. Begin cleansing the operative eyelid; cleanse the face and neck from the hairline to the shoulders; include the ear on the affected side.

Draping

See Cleft Lip Repair, p. 394.

Equipment

Headrest (e.g., doughnut)
Electrosurgical unit, monopolar or bipolar
Power source for power drill (optional)
Suction
Fiberoptic headlight and light source (optional)
Sitting stools (optional)

Instrumentation

Basic eye procedures tray
Globe and orbit procedures tray

Minor orthopedic procedures tray (available for bone graft)
Bone hook
Power drill, cord, and drill bits (for implant)

Supplies

Basin set
Needle magnet or counter
Blades (2) No. 15
Marking pen
Bulb syringe
Suction tubing
Electrosurgical pencil with needle tip or bipolar electrocoagulating forceps
Orbital floor implant material (Teflon or Silastic sheet) (available)
Local anesthetic with epinephrine (for hemostasis), syringes (2) Luer-lock control, and needles (2) 25 or 27 gauge
Cotton-tipped applicators or cellulose sponges
Antibiotic ophthalmic ointment
Ice pack (available)

Special Notes

The procedure may be performed by a plastic surgeon, ophthalmologist, or otorhinolaryngologist; equipment, instrumentation, and supplies particular to that specialty must be taken into consideration when setting up.

The table may be turned to facilitate access.

Do not allow preparation solution to pool in or around eyes and ears. Irrigate eyes from inner to outer canthus.

If cartilage or bone is to be taken for an autogenous graft, check with the surgeon regarding donor site.

RHINOPLASTY

Definition

Correction of the external appearance of the nose.

Discussion

In addition to cosmetic considerations, this procedure is performed to alleviate nasal airway problems caused by a deviated septum and nasal trauma not relieved by closed reduction. Four interrelated steps may be employed: tip remodeling, hump removal, narrowing, and septoplasty. Rhinoplasty is modified according to each patient's needs. The surgeon must endeavor to maintain proper shape, symmetry, and proportion. Mentoplasty Augmentation (see p. 409) is often performed in conjunction with rhinoplasty to achieve a more balanced appearance.

Procedure

Through the nostril an intercartilaginous incision is made along the rim of the upper lateral cartilage bilaterally, and connected, freeing the skin from over the dorsal septum and anteriorly, freeing the columella. Prominent septal, lateral, and alar cartilage are excised and after reassessment, are retrimmed as necessary. The nasal bones are then osteotomized laterally, medially (and horizontally, if necessary), and compressed to infracture the bones, creating a more normal contour. Rasping smooths any irregularity. Alignment of the septum is achieved. The anterior septum and columella are sutured; alar incisions and marginal (rim) incisions of the lower lateral cartilages are sutured as well. Intranasal packing is inserted, and an external splint is applied.

Preparation of the Patient

The patient is supine; arms may be tucked in at the patient's sides and secured by padded restraints. The patient's head may be supported on a headrest. The procedure is usually performed under local anesthesia. The surgeon often does a preliminary nasal preparation before the skin preparation. If an anesthetist is not in attendance, see circulator responsibilities, pp. 34–35.

Preliminary Nasal Preparation (on a Clean Tray)

Packing (e.g., ½″ plain gauze or cotton balls)
Cotton-tipped applicators (long; wood or metal)

Medicine cups (2)
Topical anesthetic (e.g., cocaine 4% or 5%)
Local anesthetic with epinephrine
Syringes (2) Luer-lock control, and needles (2) 25 or 27
  gauge
Atomizer
Scissors (e.g., straight Mayo)
Bayonet forceps

Skin Preparation

Check with the surgeon regarding type of preparation
solution to be used. Begin at the nose, cleanse the face
and neck extending from the hairline to the shoulders,
and down to the table at the sides of the neck.

Draping

See Cleft Lip Repair, p. 394.

Equipment

Headrest (e.g., doughnut, Shea, Richards)
Restraints, padded
Suction
Fiberoptic headlight and light source

Instrumentation

Nasal procedures tray
Beaver knife handle

Supplies

Basin set
Blades (4) No. 15
Beaver blade (e.g., No. 64)
Needle magnet or counter
Suction tubing
Syringes (2) Luer-lock control, and needles (2) 25 or 27
  gauge
Syringe, disposable (for cleaning suction tip)
Long cotton-tipped applicators
Nasal packing
Antibiotic ointment (optional)
Nasal splint

Special Notes

Do not allow preparation solution to pool in and around eyes or ears.

The table may be turned for easier access.

The table may be slightly flexed for the patient's comfort.

MENTOPLASTY AUGMENTATION

Definition

Correction of micrognathia with the insertion of a chin prosthesis.

Discussion

The indication for this procedure is to improve the cosmetic appearance of the chin. The approach is submental or intraoral.

Procedure

A short transverse incision is made in the submental region or in the labial sulcus. A supraperiosteal pocket is created just large enough to accommodate the prosthesis. The implant may be fixed with a deep mattress suture. The wound is closed. A bulky pressure dressing is applied.

Preparation of the Patient

The patient is supine; arms may be tucked in at patient's sides and secured with padded restraints. Apply electrosurgical dispersive pad if the monopolar electrosurgical unit is used. The procedure is usually performed under local anesthesia; see circulator responsibilities, pp. 34–35.

Skin Preparation

Check with the surgeon regarding the type of preparation solution to be used. Begin at the chin, cleanse the face extending from the hairline to the shoulders, and down to the table at the side of the neck.

Draping

See Cleft Lip Repair, p. 394.

Equipment

Electrosurgical unit, monopolar or bipolar

Instrumentation

Basic plastic procedures tray

Supplies

Small basin
Electrosurgical pencil with needle tip or bipolar elec-
    trocoagulating forceps
Marking pen
Blades (2) No. 15
Needle magnet or counter
Local anesthetic with epinephrine
Syringes (2) Luer-lock control, and needles (2) 25 or 27
    gauge
Implant (e.g., Silicone)

Special Notes

Do not allow preparation solution to pool in and around
the eyes.
    The table may be turned for easier access.
    The table may be slightly flexed for patient's comfort.

BLEPHAROPLASTY

Definition

Excision of a protrusion of intraorbital fat and resection of excessive redundant skin of the eyelids.

Discussion

The amount of skin resected depends upon the severity
of the deformity and the age of the patient.

Procedure

An elliptical incision is made in the recess of the or-
bitopalpebral fold of the upper lid according to previ-

ously placed markings. The orbicularis oculi muscle is incised parallel to its fibers at the apex of the bulge. The fat protrudes through the incision and is excised. The upper lid incisions may be covered with moist saline sponges while resection of a portion of the lower lids is done. The skin is undermined. The orbicularis oculi muscle is split. Fat compartments are isolated; the fat delivered, clamped at its base, and resected. The upper lids are checked for bleeding; hemostasis is obtained. Incisions in the upper lids are closed with fine interrupted sutures. The procedure is repeated for the lower lids. An occlusive (not pressure) dressing is applied.

Preparation of the Patient

The patient is supine; arms may be tucked in at patient's sides and secured with padded restraints. The surgeon may mark the eyelids prior to skin preparation and injection of the anesthetic. The procedure may be performed under general anesthesia, but local anesthesia is preferred; see pp. 34–35 for circulator responsibilities regarding local anesthesia.

Skin Preparation

Check with the surgeon regarding the type of preparation solution to be used. Begin at the eyelids; cleanse the face extending from the hairline to the shoulders, and down to the table at the sides of the neck.

Draping

See Cleft Lip Repair, p. 394.

Equipment

Restraints, padded
Electrosurgical unit (bipolar)
Sitting stools, 2 (surgeon and scrub person)
Fiberoptic headlight and light source available

Instrumentation

Basic plastic procedures tray

Supplies

Basin set
Bayonet bipolar electrocoagulating forceps
Marking pen
Blades (3 or 4) No. 15
Needle magnet or counter
Cotton-tipped applicators or cellulose sponges
Local anesthetic with epinephrine
Syringes (2) Luer-lock control, and needles (2) 25 or 27
   gauge

Special Notes

Do not allow preparation solution to pool in or around
eyes.
   The table may be turned for easier access.
   The table may be slightly flexed for the patient's comfort.

RHYTIDECTOMY

Definition

Mobilization and excision of excessive facial skin folds
and subcutaneous tissue in order to minimize wrinkles
and excessive fatty deposits.

Discussion

Rhytidectomy is often combined with blepharoplasty
(see pp. 410–411).

Procedure

The incision follows previously made markings that follow the anterior contour of the ear extending superiorly
into the scalp, inferiorly curving about the posterior aspect of the ear, and extending posteriorly to the scalp.
The skin and subcutaneous tissue are mobilized by undermining. Care is taken to avoid injury to nerves (e.g.,
the facial nerve branches, the greater auricular nerve).
After hemostasis is secured, plication sutures are
placed in the musculofascial tissues. Tension is placed
on the flap, directing it superiorly and posteriorly as

anchoring sutures are placed. Excess skin is trimmed. Wound closure is completed with fine interrupted sutures. Care is exerted not to distort the ear. A closed suction drainage unit may be placed. A pressure dressing is applied, taking care to pad the ears.

Preparation of the Patient

The patient is supine with the back slightly elevated; arms may be extended on armboards or tucked in at the patient's sides and secured with padded restraints. The head may be positioned on a headrest. The surgeon usually marks the face prior to skin preparation and injection of the anesthetic. The procedure may be performed under general anesthesia, but local anesthesia is preferred; see pp. 34–35 for circulator responsibilities regarding local anesthesia. Hair is rarely shaved, but the surgeon may request that hair around the hairline be secured.

Skin Preparation

Check with the surgeon regarding the type of preparation solution. The patient's face, ears, and neck are cleansed extending from the hairline to the shoulders, and down to the table at the sides of the neck.

Draping

See Cleft Lip Repair, p. 394.

Equipment

Headrest (e.g., doughnut, Shea, Richards) (optional)
Restraints, padded
Electrosurgical unit (bipolar)
Sitting stools, 2 (surgeon and scrub person)

Instrumentation

Basic plastic procedures tray
Deaver retractors (2) 1″

Supplies

Basin set
Bayonet bipolar electrocoagulating forceps

Marking pen
Blades (4 to 6) No. 15
Needle magnet or counter
Local anesthetic with epinephrine
Syringes (2) Luer-lock control, and needles (2) 25 or 27
    gauge
Cotton-tipped applicators
Drain (e.g., Hemovac, Jackson-Pratt) (optional)

Special Notes

See Blepharoplasty, p. 412.

DERMABRASION

Definition

Sanding of the skin to smooth scars and surface irregularities.

Discussion

This procedure removes or minimizes scars (e.g., from facial acne vulgaris and chicken pox). Dermabrasion may also be employed to remove tattoos. Fine wrinkling around the mouth can be temporarily improved with dermabrasion.

Procedure

The skin is stretched by hand and the epidermis is abraded by means of a motor-driven sanding cylinder and/or a wire brush. The area is irrigated copiously with saline during (and following) the procedure. The wound may be dressed with nonadherent gauze (e.g., Owens gauze) and gauze sponges moistened with saline. A compression bandage may be applied.

Preparation of the Patient

The patient is supine; arms may be extended on armboards or tucked in at the patient's sides and secured by padded restraints. The head may be positioned on a headrest. Anesthesia is achieved by infiltration with a local anesthetic. For circulator responsibilities regarding local anesthesia, see pp. 34–35. The surgeon may mark the scars prior to skin preparation.

Skin Preparation

Check with the surgeon regarding the type of preparation solution to be used. Begin with the area to be dermabraded. Cleanse the face, ears, and neck extending from the hairline to the shoulders, and down to the table at the sides of the neck.

Draping

See Cleft Lip Repair, p. 394.

Equipment

Headrest (e.g., doughnut)
Restraints, padded
Power unit (for dermabrader)

Instrumentation

Adson forceps
Straight Mayo scissors
Dermabrader (with wire brush and sanding cylinder) and cord, for example, Stryker

Supplies

Basin set
Local anesthetic with epinephrine
Syringes (2) Luer-lock control, and needles (2) 25 or 27 gauge
Marking pen

Special Notes

Do not allow preparation solution to pool in or around the eyes and ears.

The table may be turned to facilitate access.

The table may be slightly flexed for the patient's comfort.

This is a delicate procedure; keep distractions in the room to a minimum.

Do not leave loose sponges near the dermabrader as they may get caught in the mechanism.

OTOPLASTY

Definition

Most commonly refers to correction of a prominent ear that protrudes unduly from the side of the head; it may also refer to the correction of microtia and other congenital deformities of the ears.

Discussion

The procedure is usually performed bilaterally. The ideal time for the correction of prominent ears is 4 years of age or before the child enters school.

Procedure

A planned skin excision is marked. A new antihelical fold is marked. Several diagonal lines are marked on corresponding sides of the elliptical incision. An incision is made on the distal side, and a flap is undermined. The anterior surface of the cartilage is exposed. The anterior cartilage surface is abraded with a rasp to reduce the perichondrium, thereby subsequently reducing forward curling of the ear. A predetermined wedge may be excised and sutured with nonabsorbable suture. Mattress sutures are inserted through the previously made markings. Overlapping skin is excised. Wound closure is completed with interrupted sutures. A compression dressing is applied.

Preparation of the Patient

The patient is supine; arms may be tucked in at the patient's sides and secured with padded restraints. If the procedure is unilateral, the patient's head may be positioned on a headrest with the operative side up; adequately pad lowermost ear. For bilateral procedure the surgeon will position the head as necessary. Apply electrosurgical dispersive pad. For the pediatric patient see Pediatric General Information, pp. 518–520.

Skin Preparation

Check with the surgeon regarding the type of preparation solution to be used.

Unilateral. Begin cleansing the external ear; extend preparation from the hairline to the shoulders, beyond the midline of the face, and down to the table at the neck of the affected side.

Bilateral. Cleanse each ear; extend preparation from the hairline to the shoulders, and down to the table at the sides.

Draping

The patient is draped with a head drape with the ears exposed (drape sheet and two towels under the head with the uppermost towel wrapped around the head and clipped). A split (or drape) sheet covers the body. An additional drape sheet may be needed to cover the foot of the table.

Equipment

Headrest (e.g., Shea, doughnut) (optional)
Restraints, padded
Electrosurgical unit

Instrumentation

Basic plastic procedures tray
Small rasp

Supplies

Basin set
Blades (2) No. 15
Marking pen or methylene blue
Needle magnet or counter
Electrosurgical pencil with needle tip
Bunnell needles
Local anesthetic with epinephrine
Syringes (2), Luer-lock control, and needles (2) 25 or (2)
    27 gauge
Cotton pledgets

Special Notes

For a unilateral procedure keep lowermost ear well padded to avoid pressure injury.

The table may be turned for easier access.

Do not allow preparation solution to pool in or around the ears or eyes; a sterile cotton pledget may be placed in the ear during preparation and removed following preparation.

REPAIR OF SYNDACTYLY

Definition

Separation of webbed or fused digits.

Discussion

Syndactyly most often occurs in the hand and is commonly found bilaterally. The middle and ring finger are the most frequently webbed. Toe syndactyly does not always require surgical intervention because the movement of the toes individually is not necessary for walking. Fused digits may exist with only skin involvement, but also may occur with other digital anomalies. If webbing involves many digits, full-thickness skin grafts may be done.

Procedure

Zig-zag or Z-plasty incisions are made in the interdigital space(s) to avoid contracture and provide flaps for the web-spacing reconstruction. The neurovascular bundles are protected. Bony and ligamentous defects, if present, are corrected. The incisions are closed. Full-thickness grafts (e.g., skin from the abdomen or the medial aspect of the arm or the thigh) may be required to close defects. Stents are sutured over the grafts. A bulky dressing and splint are applied.

Preparation of the Patient

For *syndactyly of the hand,* the patient is supine; the arm on the unaffected side may be extended on an armboard, and the affected hand may be extended on a hand table. Sheet wadding and a (pediatric) tourniquet are applied to the arm on the affected side.

For *syndactyly of the foot,* the patient is supine; arms may be extended on armboards. The patient is secured to the table with the safety belt over the unaffected extremity. Sheet wadding and a tourniquet (adult or pediatric) are applied to the thigh of the affected side.

The surgeon may mark the skin prior to the skin preparation. Apply electrosurgical dispersive pad (adult or pediatric).

Skin Preparation

Syndactyly of the hand. Begin at the area(s) of syndactyly, and cleanse the hand (including interdigital spaces and nails). Extend preparation from fingertips to the arm (include the elbow).

Syndactyly of the foot. Begin at the area(s) of syndactyly, and cleanse the foot (including interdigital spaces and nails). Extend preparation from the toes to the leg (include the knee).

Draping

Syndactyly of the hand. The hand is held up in a tube (or impervious) stockinette as a sheet is draped over the hand table. A cuffed drape (or split sheet) is draped under the arm. A towel is folded (in thirds, longitudinally), wrapped around the arm, and clipped. A drape (or split) sheet is draped over the arm and shoulder and clipped under the arm. A fenestrated sheet or individual drape sheets complete the draping.

Syndactyly of the foot. The foot is held up in a tube (or impervious) stockinette as a sheet is draped over the foot of the table. A cuffed drape (or split) sheet is draped under the leg. A towel is folded (in thirds, longitudinally), wrapped around the thigh, and clipped. A drape (or split) sheet is draped over the thigh and clipped underneath. A fenestrated sheet or individual drape sheets complete the draping.

Equipment

Hand table
Tourniquet (adult or pediatric) and insufflator

Electrosurgical unit
Sitting stools, 2 to 3 (surgeon, scrub person, assistant
    surgeon)
Cast cart

Instrumentation

Minor orthopedic procedures tray

Supplies

Basin set
Sheet wadding
Esmarch bandage
Blades (2) No. 15
Electrosurgical pencil with needle tip
Needle magnet or counter
Bulb syringe
Marking pen
Stents (optional)

Special Notes

Have x-ray films in the room.

Regarding tourniquet precautions, see Open Reduction of a Carpal Bone Fracture, p. 298, for syndactyly of the hand, and Arthrotomy of the Knee, p. 336, for syndactyly of the foot.

If a skin graft is needed, check with the surgeon regarding the donor site.

DIGITAL FLEXOR TENDON REPAIR

Definition

Approximation of severed ends of a tendon caused by injury or a failed previous tendon repair.

Discussion

When a large gap exists, a graft is employed, often the palmaris longus tendon. Tendons to the digits may be severed from the forearm to the base of the distal phalanx. Injuries between the distal palmar crease and proximal interphalangeal joint should be repaired initially and treated by a tendon graft at a later time. Avoidance of tension, meticulous handling of tissue, good hemostasis, fine nonreactive sutures, and dynamic immobilization are important for success.

Procedure

The incision is made according to the site of the injury. Midlateral digital incisions are often employed. Care is taken to avoid injury to the neurovascular bundle. Pulleys are preserved when possible. The proximal tendon end is retrieved. If length is not sufficient, a graft (e.g., from the palmaris longus tendon) is prepared. The tendon ends are approximated. If the tendon insertion is involved, suture to the bond may be facilitated using fine drill holes. The suture fixing the tendon graft to the insertion is tied over a button on the dorsum of the distal phalanx to prevent soft tissue necrosis. The wound is closed. A splint is applied.

Preparation of the Patient

The patient is supine; the unaffected arm may be extended on an armboard, and the arm on the affected side may be extended on a hand table. Sheet wadding and a tourniquet are applied to the affected arm. Apply electrosurgical dispersive pad.

Skin Preparation

Begin at the repair site; cleanse the hand (including interdigital spaces and nails), extending from the fingertips to the level of the tourniquet.

Draping

The extremity is held up in a tube (or impervious) stockinette as a sheet is draped over the end of the hand table. A cuffed drape (or split) sheet is draped under the arm. A towel is folded (in thirds, longitudinally), wrapped around the arm, and clipped. A sheet is draped over the arm and shoulder and clipped under the arm. A fenestrated sheet or individual drape sheets completes the draping. If a microscope is used, a microscope drape is necessary.

Equipment

Tourniquet and insufflator
Electrosurgical unit
Hand table
Sitting stools, 2 to 3 (surgeon, scrub person, and assistant surgeon)
Loupes or microscope (available)
Cast cart
Power source for power drill (optional)

Instrumentation

Basic plastic procedures tray
Power drill and fine drill points (optional)
Microinstrumentation; see Peripheral Nerve Repair, p. 424.

Supplies

Basin set
Sheet wadding
Esmarch bandage
Tube (or impervious) stockinette
Marking pen
Blades (2) No. 15
Needle magnet or counter
Bulb syringe
Electrosurgical pencil with needle tip
Straight Keith needle and button

Special Notes

For tourniquet precautions, see Open Reduction of a Carpal Bone Fracture, p. 298.

If a graft is to be taken, check with the surgeon regarding the donor site.

PERIPHERAL NERVE REPAIR

Definition

The complete or partial anastomosis of a diseased or injured peripheral nerve.

Discussion

Peripheral nerves may be completely or partially divided by trauma, such as acts of violence, burns, or crush injury, or during the course of surgery (accidental or by intent), particularly with excision of malignant tumors. According to the patient's general condition and condition of the site of injury, it is determined whether primary or secondary repair is appropriate. If a significant length of nerve has been damaged, several methods can be employed to achieve tension-free repair including additional mobilization (avoiding injury to local blood supply), positioning adjacent joints accordingly, transposition, nerve grafting, and less often bone resection. When nerve grafting is necessary, cutaneous nerves (e.g., lateral antebrachial, sural) are used.

After areas of fibrosis or neuroma have been excised, when feasible, direct anastomosis should be effected with anatomical alignment of fascicles to improve ultimate function. The operating microscope and nerve stimulator are employed.

Procedure

For upper or lower extremity procedures, general, regional, or local anesthesia is employed. Most often a pneumatic tourniquet is utilized. The course of the involved nerve is marked on the skin, and an excision extending beyond the anticipated site of mobilization is made. The uninvolved nerve proximal and distal to the site of injury is carefully mobilized prior to dissecting the involved segment. To preserve alignment, longitudinal epineurial vessels are identified or marking sutures placed. Care is taken to avoid injury to the local branches. When necessary, endoneurolysis (dissection of the nerve trunk) is performed, disturbing uninvolved neural tissues as little as possible. Anastamosis is achieved after fascicles are rotationally aligned and approximated, employing fine nylon sutures (8-0 to 10-0 monofilament). The epineurium is sutured to add stability to the repair. Hemostatic agents such as Gelfoam and thrombin may be employed. The wounds are closed, and splinting is applied as necessary. During the course of the surgery a nerve stimulator is used to identify whether nerve tissue is functioning.

Preparation of the Patient

The patient is supine; for *upper extremity peripheral nerve repair,* the unaffected arm may be extended on an armboard, and the affected arm may be extended on a hand table. Sheet wadding and a tourniquet are applied to the affected arm.

For *lower extremity peripheral nerve repair,* a tourniquet is applied to the affected extremity, and the safety strap is secured over the thigh of the unaffected extremity.

Apply electrosurgical dispersive pad.

Skin Preparation

Upper Extremity Peripheral Nerve Repair. Begin at the repair site; cleanse the hand (including nails and interdigital spaces), extending from the fingertips to the level of the tourniquet.

Lower Extremity Peripheral Nerve Repair. Begin at the repair site; cleanse the foot (including nails and interdigital spaces), extending from the toes to the level of the tourniquet.

Draping

See Digital Flexor Tendon Repair, p. 421. If a microscope is used, a microscope drape is required.

Equipment

Hand table (upper extremity repair)
Tourniquet and insufflator
Electrosurgical unit
Cast cart
Loupes and microscope (available)

Instrumentation

Basic plastic procedures tray
Microinstrumentation, for example, Castroviejo needle holder without lock, Castroviejo needle holder with lock, von Graefe muscle hook, jewelers' forceps, and Castroviejo-Vannas scissors

Supplies

Basin set
Sheet wadding
Tube (or impervious) stockinette
Esmarch bandage
Electrosurgical pencil with needle tip
Blades (2) No. 15
Needle magnet or counter
Marking pen
Nerve stimulator (locator), for example, Concept
Bulb syringe

Special Notes

For tourniquet precautions, see Open Reduction of a Carpal Bone Fracture, p. 298.

When a nerve graft is to be taken, check with the surgeon regarding the donor site. If another site is used for the nerve graft, that extremity may have a tourniquet, and the extremity must be prepared and draped.

PALMAR FASCIECTOMY

Definition

Excision of the fascia (partial or total) of the palm.

Discussion

Dupuytren's contracture is a hereditary condition caused by hyperplasia of fibrous tissue in the palmar subcutaneous tissues with nodules fixed to the palmar fascia. Subsequent contracture results in deformity and/or contractures of the dermis or digits. The condition may also affect the plantar surface of the foot. The extent of this process is variable and does not always require surgical intervention.

Procedure

For less involved presentations, a short longitudinal palmar incision is made adjacent to the restrictive band, which is resected. For more extensive disease a longer incision with a Z-plasty arrangement is employed, resecting the palmar fascia distally. Care is taken to avoid injury to digital nerves and flexor tendons. A more extensive presentation requires excision of more tissue. Wound closure may be done by primary suture or full-thickness free skin graft (which may be taken from the medial aspect of the arm). An anterior splint is applied.

Preparation of the Patient, Skin Preparation, and Draping

See Digital Flexor Tendon Repair, p. 421.

Equipment

Hand table
Tourniquet and insufflator
Electrosurgical unit
Sitting stools, 2 to 3 (surgeon, scrub person, assistant surgeon)

Instrumentation

Basic plastic procedures tray
Basin set
Sheet wadding
Tube (or impervious) stockinette
Esmarch bandage
Electrosurgical pencil with needle tip
Blades (2) No. 15
Needle magnet or counter
Marking pen

Special Notes

For tourniquet precautions, see Open Reduction of a Carpal Bone Fracture, p. 298.

When a skin graft is to be taken, check with the surgeon regarding donor site.

REDUCTION MAMMOPLASTY

Definition

Excision of excessive breast tissue and reconstruction of the breasts.

Discussion

The principle indication for this procedure is alleviation of symptoms associated with breast weight
(greater than 0.45 kg or approximately 1 pound). The
technique employed is determined by the size of the
breast and the surgeon's preference. Proper symmetry
including nipple and areolar position must be maintained. Two categories of procedures are performed:
lateralizing, in which no scar is left medially, and procedures that result in an inverted T-scar. The nipple is
usually transplanted as a pedicle but may (with the
areola) be reapplied as a free graft.

Procedure

The incisions are marked. An incision circumscribes the
areola, which is usually left attached to underlying tissue
as a pedicle graft. Flaps are developed excising a wedge
of excessive (breast) skin and adipose tissue inferiorly; a
Freeman areola marker may be used. The breast is reconstructed by approximating the medial and lateral
breast tissue with skin flaps inferior to the nipple site,
and transversely, in the inframammary fold (creating an
inverted T). A closed suction unit may be employed. A
bulky dressing and a surgical bra may be applied.

Preparation of the Patient

The patient is either supine or in a modified sitting position with arms extended on armboards and the feet
supported by a padded footrest. Apply electrosurgical
dispersive pad.

Skin Preparation

Cleanse both breasts beginning at the nipples; extend
preparation from the neckline to the level of the iliac
crests. Cleanse the axilla well and prepare down to the
table at the sides.

Draping

Folded towels and a transverse sheet (which may be
   cut) or individual drape sheets

Equipment

Padded footrest (modified sitting position)
Electrosurgical unit
Scales (for weighing breast tissue)
Fiberoptic headlight and light source

Instrumentation

Basic/Minor procedures tray
Freeman areola marker

Supplies

Basin set
Blades (4 to 6) No. 10
Marking pen
Electrosurgical pencil
Needle magnet or counter
Drainage unit, for example, Hemovac (optional)
Surgical bra (optional)

Special Notes

Keep tissue removed from each breast separate.

Weigh and record amount of tissue taken from each breast.

The surgeon may request a surgical bra over the dressing; the nipples are left undressed for observation of viability.

AUGMENTATION MAMMOPLASTY

Definition

Implantation of breast prostheses for the purpose of enlarging the breasts.

Discussion

Indications for this procedure are micromastia (unilateral or bilateral), postpartum involution of the breasts, ptosis, and postsurgical deformity. The approach may be inframammary, periareolar, or transaxillary. The silicon rubber prostheses can be filled with gel, inflatable, or filled with gel and saline. Currently under development are endoscopic techniques to create implant pockets through minimal incisions.

Procedure

Inframammary. The line of the incision is marked. A 3 to 4 cm incision is placed just above the inframammary crease. A flap is developed inferiorly to the pectoralis fascia. A plane is developed between the pectoralis fascia and the posterior capsule of the breast. A pocket is created by blunt dissection to accommodate the implant. Care is taken to avoid intercostal nerve damage. Meticulous hemostasis is obtained; a fiberoptic lighted retractor may be employed. The implant is inserted. The subcutaneous flap is approximated. The skin may be closed using a running subcuticular closure.

Periareolar. The line of the incision is marked circumferentially. The incision is made along the inferior border of the areola. The subcutaneous tissue is dissected to the inferior border of the breast. The retromammary space is enlarged by blunt dissection to accommodate the prosthesis. Hemostasis is accomplished; a fiberoptic lighted retractor may be employed for better visualization. The prosthesis is inserted. The inferior border of the breast tissue is sutured to the pectoralis fascia. The periareolar incision may be closed with a subcuticular suture.

Transaxillary. The line of the incision is marked in the axilla. The vertical or oblique incision is carried down through the subcutaneous tissue. Using blunt dissection, a pocket over the upper pole of the sternum is dissected. Hemostasis is achieved; a fiberoptic lighted retractor may be employed. The prosthesis is inserted. The wound is closed in layers.

Preparation of the Patient

The patient is supine with arms extended on armboards. Apply electrosurgical dispersive pad.

Skin Preparation

Cleanse both breasts beginning at incisional sites (areolar, transaxillary, or inframammary). Extend preparation from the neckline to the umbilicus; cleanse the axilla and continue down to the table at the sides.

Draping

Folded towels and a transverse sheet

Equipment

Electrosurgical unit
Fiberoptic headlight and light source (optional)
Fiberoptic light source (for lighted retractor, optional)

Instrumentation

Basic/Minor procedures tray
Fiberoptic lighted retractor and cord (optional)

Supplies

Basin set
Blades (2) No. 10, (2) No. 15
Marking pen
Electrosurgical pencil
Needle magnet or counter
Skin closure strips (optional)
Surgical bra (optional)

Special Notes

The surgeon may request a surgical bra over the dressing; the nipples are left undressed for observation of viability.

ABDOMINOPLASTY / ABDOMINAL LIPECTOMY

Definition

Removal of loose, redundant abdominal skin and underlying subcutaneous fat, and the repair of the rectus muscle as necessary.

Discussion

There are variations in technique according to fat distribution and the surgeon's preference.

Procedure

A W-shaped incision approximately 2.5 cm (1 inch) above the inguinal folds may be used. The umbilicus is incised in a diamond shape and preserved for later replacement under the flap. Dissection is begun at the lower portion of the W-incision and progresses upward, leaving a fine layer of areolar tissue over the fascia. Each lateral branch of tissue is excised. The amount of tissue excised is carefully estimated before removal so that the defect can be closed with moderate tension. If there is diastasis of the rectus abdominis muscle, it is plicated. Large ventral hernias may be repaired with synthetic mesh. The wound is closed with heavy absorbable suture in the deep fat; the skin is closed with a subcuticular running suture. The vertical branch of the incision is closed first. The umbilicus is located in the vertical scar. Drains may be employed.

Preparation of the Patient

The patient is supine with arms extended on armboards. Check with the surgeon regarding slight flexion of the hips. Apply electrosurgical dispersive pad.

Skin Preparation

Begin cleansing for a low, transverse abdominal incision. Extend preparation from the midthorax to knees, and down to the table at the sides.

Draping

Folded towels and a transverse sheet (cut as necessary) or individual drape sheets

Equipment

Electrosurgical unit
Suction
Fiberoptic headlight and light source (available)
Scales (for weighing specimen)

Instrumentation

Basic/Minor procedures tray
Extra Crile and Kocher (or other grasping) clamps

Supplies

Basin set
Blades (4) No. 10
Needle magnet or counter
Marking pen
Electrosurgical pencil
Suction tubing
Drainage unit (e.g., Hemovac, Jackson-Pratt)

LIPOSUCTION

Definition

Removal of subcutaneous fat deposits employing a high-pressure vacuum-suctioning device.

Discussion

This procedure is performed for cosmetic purposes to reduce disproportionately large collections of fat in a specific area such as the hips, thighs, or abdomen; it is not performed for weight reduction. Other areas of the body for which liposuction may be employed include the chin, breasts, arms, knees, calves, buttocks, and ankles.

Procedure

The surgeon may preinject the areas where liposuction is to be employed with a solution of local anesthesia with epinephrine, to reduce bleeding, and hyaluronidase (Wydase), to minimize tissue swelling. Through a 1 cm incision, a blunt suction tip is inserted and used to tunnel under the skin, separating it from the underlying subcutaneous and connective tissues. The excess subcutaneous fat is then suctioned from the pretunneled areas using a high-pressure vacuum. The incisions are closed. Compression dressing is applied.

Preparation of the Patient

The patient is positioned as for any other surgery performed on that particular part of the body. When liposuction is employed for reducing the abdomen, hips, and thighs, the patient is supine with arms extended on armboards.

Skin Preparation

Begin at the site of the most central incision and extend the preparation appropriate distance.

Abdomen, Hips, and Thighs. Prepare from the nipples to below the knees, and down to the table at the sides. Ideally, two people are needed to elevate the lower extremities, abducting and adducting them as necessary, in order to ensure that the areas around and under each thigh and hip are adequately prepared. The pubic area is prepped last.

Draping

The patient is draped appropriately for performing surgery on that particular area of the body.

Abdomen, Hips, and Thighs. The legs are held up and abducted as each foot is grasped in a tube (or impervious) stockinette. Each stockinette is brought up over the leg covering the knee. A sheet is draped over the end of the table. A towel (folded in thirds, lengthwise) is placed over the pubic area and may be secured with a sterile, plastic adhesive drape. Cuffed drape sheets are tucked in at the patient's sides. An additional sheet is draped under the legs and thighs. The legs are lowered onto the table. A drape sheet covers the top of the field.

Equipment

High-pressure vacuum unit (e.g., Dean medical suction unit)

Instrumentation

Limited procedure tray
Blunt suction tips or blunt cannulas

Supplies

Basin set
Marking pen

Sterile, plastic adhesive drape (optional)
Tube (or impervious) stockinette (2) (optional)
Blade (1) No. 15
Suction tubing (flexible, noncollapsing)
Syringes (2) 30 mL
Needles (2) 22 gauge
Intravenous antibiotic (e.g., cefazolin sodium [Ancef])
    (optional)
Local anesthetic with epinephrine
Hyaluronidase (Wydase)
Pressure girdle

Special Notes

Prepare a local solution as directed by the surgeon (e.g.,
250 mL saline, 75 mL lidocaine [Xylocaine] 0.5% with
epinephrine, and 2 mL [300 units] Wydase).

Keep 30 mL syringes (with 22 gauge needles) filled
with the local solution.

Keep an accurate record of the total amount of solution that has been injected.

A special pressure girdle that covers the abdomen,
hips, thighs, and buttocks should be put on the patient
immediately after the wounds are dressed. The girdle
is opened on the gurney and the patient is lifted onto it.
The girdle is then hooked together.

Chapter 18

Otorhinolaryngological (ENT) Surgery

MYRINGOTOMY

Definition

Incision into the tympanic membrane to remove fluid accumulation.

Discussion

Myringotomy is indicated in acute and chronic otitis media. Myringotomy tubes of polyethylene are often implanted through the myringotomy incision to facilitate drainage of the middle ear. In children, the procedure is performed under general anesthesia.

Procedure

A speculum is inserted in the ear canal. Wax, if present, is removed. The inferior posterior portion of the drumhead is incised for acute and some chronic conditions; an incision may also be made in other positions on the drumhead for chronic otitis media. Culture may be taken. Fluid or pus is suctioned. A drainage tube may be inserted. A small amount of cotton may be placed in the ear canal.

Preparation of the Patient

The patient is supine; the head is positioned at the edge of the table with the affected ear up and the other ear

well padded. The arm on the affected side may be restrained at the patient's side and the other arm may be
extended on an armboard. For preparation of the pediatric patient, see Pediatric General Information, pp.
518–520.

Skin Preparation

The auricle and periauricular skin may be prepared;
some surgeons do not require skin preparation.

Draping

Three folded towels around the ear (optional), and a
drape (or split) sheet; usually gloves only are worn.

Equipment

Restraints, padded
Microscope
Suction

Instrumentation

Basic ear procedures tray
Handgrips for the microscope

Supplies

Small basin
Suction tubing
Myringotomy knife, disposable
Myringotomy tube, disposable (e.g., Pepparella, Shep-
    pard)
Grommet (0.045 size most frequently used)
Culture tubes (aerobic and anaerobic) (optional)
Cotton (optional)

Special Notes

The table may be turned for easier access.
  Check with the surgeon regarding whether the ear is
to be prepared and choice of preparation solution. Do
not allow preparation solution to pool in or around the
ear.

Remove wax from curettes, alligator forceps, and so on, with moistened saline sponge.

Guide suction tip and instruments into the speculum as necessary.

The scrub person grasps the drainage tube in alligator forceps to pass it to the surgeon.

MASTOIDECTOMY

Definition

Removal of bony partitions forming the mastoid air cells.

Discussion

This procedure eradicates infected tissue to obtain an aseptic dry ear. Until this is achieved, procedures to restore hearing, for example, tympanoplasty (see pp. 440–441.), are not likely to succeed.

Types
Simple. Removal of the air cells only.

Modified Radical. Removal of the air cells and the posterior external auditory canal wall. (The middle ear is not disturbed.)

Radical. Removal of the air cells and tympanic membrane and the malleus, incus, tensor tympani muscle, and mucoperiosteal lining.

Procedure

In *simple mastoidectomy* a postauricular incision is made and carried down to bone, exposing the cortex. The mastoid cells are exenterated with a burr. A drain is placed, and the incision is closed. A myringotomy may be performed.

In the *modified radical procedure,* the posterior and superior walls of the auditory canal are resected, combining the middle ear, the attic, and the mastoid cavity into a single space. Drills and burrs are employed; care is taken to avoid injury to the facial nerve and canal skin. A tympanomeatal flap is created and draped over the ossicles to partially line the mastoid cavity. A gelatin sponge may be used to pack the cavity. The incision is closed, and the wound is dressed.

In the *radical procedure* the malleus, incus, tympanic membranes, tensor tympani muscle, and the mucosa of the middle ear are excised. A strip of temporalis muscle may be used to fill the cavity. The cavity may be left to heal by secondary intention. The wound is packed and dressed.

Preparation of the Patient

The patient is supine; the head is positioned on a head-rest and turned to the side with the operative ear up; the other ear is well padded. The arm on the affected side may be tucked in at patient's side, and the arm on the other side may be extended on an armboard; both arms may be secured with padded restraints. Hair is secured out of the field. Apply electrosurgical dispersive pad if electrosurgical unit is to be used. Local anesthetic may be administered before the skin preparation; see pp. 34–35 for circulator responsibilities regarding local anesthesia.

Skin Preparation

Begin cleansing the operative ear extending from the hairline to the shoulder and well beyond midline of the face. Prepare well behind the ear on the operative side.

Draping

Before scrubbing, the surgeon adjusts the microscope. The scrub person drapes the microscope with a sterile cover. The patient may be draped with three or four towels placed around the ear followed by a sterile, plastic adhesive drape (optional). The head is draped with a disposable sheet, placing the adhesive strip at the forehead. Two folded towels (V-shape) are draped at the patient's neck. The patient's body is covered with a split (or drape) sheet.

If disposable drapes are unavailable, the patient is draped with a head drape (drape sheet and two towels under the head with the uppermost towel wrapped around the head and clipped). Three or four towels are draped around the ear followed by a sterile, plastic adhesive drape (optional). Two folded towels are draped at the patient's neck, and the patient's body is covered with a drape sheet.

Equipment

Headrest (e.g., Shea)
Restraints, padded
Microscope
Suction
Power source for power drill
Electrosurgical unit (optional)

Instrumentation

Limited procedure tray
Basic ear procedures tray
Drill (e.g., micro Stryker), burrs, and cord
Suction-electrocoagulator and cord (optional)

Supplies

Basin set
Sterile, plastic adhesive drape (optional)
Blades (2) No. 15
Needle magnet or counter
Suction tubing (latex preferred because of flexibility)
Gelfoam (cut 1 × 1 mm)
Local anesthetic (e.g., lidocaine [Xylocaine] with epinephrine)
Control syringes (2) 5 mL
Needles, for example, 27 gauge (1½″), 25 gauge (1⅛″)
Bulb syringe
Eye patch (available)

Special Notes

The table may be turned to facilitate access.

Check with the surgeon regarding necessity for shaving any hair around the ear.

Check with the surgeon regarding the choice of preparation solution.

Do not allow preparation solution to pool in or around eyes and ears.

Some surgeons use continuous irrigation. Equipment needed includes irrigation solution (e.g., Physiosol), suction tubing, small Y-connector, irrigation set, and straight polyethelene tubing.

TYMPANOPLASTY

Definition

Refers to a variety of reconstructive procedures of the tympanic membrane and middle ear structures.

Discussion

Tympanoplasty restores or improves hearing in patients with a conductive-type hearing loss. This procedure may be performed for chronic otitis media, adhesive otitis, tympanosclerosis, and in conjunction with mastoidectomy (see pp. 437–438), as necessitated by the disease process. Often a flap of atrophic epithelium has retracted into the middle ear; this must be excised along with any infected or questionably infected tissue.

Tympanoplasty is classified according to the condition of the ossicles.

Types
I   Malleus, incus, and stapes are intact and mobile.
II   Malleus is eroded.
III Malleus and incus are absent; stapes intact and mobile.
IV All ossicles are absent, except a mobile stapes footplate.
V   All ossicles are absent, except an immobile stapes footplate.

Procedure

An endaural approach is employed. The tympanic membrane, if not widely perforated, is incised and reflected. The pathology within is assessed; mastoidectomy (see pp. 437–438) may be required. Diseased tissues including atrophic epithelium, fibrotic tissue, and damaged ossicles or any portions thereof are excised. The ossicular chain is reconstructed using artificial materials, homograft, ossicular bone, or fragments of the ossicles. Myringoplasty is performed utilizing temporalis fascia, perichondrium, vein, or periosteum. The edges of the perforation are separated, and the graft is placed on the inner surface of the drum remnant. The middle ear is filled with gelatin sponge fragments combined with blood, which support and nourish the graft. Skin flaps, if employed, may be sutured. A protective dressing is applied.

Preparation of the Patient, Skin Preparation, and Draping

See Mastoidectomy, pp. 438–439.

Equipment

Microscope
Rigid endoscopic telescope (2.7 mm 0° and 70°) available
Suction
Power source for power drill

Instrumentation

Basic ear procedures tray
Drill (e.g., micro Stryker), burrs, and cord

Supplies

Basin set
Blades (3) No. 15
Needle magnet or counter
Suction tubing (latex preferred because of flexibility)
Gelfoam (cut 1 × 1 mm)
Control syringes (2) 5 mL
Local anesthetic with epinephrine
Needles 27 gauge (1½″), 25 gauge (1″)
Sterile, plastic adhesive drape (optional)
Bulb syringe
Tongue blade (to smooth graft)

Special Notes

The table may be turned to facilitate access.
   Do not allow preparation solutions to pool in or around eyes and ears.

New blades are used on a graft.

The graft may be smoothed over a flat surface such as an overturned basin.

STAPEDECTOMY

Definition

Removal of the stapes and the establishment of a linkage between the incus and the oval window by placement of a prosthesis.

Discussion

Stapedectomy reestablishes the chain of sound transmission in otosclerosis. Part or all of the stapes footplate may be removed. The oval window can be covered with vein, mucous membrane, connective tissue, collagen, or Gelfoam. Sound transmission may be reestablished with a large variety of materials including the crus of the stapes, Teflon, stainless steel wire, platinum prosthesis, fat, and carved autogenous bone prosthesis.

Procedure

An incision is made in the posterior and superior auditory canal wall above the annulus, creating a skin flap. Bone is excised, to visualize the oval window, using burrs or curettes. The tympanic membrane is reflected. Care is taken to avoid injury to the chorda tympani nerve. The extent of the pathologic process is assessed to determine the extent of the stapes excision. The type of prosthesis to be used is based on the dimensions and the degree of sclerosis. The crus of the stapes and the footplate are transsected and removed (completely or partially). The stapedius tendon is sectioned. The remaining footplate is distracted and the oval window is sealed by connective tissue and the stapes replaced. In total stapedectomy, after the stapes is separated from the incus and removed, a wire (or other prosthesis) is attached to the incus and placed on the oval window graft. A dry field is aided by the use of epinephrine-soaked Gelfoam pledgets. The skin flap is replaced. Gelfoam is placed over the flap, and cotton is placed in the canal. Antibiotic irrigation and/or systemic antibiotics may be used.

Preparation of the Patient, Skin Preparation, Draping, and Equipment

See Mastoidectomy, pp. 438–439.

Instrumentation

Basic ear procedures tray
Power drill (e.g., micro Stryker), burrs, and cord
Suction-electrocoagulator and cord

Supplies

Basin set
Blade (1) No. 15
Suction tubing (latex preferred for flexibility)
Gelfoam (cut 1 × 1 mm)
Local anesthetic with epinephrine
Control syringe (e.g., 5 mL), and needle (e.g., 25 or 27 gauge [1½″])
Bulb syringe
Syringe (to flush suction)
Prostheses (variety available)
Antibiotic irrigation (optional)

Special Notes

Do not allow preparation solution to pool in or around eyes and ears.

Gelfoam may be moistened with epinephrine, for example, 1:1000

The prosthesis packaging is not opened until the surgeon determines the type and size.

If a graft is needed, check with the surgeon regarding the donor site.

SUBMUCOUS RESECTION OF THE NASAL SEPTUM (SMR)

Definition

Excision of a portion of the cartilaginous or osseous nasal septum beneath flaps of mucous membrane, perichondrium, and/or periosteum.

Discussion

The procedure is performed to provide a clear airway by establishing an adequate partition between the left and right nasal cavity. The procedure may be combined with rhinoplasty (see pp. 406–409). Numerous anatomic configurations of the intranasal structure may be responsible for the obstructive airway.

Procedure

An incision is made anteriorly over the septum to include the mucous membrane and perichondrium, which is then reflected with elevators beyond the septal area to be resected. The septal cartilage is excised carefully, avoiding penetration of the opposite mucoperichondrium. The mucoperichondrium of the opposite side is elevated (not contiguous with the first side) to avoid later communication that may result in fistula. Retracting the flaps, the cartilage is excised. Excessive cartilage should not be removed to prevent postoperative deformity. Occasionally, a cartilage graft may be placed within the flaps. A punch, rongeur, or cutting forceps is used to excise bony fragments of the ethmoid and deviated vomer. A gouge and mallet maybe used for the vomer. The intranasal incisions are sutured. A petrolatum gauze packing is inserted to join the membranes in the midline and aid in hemostasis. An external splint may be applied. A dressing is placed under the nose.

Preparation of the Patient, Preliminary Nasal Preparation, Skin Preparation, Draping, Equipment, Instrumentation, Supplies, and Special Notes

See Rhinoplasty, pp. 407–409.

INTRANASAL ANTROSTOMY/INTRANASAL FENESTRATION OF THE NASOANTRAL WALL

Definition

An opening made into the maxillary sinus though the nasoantral wall beneath the inferior turbinate.

Discussion

The indication for this procedure is chronic purulent maxillary sinusitis.

Procedure

A mucosal incision is made over the inferior turbinate, which is then elevated superiorly with a periosteal elevator. The nasoantral wall and the inferior turbinate are fenestrated, and the opening is enlarged with a rongeur. The inferior meatus of the nasal wall is removed down to the level of the floor of the nasal cavity. Polyps and diseased mucosa are excised, if present. The sinus may be irrigated with saline and suctioned. The sinus cavity is inspected by direct vision. If the disease process appears irreversible, a Caldwell-Luc procedure (see p. 447) is performed. Intranasal packing is indicated only for hemostasis as necessary. A dressing is placed under the nose.

Preparation of the Patient

The patient is supine; the arm on the affected side may be tucked in at the patient's side, and the other arm may be extended on an armboard. Arms may be restrained by padded restraints. The procedure is usually performed under local anesthesia. The surgeon does a preliminary nasal preparation even if general anesthesia is administered. For circulator responsibilities regarding local anesthesia, see pp. 34–35.

Preliminary Nasal Preparation (on a Clean Mayo Stand)

Bayonet forceps
Nasal speculum
Scissors
Atomizer
Packing of choice
Cups (2) medium
Cotton-tipped applicators
Local anesthetic (e.g., lidocaine [Xylocaine] 1% with epinephrine)
Topical anesthetic (e.g., Cocaine 4% or 5%)

Skin Preparation

Check with the surgeon regarding choice of preparation solution. Begin preparing the nose extending from the hairline to the shoulders, and down to the table at the sides of the neck. The surgeon may prepare the inside of the nose and mouth.

Draping

The patient is draped with a head drape (a drape sheet and two towels under the head; the uppermost towel may be wrapped around the head, over the eyelids, and clipped). The patient's body is covered with a split (or drape) sheet.

Equipment

Restraints, padded
Fiberoptic headlight and source
Suction
Electrosurgical unit (bipolar)

Instrumentation

Nasal procedures tray
Limited procedure tray
Metal tongue depressor
Polyp forceps
Nasal snare with wires

Supplies

Basin set
Blades (2) No. 15
Needle magnet or counter
Bulb syringe
Bayonet bipolar electrocoagulating forceps
Nasal packing, for example, ½" Iodoform gauze or petrolatum-impregnated gauze (for bleeding)

Special Notes

The table may be turned to facilitate access.
    Do not allow preparation solution to pool in and around the eyes.

Eyes may be protected with eye patches prior to draping.

CALDWELL-LUC PROCEDURE (RADICAL DRAINAGE OF THE ANTRUM OF THE MAXILLARY SINUSES)

Definition

Creation of an opening into the antrum of the maxillary sinus through the canine fossa.

Discussion

This procedure permits evacuation of diseased sinus and scar tissue under direct vision when intranasal antrostomy alone is inadequate to accomplish satisfactory drainage.

Procedure

An incision is made above the canine and second molar teeth. The periosteum is elevated. The infraorbital nerve is identified and protected. The anterior wall of the sinus is fenestrated with a burr or osteotome, and the opening is enlarged with a rongeur. The pathologic process is assessed. Diseased mucosa, cysts, polyps, and so on are excised. The nasoantral wall in the inferior meatus is perforated, for example, with a trocar. The opening is enlarged under direct vision from the antral incision. The gingival incision is closed with absorbable suture. Intranasal packing is used only for hemostasis as necessary. An ice pack is applied to the cheek.

Preparation of the Patient

The patient is supine; the arm on the affected side may be tucked in at the patient's side, and the other arm may be extended on an armboard. Arms may be restrained by padded restraints. The procedure may be performed under local or general anesthesia. The surgeon usually does a preliminary nasal preparation.

Preliminary Nasal Preparation, Skin
Preparation, Draping, Equipment,
Instrumentation, Supplies, and Special
Notes

See Intranasal Antrostomy, pp. 445–447.

Additional Special Notes

Have ice pack ready at the conclusion of the procedure.

NASAL POLYPECTOMY

Definition

Excision of an edematous hypertrophy of the nasal mucosa resulting from a chronic edematous inflammatory process.

Discussion

Nasal polyps, usually located in the middle meatus, may occur singly or in numbers, and may be pedunculated or sessile. The antrochoanal polyp arises from the mucosa of the maxillary sinus near the posterior sinus wall; these polyps may grow large enough to obstruct the entire nasopharynx. The antrochoanal polyp may recur unless a Caldwell-Luc procedure (see p. 447) is performed.

Procedure

Each polyp is individually encircled with the wire of a nasal polyp snare, grasped with forceps, and amputated. The nasal cavity is packed with a petrolatum-impregnated gauze. The choanal polyp is removed under general anesthesia. The snare wire is passed into the nasal cavity and into the nasopharynx. The wire is looped around the polyp. The polyp is grasped by forceps introduced through the oropharynx and amputated with the snare.

Preparation of the Patient, Preliminary
Nasal Preparation, Skin Preparation,
Draping, and Equipment

See Rhinoplasty, pp. 407–408.

Instrumentation

Nasal procedures tray
Limited procedure tray
Metal tongue depressor
Polyp forceps
Nasal snare, with wires

Supplies

Basin set
Blade (1) No. 15
Cotton-tipped applicators (long)
Nasal packing (e.g., petrolatum-impregnated gauze)

Special Notes

Check with the surgeon regarding the choice of preparation solution. Do not allow preparation solution to pool in or around the eyes.

The table may be turned to facilitate access.

The table may be slightly flexed for the patient's comfort.

DRAINAGE OF THE FRONTAL SINUS

Definition

Permits drainage of the infected frontal sinus by incision through its bony envelope by any of several approaches.

Discussion

This procedure is indicated for chronic infection not responsive to antibiotics or antihistamines and for a spreading acute infection. Drainage is directed externally, with obliteration of the sinus cavity, or intranasally.

Procedure

An incision is made along the inferior margin of the eyebrow to the anterolateral aspect of the nasal bone. The periosteum is reflected. The lacrimal crest is identified. Ethmoidal vessels are controlled and the ethmoid sinus entered; the frontal sinus is then likewise entered after bone is rongeured, removing the floor of the sinus. Diseased mucous membrane is excised using curettes, periosteal elevators and pituitary forceps. Care is taken to remove all involved membrane to avoid later mucocele formation and recurrent infection. Additional ethmoidal cells may be removed. A nasofrontal passage is made by removing a portion of the middle turbinate. Drains are placed to maintain the passage. The external wound is closed and dressed.

Preparation of the Patient

The procedure is usually performed under general anesthesia. The patient is supine; the arm on the affected side may be tucked in at the patient's side, and the other arm may be extended on an armboard. The surgeon usually does a preliminary nasal preparation. Apply electrosurgical dispersive pad.

Preliminary Nasal Preparation (on a Clean Mayo Stand)

Bayonet forceps
Nasal speculum
Packing of choice
Scissors
Atomizer
Cups (2) medium
Cotton-tipped applicators
Local anesthetic (e.g., lidocaine [Xylocaine] 1% with epinephrine)
Topical anesthetic (e.g., cocaine 4% or 5%)

Skin Preparation

Check with the surgeon regarding the choice of preparation solution. The patient's face is cleansed beginning at the eyebrow on the affected side, extending from the hairline to the shoulders, and down to the table at the sides of the neck.

Draping

See Intranasal Antrostomy, p. 446.

Equipment

Suction
Fiberoptic headlight and light source
Electrosurgical unit
Power source for saw

Instrumentation

Limited procedure tray
Nasal procedures tray
Weitlaner self-retaining retractor
Power saw (e.g., Stryker), with oscillating blade and
    cord

Supplies

Basin set
Suction tubing
Blades (2) No. 15
Needle magnet or counter
Bulb syringe
Drain (e.g., small Penrose)
Electrosurgical pencil
Nasal packing

Special Notes

The table may be turned to facilitate access.
    Do not allow preparation solution to pool in or around
the eyes.
    The table may be slightly flexed for the patient's com-
fort.
    Cultures may be taken.

SINUS ENDOSCOPY

Definition

Endoscopic examination of the nasal and paranasal sinuses.

Discussion

Most infections of the nasal sinuses are thought to be
rhinogenic. Sinus endoscopy permits the diagnosis and

treatment of diseases of the nose and paranasal sinuses under direct visualization. Evaluation of the conditions of the lateral nasal wall that usually underlie acute or chronic sinusitis permits the removal of tissue in the ethmoidal prechambers. If necessary, diseased ethmoidal tissue can be excised using endoscopic guidance and radiologic studies (performed preoperatively). Partial or total resection of the middle turbinate as well as more radical procedures such as total sphenoethmoidectomy can be performed, although the more radical procedures are avoided if possible.

Procedure

The procedure is usually performed under general anesthesia, but it may be performed under local anesthesia with IV sedation. The surgeon inserts cotton balls that have been soaked in topical anesthetic (e.g., cocaine 5%), with the excess squeezed out, into the nares. After several minutes the cotton balls are removed, and the endoscope is inserted through each nostril successively. The surgeon injects a local anesthetic with epinephrine into the ethmoidal prechambers bilaterally through a small-gauge spinal needle. The ethmoidal prechambers are examined. The procedure performed depends entirely on the pathology encountered. Diseased tissue (infected hypertrophic mucosa) is excised as necessary (including the ucinate processes and the middle turbinates). Ethmoidectomy may be performed and infrequently total sphenoethmoidectomy. The maxillary sinus ostia are not routinely enlarged. Merocel sinus-pak or nasal packing with topical anesthetic with epinephrine may be employed. Tincture of benzoin may be applied to the face to secure the strings from the packing. A moustache dressing is not required.

Preparation of the Patient

Anesthesia is usually general (with supplementary topical and local), and the patient is intubated (a Rae tube may be preferred). The table is in reverse Trendelenberg, and the patient's head is stabilized with a headrest. The arms may be tucked in at the patient's sides.

Preliminary Nasal Preparation

Packing (e.g., cotton balls)
Medicine cup
Iodine cup
Topical anesthetic (e.g., cocaine 5%)
Nasal speculum (small, medium, large)
Bayonet forceps

Skin Preparation

Check with the surgeon regarding the type of preparation solution to be used. Begin at the nose, and cleanse the face and neck extending from the hairline to the shoulders, and down to the table at the sides of the neck.

Draping

The patient may be draped with three towels placed around the head. A split (or drape) sheet covers the patient's body.

Equipment

Headrest (e.g., doughnut)
Suction
Electrosurgical unit
Fiberoptic headlight and light source
Fiberoptic light source (for endoscopes)
Camera screen (optional)

Instrumentation

Nasal procedures tray
Nasal endoscopy tray
Light cords for endoscopes
Camera, coupler, and cord

Supplies

Basin set
Electrosurgical pencil

Topical anesthetic (e.g., cocaine 5%)
Local anesthetic (e.g., 1% Xylocaine with epinephrine)
Spinal needle (e.g., 25 gauge)
Cotton balls
Defogger (e.g., fog reduction-elimination device)
Sinus packing (e.g., Merocel)
Tincture of benzoin (optional)
Pitcher, suction tubing, 3 ring syringe, 5 mL syringe

Special Notes

Do not allow preparation solution to pool in and around the eyes.

All cords, camera, coupler, and light cords may be soaked in aqueous glutaraldehyde solution (see p. 18).

Room lights may be turned off during procedure. Light from the x-ray viewbox may be used.

Have available suction-cautery.

Have available sterile IV tubing.

Be prepared for specimens to be sent to laboratory (e.g., right and left turbinates and ethmoids).

Keep fog elimination device on the field for the surgeon's convenience.

TONSILLECTOMY AND ADENOIDECTOMY (T & A)

Definition

Tonsillectomy is the excision of the faucial (palatine) tonsils. Adenoidectomy is the excision of the nasopharyngeal tonsils (adenoids).

Discussion

The faucial tonsils and the nasopharyngeal tonsils are aggregates of lymphoid tissue in the posterior nasopharynx that hypertrophy secondary to infection. In children tonsillectomy is relatively simple, whereas in adults, because of long standing fibrosis, the procedure is more difficult. The adenoids are usually atrophied by age 15.

Procedure

The mouth is retracted open with a self-retaining mouth gag. The tongue is depressed with a tongue blade. Adenoids are removed with an adenotome and/or a curette. A tonsil is grasped, and the mucosa is dissected free, preserving the posterior tonsil pillar. The capsule of the tonsil is separated from its bed. A forceps is passed through the loop of the snare and the tonsil is seized. The snare loop is passed over the free portion of the tonsil, and the tonsil is amputated. The fossa may be packed with a tonsil sponge. Bleeding may be controlled with cautery, ties (slip knot), and/or suture. The procedure is repeated on the opposite tonsil.

Preparation of the Patient

The patient is supine; arms may be extended on armboards or tucked in at the patient's side and restrained with padded restraints. A rolled towel may be placed under the shoulders to extend the neck. General anesthesia is given to all children and some adults. Apply electrosurgical dispersive pad if the suction-electrocoagulator is used.

Skin Preparation

None usually required.

Draping

A sheet may be draped over the patient's body.

Equipment

Restraints, padded
Fiberoptic headlight and light source
Footrest, padded (local, adult)
Suction
Electrosurgical unit (monopolar or bipolar)

Instrumentation

Tonsillectomy and adenoidectomy tray
Suction-electrocoagulator and cord (optional)
Bayonet electrocoagulating forceps and cord (optional)

Supplies

Basin set
Suction tubing

Blade (1) No. 12

Tonsil sponges

Anesthetic with epinephrine (for local procedure); syringes (2) Luerlock control, needles (2) 25 gauge spinal

Special Notes

Have alternate suction available.

The table may be turned.

Have ties mounted on a tonsil clamp ready in advance.

Keep tonsils separate, and identify specimens as right and left.

Do not dismantle suction or remove instruments until the patient leaves the room so that they are available in case of sudden bleeding.

LARYNGOSCOPY

Definition

Endoscopic examination of the larynx.

Discussion

Laryngoscopy is performed for diagnosis, biopsy, and/or treatment of laryngeal lesions, for aspiration of secretions, to assess laryngeal trauma, or to remove a foreign body. Use of a microscope facilitates visualization. In suspension laryngoscopy, a self-retaining laryngoscope holder gives the surgeon bimanual freedom. A carbon dioxide laser (see laser precautions in Appendix, pp. 619–624) may be used in conjunction with microlaryngoscopy to remove benign lesions and early malignant tumors of the larynx. With the carbon dioxide laser, excision is facilitated, hemostasis is readily achieved, and there is rapid wound healing with a minimum of postoperative pain and swelling. Lesions removed by laser energy are vaporized by intense heat, leaving a small crater. One disadvantage of using the laser is that tissue can be biopsied, but vaporized tissues are unavailable for histologic examination.

Procedure

The patient's head is tipped back, and the laryngoscope is inserted. The oropharynx and the larynx are inspected; the scope is lifted as necessary. Care is taken not to use the teeth as a fulcrum; a bite block may be used. A self-retaining laryngoscope holder may be employed. The microscope may be used. Lesions may be biopsied, secretions may be aspirated, and so on. For carbon dioxide laser microlaryngoscopy, a micromanipulator, used to direct the laser beam, is coupled to a standard microscope. Stainless steel mirrors reflect the beam to inaccessible areas. A special vocal cord retractor with suction attachments is used to clear smoke from tissue evaporation. Two suctions are employed when performing cancer surgery for rapid clearing of the plume.

Preparation of the Patient

Anesthesia may be general or topical. *General anesthesia:* The patient is supine; arms may be tucked in at the patient's sides. Following intubation with a small endotracheal tube, the table is turned so that the surgeon is at the head of the table. General anesthesia is required for microlaryngoscopy.

Topical Anesthesia: The patient is usually sitting up while the anesthetic is administered; the patient is supine for the procedure. To facilitate passage of the laryngoscope, the patient's head is tilted backward; the neck may be supported with a roll or small sandbag.

Topical Anesthesia Preparation (on a Clean Mayo Stand)

Laryngeal spatulas
Laryngeal mirror
Small basin with very warm water (for mirror)
Topical anesthetic spray (e.g., Cetacaine)
Gauze sponges
Laryngeal syringe with straight and curved cannulas
Cup, medium (medication)
Topical anesthetic (e.g., cocaine 4% or 5%)
Cotton-tipped applicators

Cotton
Tissues

Skin Preparation

None required.

Draping

The patient may be covered with a drape sheet. The
back table is covered with a drape sheet. Folded towels
are used to stabilize the laryngoscope holder. Gloves
are worn.

Equipment

Small roll or sandbag
Fiberoptic headlight and light source
Fiberoptic light source (for laryngoscope)
Suction
Footstool
Microscope and 400mm lens (microlaryngoscopy)
Carbon dioxide laser (optional); see Appendix, pp.
    619–624, for laser precautions.

Instrumentation and Supplies

Bite block
Laryngoscope and cord (e.g., Jackson)
Laryngoscope holder (e.g., Lewy)
Suction tubing
Aspirating tubes (2) (Lukens)
Biopsy forceps (assorted)
Suction tip
Sponge carriers (2), loaded with sponges
Telfa and needle, 25 gauge (for specimen removal)
Small basin with saline
Toluidine blue (stain to detect carcinoma)

Add for Microlaryngoscopy

Double-barrel scope (e.g., Dedo, Jako) and cord
    (use with laryngoscope holder)
Microlaryngeal forceps (assorted), scissors, knife,
    hook, aspiration tube, vocal cord retractor (with
    suction attachments)

Special Notes

Protective eye goggles should be worn.

Have sitting stool available for surgeon.

Very small amount of toluidine blue is needed (approximately 1 mL).

The scrub person works directly from the back table without the Mayo stand.

Pass biopsy forceps with tip closed.

Guide suction tip, forceps, and so on into the scope as necessary.

The biopsy specimen may be removed from forceps with a needle and placed on Telfa; do not crush specimen.

TRACHEOSTOMY

Definition

An opening made into the trachea with the insertion of a cannula to facilitate breathing.

Discussion

The procedure may be done as an emergency, or electively, in order to maintain an airway. Several techniques are used; numerous cannulas are available including those adapted for anesthesia and/or the respirator.

Procedure

A transverse (or longitudinal) incision is made overlying the proximal trachea. The platysma and deep fascia are incised; the thyroid isthmus is retracted superiorly, and the superior tracheal rings are exposed. An anterior disc of the third and fourth tracheal rings is excised (or incised). Stay sutures may be used to mark the stoma, and for retraction, in case of the need to replace the cannula. Several sutures approximate the skin. The tracheostomy tube is held in place with umbilical tapes tied into a square knot behind the neck. A gauze dressing split around the tube is applied to the wound.

Preparation of the Patient

The patient is supine with a folded sheet behind the shoulders to extend the neck; arms may be tucked in at the patient's sides. The procedure may be performed under local or general anesthesia.

Skin Preparation

Begin cleansing entire neck extending from the infra-auricular border to the axillae, and down to the table at the neck and shoulders.

Draping

Folded towels and a sheet with a small fenestration

Equipment

Suction
Electrosurgical unit

Instrumentation

Tracheostomy tray

Supplies

Basin set
Suction tubing
Blades (1) No. 10, (2) No. 15, and (1) No. 11
Tracheostomy tubes, silicone or Portex (preferred), adults size No. 6 to No. 8
Catheters (2) for suctioning tracheostomy tube (e.g., Robinson 14 Fr or 16 Fr)
Electrosurgical pencil
Umbilical tapes
10 mL syringe (to inflate cuff)
Local anesthetic, syringe (Luerlock control), and needles, 25 or 27 gauge
Marking pen (optional)

Special Notes

If the procedure is performed under general anesthesia, an endotracheal tube is inserted. As the tracheostomy tube is placed, the endotracheal tube is withdrawn.

A gauze dressing split around the tube is the customary dressing.

The obturator for the tracheostomy tube must accompany the patient out of the room. It will be needed to reinsert the tube if it becomes dislodged. Tape the obturator to the top of the gurney.

Be certain the cardiac arrest cart is nearby.

The scrub person needs to test the tube cuff for leakage.

EXCISION OF THE SUBMAXILLARY (SUBMANDIBULAR) GLAND

Definition

Excision of the submaxillary gland.

Discussion

The procedure is performed most often for benign disease such as chronic inflammation (sialadenitis), stone (sialolithiasis), or ductal stricture. Tumor, including malignancy, is less often encountered.

Procedure

A transverse incision is made over the gland below the lower edge of and parallel to the mandible. Structures to be protected during dissection are the mandibular branch of the facial nerve, the lingual nerve and hypoglossal nerve. The anterior facial vein is divided and the fascial envelope about the gland incised. The gland is dissected free of surrounding tissues. The facial artery is ligated. Wharton's duct is identified adjacent to the lingual nerve, ligated, and divided. The wound is closed in layers. A closed suction drain is employed.

Preparation of the Patient

The patient is supine with the head turned and the affected side up. A folded sheet may be placed under the shoulders to facilitate access. The procedure is usually performed under general anesthesia. Apply electrosurgical dispersive pad.

Skin Preparation

Begin under the chin extending from the infra-auricular border to the axilla. Prepare beyond the midline and down to the table at the neck and shoulder.

Draping

Four folded towels and a sheet with a small fenestration

Instrumentation

Basic plastic procedures tray
Extra mosquito clamps
Lacrimal duct probes available (exploration submaxillary duct)

Supplies

Basin set
Suction tubing
Blades (2) No. 15
Needle magnet or counter
Electrosurgical pencil
Dissectors (e.g., peanut)
Drainage unit (e.g., Hemovac)
Bulb syringe
Nerve stimulator (locator) (optional)

PAROTIDECTOMY

Definition

Excision of all or a portion of the largest salivary gland.

Discussion

The procedure is performed for inflammatory disease and benign and malignant tumors. Most significant in parotid gland surgery is the course of the facial nerve through the gland dividing the larger superficial portion from the deeper portion. In malignancy, if suspicious lymph nodes are encountered, a radical neck dissection (see pp. 467–468) may be done.

Procedure

An incision is made in the preauricular region, continued inferiorly around the earlobe, and then anteriorly toward the hyoid bone. The fascia is incised. Careful exposure of the facial nerve is necessary; a nerve stimulator can be used to help in its identification. The superficial portion of the gland may be resected after blunt and sharp dissection; removal of the deeper portion may be necessary for malignancy. If a major nerve branch courses through the tumor, it must be sacrificed and a nerve graft substituted. The graft may be obtained from the great auricular nerve or superficial branches of the cervical plexus. Stenson's duct is ligated and divided. The wound is closed, often employing a drain.

Preparation of the Patient

The patient is supine with the operative side of the face uppermost. A headrest may be used. The arms may be tucked in at the patient's sides. Apply electrosurgical dispersive pad.

Skin Preparation

Check with the surgeon regarding choice of preparation solution. Begin with the affected cheek; cleanse the entire side of the face well beyond the midline including the ear, extending from the hairline to the axilla. Some surgeon's request that the ear canal be dried and a cotton ball be placed in the ear.

Draping

Folded towels, sterile, plastic adhesive drape (optional), and a sheet with a small fenestration

Equipment

Suction
Electrosurgical unit

Fiberoptic headlight and light source
Headrest (e.g., Richards) (optional)

Instrumentation

Basic/Minor procedures tray
Thyroid tray
Extra right-angle clamps
Nerve hooks

Supplies

Basin set
Blades (1) No. 10, (3) No. 15
Suction tubing
Electrosurgical pencil (needle tip available)
Dissector (e.g., peanut)
Bulb syringe
Marking pen
Drain (e.g., ¼″ Penrose, Hemovac)
Sterile, plastic adhesive drape (optional)
Nerve stimulator (locator)

Special Notes

The table may be turned to facilitate access.
    Do not allow preparation solution to pool in or around
the eyes and ears.
    A sterile magnetic instrument pad may be helpful.

LARYNGECTOMY

Definition

Complete or partial removal of the larynx.

Discussion

Laryngectomy is primarily performed for malignancy.
Cancers of the larynx are classified according to
anatomic position.
Supraglottic: From the epiglottis to and including the
    false cords
Glottic: Floor of the ventricle to below the glottis in-
    cluding the true cords

Infraglottic: From below the true vocal cords to the cricoid cartilage

Transglottic: Lesions that extend from above the ventricle to true and false cords and subglottically

Associated with these cancers are those of the hypopharynx and pyriform sinus. Numerous presentations may occur from small unilateral lesions to extensive ones, invading widely, with cervical lymph node metastasis. Treatment modalities include radiation, surgery, laser surgery, and palliative measures and chemotherapy in advanced lesions. Hemilaryngectomy, partial or total laryngectomy, local lesion excision, laser treatment, or adjunctive radical neck dissection will be determined by the clinical extent of the malignancy and the patient's general status.

Procedure

For more extensive lesions involving both cords, transglottic lesions, or when laryngeal cartilage is involved, total laryngectomy is done. A curvilinear incision is made above the suprasternal notch. The strap muscles are divided, as is the isthmus of the thyroid gland. The trachea may be divided between rings 2 and 3, and the endotracheal tube replaced in the distal trachea, with the infraglottic area packed to prevent secretions from filling the wound or entering the airway. Skin flaps are elevated. The larynx is sutured closed inferiorly. The superior cornua of the thyroid cartilage and hyoid bone are freed from strap and supraglottic muscles (which may also be excised). A portion of the thyroid may be excised. The constrictor muscles are divided posterolaterally. The posterior aspect of the cricoid cartilage is entered. Dissection continues to the base of the tongue. With traction on the epiglottis and the severed end of the trachea, dissection is completed. The pharynx is closed. The tracheostomy stoma is matured to the surrounding skin, and a trachcostomy tube is placed. The wound flaps are approximated over a closed suction catheter. A moderate pressure dressing is placed.

Preparation of the Patient

The patient is supine; arms may be tucked in at the patient's sides. A folded sheet may be placed under the shoulders to facilitate exposure. Apply electrosurgical dispersive pad.

Skin Preparation

Begin at the neck extending from the inferior auricular border to the axilla, and to the table at the sides.

Draping

Folded towels, sterile, plastic adhesive drape (optional), and a sheet with a small fenestration

Equipment

Suction
Electrosurgical unit

Instrumentation

Basic/Minor procedures tray
Thyroid tray
Tracheostomy tray (available)
Right-angle clamps (finely pointed)
Small Yankauer suction

Supplies

Basin set
Blades (2) No. 10, (3) No. 15
Needle magnet or counter
Dissectors (e.g., peanut)
Marking pen
Suction tubing
Sterile plastic adhesive drape (optional)
Umbilical tape
Electrosurgical pencil (with needle tip)
Catheters (2) flexible, open ended for suctioning tracheostomy tube
Tracheostomy tubes (assorted types and sizes)

Special Notes

Have alternate suction available.
    A sterile magnetic instrument pad may be helpful.

A cuffed tracheostomy tube is inserted in the tracheal stoma until the edema subsides (about 48 hours). It is then replaced with a laryngectomy tube.

RADICAL NECK DISSECTION

Definition

Excision of cervical lymph-node bearing tissue and adjacent muscular and vascular structures.

Discussion

The procedure is done for malignancy of the head and neck region. It may be performed as an independent procedure or in conjunction with primary tumor resection of local structures whose lymphatics drain to the cervical lymph nodes, for example, thyroid, larynx, and jaw. When combined with more extensive resections about the pharynx and larynx, a tracheostomy (see p. 459) is performed as well. Radiation therapy may be performed in conjunction with this procedure.

Procedure

An incision (Y, double Y, T, parallel-transverse, Z) is made in the lateral neck usually from beneath the jaw to the supraclavicular region. Skin flaps are mobilized. The external jugular vein is severed, the deep cervical fascia is incised (including some cutaneous nerve branches), and the sternoclavicular origins of the sternomastoid muscle are divided. The internal jugular vein is isolated and divided. The omohyoid muscle is transsected. Fatty tissues bearing lymph nodes are dissected from underlying structures in continuity with other transsected structures. The insertion of the sternomastoid muscle is divided, as is the lower pole of the parotid gland avoiding injury to branches of the facial nerve. The facial artery and vein are divided, and the submaxillary gland and proximal end of the internal jugular vein are divided after dissecting additional fatty tissues from under the jaw. The tissue bloc is then excised. The accessory nerve may be preserved, and the thoracic duct is protected. The flaps are closed over suction drains. A moderate pressure dressing is applied.

Preparation of the Patient

The patient is supine; the arm on the operative side may be tucked in at the patient's side, and the other arm may be extended on an armboard. Following intubation, the patient's head is turned with the face and neck on the operative side facing uppermost. Pad the lowermost ear to prevent pressure injury. A folded sheet may be placed under the shoulder to facilitate access. A Foley catheter may be inserted in the patient's bladder. Apply electrosurgical dispersive pad.

Skin Preparation

Check with the surgeon regarding choice of preparation solution. Begin by cleansing the neck and face extending from the hairline to the nipples, and down to the table at the sides.

Draping

The patient may be draped with a head drape (drape sheet and two towels under the head with the uppermost towel wrapped around the head and clipped). The neck is draped with folded towels secured with a sterile, plastic adhesive drape or sutured or stapled to the skin. The field is covered with a fenestrated sheet.

Equipment

Suction
Electrosurgical unit
Scales (to weigh sponges)

Instrumentation

Basic/Minor procedures tray
Thyroid tray
Tracheostomy tray (available)
Extra mosquito clamps (24)
Extra towel clips (8)
Right-angle clamps (finely pointed)
Andrews suction

Supplies

Foley catheter and urimeter
Basin set
Marking pen
Suction tubing
Electrosurgical pencil
Blades (2) No. 10, (3) No. 15
Needle magnet or counter
Graduate
Bulb syringes (2)
Dissectors (e.g., peanut)
Umbilical tapes, vessel loops
Nerve stimulator (locator)
Suction drainage unit (e.g., Hemovac)

Special Notes

A sterile magnetic instrument pad may be helpful.
Check with the blood bank that blood is ready and available as ordered.
Weigh sponges.
Measure irrigation fluids accurately.

EXCISION OF LESIONS OF THE ORAL CAVITY (PARTIAL GLOSSECTOMY WITH MARGINAL RESECTION OF THE MANDIBLE)

Definition

Excision of a portion of the mandible and lymphoid bearing tissues of the ipsilateral neck.

Discussion

Lymph channels drain the tongue and floor of the mouth into the cervical glands. Tumor cells may extend directly into the periosteum and cortex of the mandible. When the lesions of the oral cavity (i.e., tongue and floor of the mouth) are excised, lymphoid-bearing tissues as well as a portion of the mandible must also be excised. If inadequate tissue remains for closure, a flap may be transposed (e.g., from the forehead or deltopectoral area), which allows some degree of mobility for the remaining tongue and cheek. The mandible may be transsected for exposure and later repaired with stainless steel wire. Radiation therapy may be combined with surgical treatment.

Procedure

A tracheostomy (see p. 459) is performed under local anesthesia. Following induction of general anesthesia, a radical neck dissection is done (see pp. 467–468). The lower lip is transsected in the midline. The submental region is dissected, excising adipose tissue and lymph nodes. The outer cortex of the mandible is exposed and transsected with a Gigli saw. The tongue is split in the midline to the posterior third and a cheek flap is mobilized behind the last molar. The inner cortex of the mandible including the alveolar ridge is transsected from the outer cortex with a power saw, preserving the latter. The outer cortex is retracted, and the intrinsic muscles of the tongue and muscles attached to the hyoid bone are further transsected in continuity with the remainder of the specimen. The anterior and posterior bellies of the digastric muscle, submaxillary gland, and hypoglossal and lingual nerves are included in the specimen. Reconstruction is begun by stabilizing the remaining mandible with a short Kirschner wire centrally and stainless steel wires passed through drill holes and tightened. Soft tissues are approximated from the tongue to tissue above the hyoid bone and platysma, tying those sutures over the mandible. Additional coverage may be obtained from mobilization of the forehead or a deltopectoral flap. The tongue is again sutured to the platysma. The remaining exposed mandible is covered by tissues of the floor of the mouth and skin. Mucosal sutures complete the repair of the floor of the mouth. The lip is repaired in layers, snugly, to prevent excessive drooling. The neck incisions are closed over suction drains.

Preparation of the Patient

The patient is supine; arms may be tucked in at the patient's sides. A folded sheet may be placed under the patient's shoulders to facilitate exposure. Apply electrosurgical dispersive pad.

Skin Preparation

Check with the surgeon regarding choice of preparation solution and the area to be prepared, particularly regarding the mouth. The entire face and neck may be prepared extending from the hairline to nipples, and down to the table at the sides around the neck and shoulders. The inside of the mouth may be painted with swabs.

Draping

The patient may be draped with a head drape (drape sheet and two towels under the head with uppermost towel wrapped around the head and clipped). The neck is draped with folded towels secured with a sterile, plastic adhesive drape, staples, or sutures. The field is covered with a fenestrated sheet.

Equipment

Scales (to weigh sponges)
Suction
Electrosurgical unit
Fiberoptic headlight and light source
Power source for power saw

Instrumentation

Tracheostomy tray
Basic/Minor procedures tray
Thyroid tray
Tonsillectomy and adenoidectomy tray
Andrews suction
Right-angle clamps (4), finely pointed
Tonsil clamps (4)
Gigli saws, wire cutters, nerve hook
Power saw and cord (e.g., Stryker)

Supplies

Basin set
Marking pen
Suction tubing
Electrosurgical pencil

Blades (2) No. 10, (3) No. 15
Needle magnet or counter
Sterile, plastic adhesive drape
Graduate
Bulb syringes (2)
Umbilical tapes, vessel loops
Nerve stimulator (locator)
Dissectors (e.g., peanut)
Bone wax
Stainless steel wire
Local anesthetic, syringe (Luerlock, control), and nee-
  dles 25 or 27 gauge
Tracheostomy tubes, silicone or Portex (preferred),
  adults sizes No. 6 to No. 8
Syringe, 10 mL (to inflate cuff)
Magnetic instrument pad (optional)
Suction drainage unit (e.g., Hemovac)

Special Notes

Check with the blood bank that blood is available as ordered.

Measure irrigation used for accurate assessment of
blood loss.

Weigh sponges.

Be certain cardiac arrest cart is nearby.

Test tracheostomy cuff for leakage.

Tape the obturator to the top of the gurney when patient is transferred to the recovery room; it will be
needed to reinsert the tube if the tube becomes dislodged.

Chapter 19

Ophthalmic Surgery

GENERAL INFORMATION

Ophthalmic surgery requires close attention to detail. A minor breach of technique could potentially lead to complete or partial loss of vision of the operated eye. Preparation and protection of the operative site and prevention of infection are of paramount importance.

In order to avoid undue repetition, the following will apply to all procedures in this section unless otherwise stated.

Anesthesia

Anesthesia for ophthalmic surgery may require immobility (akinesia) of the globe and lids, anesthesia of the globe and adnexae, control of intraocular pressure, general relaxation of the patient, and prevention of retching, coughing, and blood pressure fluctuations, even after the procedure is completed. The choice of anesthetic depends upon the nature of the procedure, the surgeon's (and patient's) preference, and the general status and level of anxiety of the patient.

Topical anesthesia is effected by the instillation of the agent (e.g., tetracaine 0.5%) into the conjunctival sac. This method may suffice for superficial procedures (e.g., excision of a pterygium) or may precede administration of local anesthesia. Infiltration anesthesia is the direct injection of an agent into the surgical site (as

473

in surgery of the lids). For more involved procedures, a regional block of cranial nerve branches can be employed. For procedures requiring immobilization of the globe, a retrobulbar block and an O'Brien and/or Van Lint block (or their modifications) are performed to provide akinesia of the lids and extraocular muscles. In a retrobulbar block the anesthetic agent is injected into the muscle cone (behind the globe) blocking cranial nerves III, IV, and VI to immobilize the extraocular muscles and to produce anesthesia of the conjunctiva, cornea, and uvea by blocking the ciliary nerve branches. The O'Brien block deposits the anesthetic about branches of the facial nerve (over the condyle of the mandible, inferior to the posterior zygomatic process) to paralyze the orbicularis oculi muscle. The Van Lint block similarly produces paralysis of the orbicularis muscle, anesthetizing facial nerve branches over the periosteum just lateral to the orbital rim. Combining these blocks ensures complete akinesia. General anesthesia or heavy sedation may be preferred and/or combined with conduction anesthesia.

Skin Preparation

Unilateral. Prepare the affected eye extending from the hairline to the inferior border of the mandible (the preparation may extend only to the superior border at some hospitals), and at the sides from the anterior auricular border to well beyond the midline. Begin by cleansing the eyelid, eyelashes, eyebrow, and skin around the operative eye. Do not allow preparation solution to pool in the eye. Using applicator sticks, carefully cleanse the lid margins. Irrigate the eye from the inner to outer canthus using a bulb syringe containing normal saline.

Bilateral. Prepare the eyes extending from the hairline to the inferior border of the mandible. Cleanse both eyes in the manner employed for a unilateral preparation as just described.

Draping

In an attempt to eliminate lint on the field, most ophthalmic surgeons use disposable drapes.

Unilateral. The adhesive-backed strip of a sheet is placed on the forehead. A split sheet is then draped so that the operative eye and the surrounding area fits into the split (V) of the drape; the adhesive-backed tails of the split sheet are secured at the top of the head, and the remainder of the split sheet is draped over the patient's body. A sterile, plastic adhesive drape is placed over the operative eye and the surrounding field.

Bilateral. The adhesive-backed strip of a sheet is placed on the forehead. A split sheet is then draped so that the bridge of the nose fits into the split (V) of the drape; the adhesive-backed tails of the split sheet are secured at the top of the head, and the remainder of the split sheet is draped over the patient's body. A sterile, plastic adhesive drape is placed over both eyes and the surrounding field.

Special Notes

Keep talking and movement in the room to a minimum. Remember that the patient is often awake. Distractions can interfere with the surgeon's concentration and performance.

For procedures in which local anesthesia is used without the presence of an anesthetist, see circulator responsibilities, pp. 34–35.

Local anesthesia (infiltration or block) may be administered prior to final skin preparation and draping.

Hyaluronidase (Wydase) may be added to the local anesthetic solution to enhance absorption and dispersion of the agent.

Eyelashes are not routinely clipped; if lashes are trimmed, it is done prior to the skin preparation. Coat the scissors with a thin layer of petrolatum so that the severed lashes adhere to the scissors (rather than fall into the eye).

Eyes are *always* irrigated from inner to outer canthus.

Powderless gloves are used.

The scrub person may be required to irrigate the eye frequently during the procedure to keep the cornea moist and clear.

Extreme care is taken to protect instruments, especially microsurgical instruments, from damage, particularly the tips and cutting surfaces.

Precautions are taken to keep lint off the instruments and the surgical field.

Ophthalmic drops are instilled into the conjunctival sac.

EXCISION OF A CHALAZION

Definition

Incision and curettage of a granulomatous swelling of the Meibomian gland(s).

Discussion

A chalazion can be a single swelling or multiple swellings, either noninfected or infected, which may sometimes subside sponaneously but otherwise is excised through a conjunctival or skin approach.

Procedure

A *conjunctival approach* is employed when the chalazion is pointing through the conjunctiva. The chalazion is centered in a chalazion clamp, and the lid is everted. The chalazion is incised at right angles to the lid margin, and its contents are evacuated with a curette. The clamp is slowly removed when hemostasis has been effected. For the *skin approach* the chalazion is centered in a chalazion clamp. An incision is made parallel to the lid. The orbicularis oculi muscle is cut exposing the Meibomian gland. The gland is incised and its contents thoroughly curetted. The wound is appoximated. Antibiotic ophthalmic ointment may be instilled, and an eyepad is applied.

Preparation of the Patient

The patient is supine; one arm may be extended on an armboard; the other arm may be tucked in at the patient's side. The head may be supported by a headrest with the head turned (affected side up). The procedure is usually performed under local anesthesia. Topical anesthetic eye drops may be instilled. See pp. 34–35 for circulator responsibilities regarding local anesthesia.

Skin Preparation and Draping

See Ophthalmic Surgery, General Information, pp. 473–476.

Equipment

Headrest (e.g., horseshoe) (optional)
Sitting stools

Instrumentation

Basic eye procedures tray
Eyelid and conjunctival procedures tray

Supplies

Basin set
Sterile, plastic adhesive drape
Cotton-tipped applicators or cellulose sponges
Blade (1) No. 15 or (1) No. 11
Cautery (wet field or disposable)
Balanced salt solution (BSS), tear substitute
Topical anesthetic eye drops, for example, tetracaine (optional)
Local anesthetic (e.g., lidocaine [Xylocaine] 2% with epinephrine)
Dye (e.g., methylene blue) (optional)
Antibiotic ophthalmic ointment (optional)

CANTHOTOMY

Definition

Incision of the canthus.

Discussion

The procedure is indicated when there is an adhesion of the eyelids or when exposure to the globe is inadequate. Canthotomy may be performed prior to cataract extraction or in conjunction with other procedures.

Procedure

A straight mosquito hemostat is clamped over the outer canthus for at least 60 seconds to effect hemostasis. The skin and conjunctiva are incised. Antibiotic ophthalmic ointment may be instilled and an eye patch applied.

Preparation of the Patient

The patient is supine. One arm may be extended on an armboard; the other arm may be tucked in at the patient's side. The head may be supported on a headrest. The procedure is usually performed under local anesthesia. Topical anesthetic eyedrops may be instilled. See pp. 34–35 for circulator responsibilities regarding local anesthesia.

Skin Preparation and Draping

See Excision of a Chalazion, p. 477.

Instrumentation

Basic eye procedures tray

Equipment

Headrest (e.g., horseshoe) (optional)
Sitting stools

Supplies

Basin set
Sterile, plastic adhesive drape
Cotton-tipped applicators or cellulose sponges
Blade (1) No. 15
Cautery (wet field or disposable)
Balanced salt solution (BSS), tear substitute
Anesthetic drops (e.g., tetracaine) (optional)
Local anesthetic (e..g., lidocaine [Xylocaine] 2% with epinephrine)
Antibiotic ophthalmic ointment (optional)

TARSORRHAPHY/CANTHORRHAPHY

Definition

Tarsorrphaphy is the approximation of the margins of the eyelids. *Canthorrhaphy* refers also to approximation of the lid margins, but with a partial excision of the lateral or medial canthus.

Discussion

In cases of chronic corneal ulceration or after the removal of a globe when a prosthesis is not utilized or when the palpebral fissure is abnormally widened as in facial nerve palsy (e.g., Bell's palsy or secondary to surgery or trauma) or in ptosis secondary to Grave's disease, the lids cannot adequately protect the cornea and prevent undue drying of the conjunctival membranes. Tarsorrhaphy is indicated when the condition is either temporary or permanent and can be reversed with a minimal procedure. Permanent reduction of the palpebral fissure is achieved by lateral (and less often medial) canthorrhaphy. Numerous modifications and alternative procedures have been described including tarsoconjunctival flap rotation from the upper lid to the lower lid, and the implantation of a gold weight beneath the orbicularis oculi muscle, and so on.

Procedure

Tarsorrhaphy. Employing topical anesthetic drops and infiltration of local anesthetic into the lids. The lids are grasped and manipulated to determine the extent of closure necessary. The lateral (or medial) lid margins are approximated by placement of mattress sutures passed through the lid margins avoiding the eyelash bearing surfaces. If any tension is created, the sutures are tied over silicone pegs (or other stent material). For a more permanent union a section of conjunctiva is excised prior to suture placement. For reversal (if the underlying condition necessitating the procedure is corrected or resolved), the tarsorrhaphy is incised and the wound surfaces sutured to prevent readhesion.

Canthorrhaphy. After anesthesia is instituted, the extent of the canthorrhaphy is determined (and marked). The lid margin is split to the canthal angle, and a segment excised including the lash follicles; the mucosa adjacent is abraded. Sutures approximate the lid margins and are tied over stents (e.g., silicone pegs). When performed medially, the caruncle canaliculi are preserved. If further support is required, the canthal tendon (palpebral ligament) is shortened and/or sutured to adjacent orbital periosteum.

Preparation of the Patient, Skin
Preparation, Draping, Instrumentation, and
Equipment

See Canthotomy p. 478.

Supplies

Basin set
Sterile, plastic adhesive drape
Cotton-tipped applicators or cellulose sponges
Blade (1) No. 11
Cautery (wet field or disposable)
Balanced salt solution (BSS)
Silicone tubing cut in 3 mm pieces
Anesthetic drops (e.g., tetracaine) (optional)
Local anesthetic (e.g., lidocaine [Xylocaine] 2% with epinephrine)
Antibiotic ophthalmic ointment (optional)

CORRECTION OF ECTROPION

Definition

Correction of an eversion and drooping of the lower eyelid.

Discussion

The method of correction employed depends on the type and severity of the deformity. Ectropion usually occurs bilaterally.

Types

Involutional, the most common type, caused by a relaxation of the orbicular muscle, may occur as a result of aging.

Congenital, associated with Down's syndrome, is the result of an elongation of the lower lid.

Paralytic, in which the orbicularis oculi has lost its tone caused by cranial nerve VII paralysis.

The Byron-Smith procedure, a modification of the Kuhrt-Szymanowski procedure, is employed for involutional ectropion.

Procedure

Byron-Smith Procedure. A skin incision is made below the lid margin extending from the punctum to just beyond the lateral canthus. A second incision (an extension of the first) is made in the direction of the earlobe. A skin-muscle flap is developed and elevated across the lower lid. A vertical incision is made through the tarsus (in the lateral third of the eyelid) and angled into the inferior cul-de-sac. The two free edges of the lid are overlapped until tight, and the redundant portion excised. The two lid edges are approximated. The orbicularis oculi muscle is approximated. The skin is pulled laterally; redundant skin is resected. The skin is approximated. In younger patients, if the punctum is still everted, a tarsal-conjunctival resection may be necessary. Antibiotic ophthalmic ointment may be instilled and an eye pad placed.

Preparation of the Patient

The patient is supine; the arm on the side of operative eye may be tucked in at the patient's side, and the other arm may be extended on an armboard. A headrest may be used. The procedure may be performed under local or general anesthesia. See circulator responsibilities regarding local anesthesia, pp. 34–35. Tetracaine drops may be instilled.

Skin Preparation and Draping

See Ophthalmic Surgery, General Information, pp. 473–476.

Equipment

Headrest (e.g., horseshoe) (optional)
Sitting stools

Instrumentation

Basic eye procedures tray
Eyelid and conjunctival procedures tray

Supplies

Basin set
Sterile, plastic adhesive drape
Cotton-tipped applicators or cellulose sponges
Blade (1) No. 15 or (1) No. 11
Cautery (wet field or disposable)
Balanced salt solution (BSS), tear substitute
Topical anesthetic drops (e.g., tetracaine) (optional)
Local anesthesia (e.g., lidocaine [Xylocaine] 2% with epinephrine)
Marking pen
Antibiotic ophthalmic ointment (optional)

CORRECTION OF ENTROPION

Definition

Correction of an inversion of the lid margins and eye-lashes.

Discussion

Entropion usually affects the lower lid. The condition may be corrected by various procedures.

Types

Congenital is due to hypertrophy of the marginal and pretarsal orbicularis oculi muscle, which causes the eyelid margin to be pushed up and against the globe.

Involutional (most common) occurs when canthal tendons retain their rigidity but the apposition of the lid to the globe is changed (e.g., from senile atrophy of orbital fat) resulting in the inversion of the eyelid, or it may occur as the result of weakness of the retractor muscles of the lower lid.

Procedure

Internal Tarsal-Orbicularis Resection. The lower lid is everted with a chalazion clamp. The line of incision may be marked inside the eyelid. A base-down triangle of skin, orbicularis oculi muscle, and tarsus is excised. The edges are sutured together, and the "dog-ear" edge of remaining tissue is excised. In an alternate method (skin-tarsal fixation), the orbicular muscle is divided and sutured to the lower border of the tarsus.

Preparation of the Patient, Skin
Preparation, Draping, Equipment,
Instrumentation, and Supplies

See Correction of Ectropion, pp. 481–482.

BLEPHAROPTOSIS REPAIR

Definition

Correction of a drooping upper eyelid.

Discussion

The condition may be unilateral or bilateral. Any one of a number of techniques may be employed depending on the type and severity of the deformity.

Types

Congenital: Mild to severe (eyelid droops 1.5 mm to 4 mm or more)

Acquired: May be neurogenic or due to myogenic and aponeurosis defects

Traumatic: Also as a result of ocular surgery

Mechanical: Blepharochalasis or enophthalmos may be the cause

External levator resection is indicated in patients with moderate to severe ptosis and fair to poor levator function.

Procedure

External Levator Resection. A traction suture is placed in the lid to permit downward traction. An incision is made from canthus to canthus and carried through the orbicularis oculi to the superior border of the tarsus. The upper half of the tarsus is exposed. The upper skin edge is grasped, and the orbicularis is separated from the orbital septum. The fat is retracted posteriorly, and the levator aponeurosis is excised. The eyelid is everted, and the conjunctiva is incised. The aponeurosis is buttonholed at its medial and lateral border, a straight hemostat is placed across it, and Müller's muscle and the tissues are transsected. The conjunctiva is reapproximated. Müller's muscle and the levator are sutured to the tarsus. The excess levator is excised. Lid crease skin sutures are placed. The lower lid is pulled up over the globe by sutures placed in the lower lid through a silicone peg or bolster, which are taped to the forehead. These sutures are removed the next day.

Preparation of the Patient, Skin Preparation, Draping, Equipment, Instrumentation, and Supplies

See Correction of Ectropion, pp. 481–482.

LACRIMAL DUCT PROBING

Definition

Opening of the nasolacrimal duct.

Discussion

The procedure is done to prevent acute infection of the lacrimal drainage system. If conservative management of a lacrimal duct obstruction is unsuccessful, probing is indicated. When repeated probings are technically successful but have otherwise failed, an indwelling silicone tube is inserted.

Procedure

The upper canaliculus is dilated with a lacrimal dilator. A lacrimal probe (e.g., size 000) is inserted and passed through the imperforate opening into the nose. The procedure may be repeated with the next larger size lacrimal probe, and so on. A lacrimal cannula is used to irrigate through the upper canaliculus into the nose. Antibiotic ophthalmic drops may be instilled.

Preparation of the Patient

In infants (up to 6 months), the procedure may be performed using a topical anesthetic. The patient is positioned in a mummy-like wrap. The procedure is usually performed under general anesthesia for the child over 6 months. The child is supine. The head and foot of the table may be dropped to provide closer access to the patient. Extremities are restrained using padded restraints. For preparation of the pediatric patient, see Pediatric General Information, pp. 518–520.

Skin Preparation

See Ophthalmic Surgery, General Information, pp. 473–476.

Draping

The patient is usually draped very simply with folded towels around the eye; a body sheet may be used.

Equipment

Sitting stools (optional)
Restraints, padded or mummy wrap (optional)

Instrumentation

Basic eye procedures tray
Lacrimal dilators (e.g., Bowman)
Lacrimal probes
Lacrimal cannula
Safety pins

Supplies

Small basin
Balanced salt solution (BSS), tear substitute
Cotton-tipped applicators or cellulose sponges
Antibiotic ophthalmic drops (optional)

Special Notes

Gloves only may be worn.
    Fluorescein dye may be requested to test the patency of the duct.

EXCISION OF EYELID LESIONS

Definition

The repair of an eyelid defect due to excision of a lesion.

Discussion

Repair of these wounds includes the orientation of the tissue according to skin lines without tension. For additional information see Blepharoplasty, pp. 410–412.

Procedure

In the excision of lid margin tumors, the lesion is removed in a pentagon-shaped pattern, taking care to include adequate tumor margins. Lateral canthotomy is done to effect closure without undue traction. Sutures are placed through the lid margins to restore continuity. The tarsal plate is closed separately with absorbable sutures. The skin is closed with nonabsorbable suture as is the canthus.

Preparation of the Patient

The patient is supine; the arm on the side of the operative eye may be tucked in at the patient's side, and the other arm may be extended on an armboard. A headrest may be used. The procedure may be performed under local or general anesthesia. See circulator responsibilities regarding local anesthesia, pp. 34–35. Tetracaine drops may be instilled.

Skin Preparation and Draping

See Ophthalmic Surgery, General Information, pp. 474–475.

Equipment

Headrest (e.g., horseshoe) (optional)
Sitting stools

Instrumentation

Basic eye procedures tray
Eyelid and conjunctival procedures tray

Supplies

Basin set
Sterile, plastic adhesive drape
Cotton-tipped applicators or cellulose sponges

Blade (1) No. 15 or (1) No. 11
Cautery (wet field or disposable)
Balanced salt solution (BSS), tear substitute
Topical anesthetic drops (e.g., tetracaine) (optional)
Local anesthesia (e.g., lidocaine [Xylocaine] 2% with
  epinephrine)
Marking pen
Antibiotic ophthalmic ointment (optional)

EYELID LACERATION REPAIR

Definition

The repair of an eyelid defect due to traumatic laceration.

Discussion

If the canaliculus is not involved, the defect through
the lid margin is repaired like the incision of a lid tumor; see pp. 485–487.

Procedure

When the canaliculus is injured, especially with children, dog bites and claw injuries, a special Veirs rod
may be placed through the cut end. A nonabsorbable
suture (e.g., 10-0 nylon) is used to reapproximate the
canaliculus around the rod. The subcutaneous tissue
and skin are closed.

Alternatively, a silicone tube with lacrimal probes at
each end pass through the upper canaliculus and the
cut end of the lower canaliculus. The tubes are then
passed down into the nose with the tubes untied. The
rods are removed.

Preparation of the Patient,
Skin Preparation, Draping, Equipment,
and Supplies

See Excision of Eyelid Lesions, pp. 486–487.

Instrumentation

Basic eye procedures tray
Eyelid and conjunctiveal procedures tray

Veirs rod, available
Silicone tube with lacrimal probes, available

DACRYOCYSTORHINOSTOMY

Definition

Reestablishment of a passageway between the lacrimal duct and the nasal cavity.

Discussion

This procedure is indicated in patients with chronic dacryocystitis who have not responded to probing, irrigation, and silicone intubation.

Procedure

An incision is made along the side of the nose 1 cm from the canthus to just above the level of the alar cartilages. Traction is placed on the skin so the deeper incision does not lie directly under the skin incision, avoiding a direct cutaneous-osseous scar. The periosteum is incised and separated from the bone with a periosteal elevator. The sac is separated from the fossa and the superior punctum is probed to identify its location. An H-incision is made in the sac, which is retracted laterally as a power drill is used to remove the lacrimal crest. The nasal packing (from the preliminary nasal preparation) is removed. The nasal mucosa is exposed, and a Kerrison rongeur is employed to enlarge the opening. Care is taken to protect the corneas. An H-incision is made in the nasal mucosa. The flaps of the lacrimal sac and the flaps of the nasal mucosa are reapproximated. Hemostasis is achieved. The nose is packed with thrombin-soaked Gelfoam pledgets or gauze packing (e.g., Adaptic, Iodoform, or petrolatum-impregnated gauze). The subcutaneous and skin layers are closed. A catheter may be passed through the nasolacrimal duct for postoperative irrigation. A folded eye pad may be placed over the incision only.

Preparation of the Patient

The patient is supine; the arm on the side of the operative eye is tucked in at the patient's side, and the other arm may be extended on an armboard. The table is placed in reverse Trendelenburg; a padded footboard is used. The procedure is performed under general anesthesia; however, the surgeon does a preliminary nasal preparation prior to the skin preparation, and local anesthesia with epinephrine may be administered during the procedure.

Preliminary Nasal Preparation (on a Clean Mayo Stand)

Topical anesthetic (e.g., cocaine 4% or 5% or phenylephrine [Neo-Synephrine] 0.25% or 0.5%)
Bayonet forceps
Nasal speculum
Packing material
Medicine cup

Skin Preparation

See Ophthalmic Surgery, General Information, p. 474; prepare for a bilateral eye procedure.

Draping

See Ophthalmic Surgery, General Information, pp. 474–475. Drape as for a unilateral eye procedure. In addition to the eye, the entire nose is draped into the field.

Equipment

Footboard, padded
Suction
Power source for power drill
Sitting stools

Instrumentation

Limited procedure tray
Basic eye procedures tray
Dacrocystorhinostomy tray
Kerrison rongeurs
Power drill (e.g., Stryker), burrs, and cord

Supplies

Basin set
Balanced salt solution (BSS), tear substitute
Cotton-tipped applicators or cellulose sponges
Blades (1) No. 15, (1) No. 11
Needle magnet or counter
Suction tubing
Local anesthetic (e.g., lidocaine [Xylocaine] 1% with epinephrine)
Bulb syringe
Topical anesthetic (e.g., cocaine, 4% or 5%, or phenylephrine [Neo-Synephrine] 0.25% or 0.5%)
Catheter (e.g., 10 Fr Robinson) or infant feeding tube (optional)
Packing (e.g., ¼″ gauze and Adaptic)
Cautery, disposable
Thrombin (e.g., 5000 units)
Gelfoam (cut into pledgets 2 × 1 cm)

Special Notes

Local anesthesia with epinephrine may be administered during the procedure to aid in hemostasis.

Protective goggles may be worn.

The area being drilled is lightly irrigated with saline to minimize friction and buildup of heat; saline and bone fragments are suctioned.

CORRECTION OF STRABISMUS

Definition

Alignment of the visual axes of the eyes.

Discussion

When medical treatments (glasses, patching, and fusion exercises) fail to align the axes of the eyes, surgical treatment is indicated. Complete restoration to normal alignment cannot always be achieved.

Types

Lateral rectus resection is the shortening of this extraocular muscle by removing a portion of it and the reanastomosis of the cut ends.

Medial rectus recession is the lengthening of this extraocular muscle by detaching it from its original insertion and reattaching it more posteriorly on the sclera.

Procedure

Lateral Rectus Resection. An eye speculum is inserted. An incision is made in the conjunctiva at the limbus to expose the lateral rectus muscle. The eye is rotated medially as far as possible. Two traction sutures are placed in the conjunctiva. The conjunctiva is freed from underlying tissue. A muscle hook is passed under the muscle insertion. The amount of muscle to be resected is measured with a caliper (previously adjusted). A muscle clamp is clamped over the muscle and the measured portion (specimen) is excised. The end of the muscle is reattached to the original point of insertion. Hemostasis is achieved. The conjunctiva is closed. Antibiotic ophthalmic ointment may be instilled, and an eye pad is applied.

Medial Rectus Recession. An eye speculum is inserted. An incision is made in the conjunctiva at the limbus; the conjunctiva is undermined. The distance from the original point of insertion to the new one is measured with a caliper (previously adjusted). The new point of insertion may be marked. Two absorbable sutures are placed in the end of the muscle (and left untied with the needles attached). A straight mosquito hemostat is clamped across the muscle (between the sutures and the insertion) in order to compress small blood vessels and discourage oozing. The clamp is removed, and a muscle hook is passed under the muscle. The muscle is incised, and the cautery is employed as necessary to achieve hemostasis. The muscle is reattached at the new point of insertion further back on the globe with the previously placed sutures. The conjunctiva is closed. Antibiotic ophthalmic ointment is instilled, and an eye pad is applied.

Preparation of the Patient

The procedure is usually performed under general anesthesia. A retrobulbar injection may be administered prior to the skin preparation. The patient is supine; the arm on the side of the affected eye may be tucked in at the patient's side, and the other arm may be extended on an armboard.

Skin Preparation and Draping

See Ophthalmic Surgery, General Information, pp. 474–475.

Equipment

Headrest
Loupes (optional)
Sitting stools

Instrumentation

Basic eye procedures tray
Basic eye muscle procedures tray

Supplies

Basin set
Cotton-tipped applicators or cellulose sponges
Cautery (disposable)
Balanced salt solution (BSS), tear substitute
Needle magnet or counter
Antibiotic ophthalmic ointment
Marking pen (optional)

EVISCERATION OF THE EYE

Definition

Removal of the entire contents of the eye within the scleral shell.

Discussion

The sclera and muscles attached to the sclera remain intact to accommodate a prosthesis. Indication for evisceration is a hopelessly traumatized eye in a young person with no history of previous eye disease. The cosmetic result is superior to the result of enucleation because the extraocular muscles still attached to the scleral shell result in a moveable implant.

Procedure

A peritomy is made superiorly from 3 o'clock to 9 o'clock position. An incision (same length) is made in the exposed sclera through to the uvea. The entire uvea is separated from the sclera by an evisceration spoon and is completely removed. The remaining uvea may be removed with a gauze sponge on a hemostat rotated within the scleral shell or with a chalazion curette. The wound is irrigated. Hemostasis is achieved. Scleral edges are held open by tagged sutures while implant is inserted by a sphere introducer. The posterior surface of the cornea is removed to reduce its sensitivity. The sclera is closed with interrupted sutures. The conjunctiva is approximated with interrupted sutures. A conformer is placed in the cul-de-sac. Antibiotic ophthalmic ointment is instilled, and an eye patch is applied.

Preparation of the Patient

The patient is supine; the arm on the side of the operative eye may be tucked in at the patient's side, and the other arm may be extended on an armboard.

Skin Preparation and Draping

See Ophthalmic Surgery, General Information, pp. 474–475.

Equipment

Suction
Sitting stools

Instrumentation

Basic eye procedures tray
Globe and orbit procedures tray
Curettes
Sphere prosthesis and conformer

Supplies

Basin set
Balanced salt solution (BSS), tear substitute

Cautery (wet field or disposable)
Cotton-tipped applicators or cellulose sponges
Blade (1) No. 11
Suction tubing
Antibiotic ophthalmic ointment

Special Notes

Have prosthesis ready to implant.

Follow hospital policy for recording the insertion of a prosthesis.

Complete the manufacturer's forms.

ENUCLEATION OF THE GLOBE

Definition

Removal of an eye (without rupture of the globe).

Discussion

The procedure is indicated in certain instances of severe trauma, intraocular malignancy, intolerable pain, and unsightly appearance. A plastic or silicone sphere is placed within Tenon's capsule. A conformer is placed over the sphere. The conformer is replaced with an artificial eye 8 weeks postoperatively.

Procedure

A peritomy is made at the limbus circumferentially separating the conjunctiva and Tenon's capsule from the globe. The superior oblique tendon is grasped with a muscle hook and divided. The inferior oblique muscle is double-clamped with hemostats for hemostasis; the muscle is cut. Hemostats are released after several minutes. All attachments to the globe are separated, permitting the globe to move freely. The eye is held steady by the medial rectus insertion. The location of the optic nerve is identified. The optic nerve is transsected, the globe delivered, and the remaining attachments are separated. Hemostasis is achieved. A sphere implant is sutured into Tenon's capsule. The conjunctiva is approximated. A conformer is placed over the sphere in the cul-de-sac. An intermarginal suture is placed to produce a mild pressure effect. Antibiotic ointment may be instilled, an eye pad is placed, and a pressure dressing is applied.

Preparation of the Patient

The patient is supine; the arm on the side of the operative eye may be tucked in at the patient's side, and the other arm may be extended on an armboard.

Skin Preparation and Draping

See Ophthalmic Surgery, General Information, pp. 474–475.

Equipment

Suction
Sitting stools

Instrumentation

Basic eye procedures tray
Globe and orbit procedures tray
Sphere prosthesis and conformer

Supplies

Basin set
Balanced salt solution (BSS), tear substitute
Cautery (wet field or disposable)
Cotton-tipped applicators or cellulose sponges
Suction tubing
Antibiotic ophthalmic ointment

Special Notes

Have prosthesis ready to implant.
   Follow hospital policy for recording the insertion of a prosthesis.

ORBITAL EXENTERATION

Definition

Removal of the eye and a significant portion of the orbital tissues.

Discussion

The amount of tissues removed beyond the globe depends upon the origin and extent of the disease process. Exenteration is usually performed for neoplasms, but may also be performed for benign disease such as phycomycosis.

Classification
1. *Subtotal:* Eye and epibulbar tissues excised
2. *Total* (with or without eyelid skin): Removal of all tissues within the bony orbit, including periorbita
3. *Radical:* Removal of one or more bony orbital walls in addition to soft tissues and periosteum.

The subtotal procedure is used to remove tumors involving the anterior portion of the eye and the conjunctiva. The total procedure is indicated when intraocular tumor (e.g., melanoma) extends into the orbit. Malignant tumors not involving bone that do not respond to radiation may require total exenteration. Radical exenteration is indicated when a malignant sinus tumor invades the orbit or when a malignant skin tumor involves the orbital bones. After the wound has healed, the cavity may be covered with a black patch or a cosmetic plastic prosthesis.

Procedure

For *total exenteration,* with preservation of eyelid skin, an incision is made circumferentially around the palpebral fissure. The skin is dissected to the orbital rim. Orbicularis muscle may be incised with the cutting blade of an electrosurgical pencil. The periosteum is separated from the orbital rim and walls; care is taken to avoid perforation of bony walls. The eye and soft tissues within the orbit are removed. The skin is undermined and closed over the lateral orbital rim. A split-thickness skin graft may be used to cover denuded orbital walls. The orbital cavity is packed with gauze impregnated with antibiotic ointment, and a moderate pressure dressing is applied. Alternatively, the bone surfaces may be permitted to heal by spontaneous epithelialization.

Preparation of the Patient

The patient is supine; the arm on the side of the operative eye may be extended on an armboard and the other arm may be tucked in at the patient's side. Apply electrosurgical dispersive pad.

Skin Preparation and Draping

See Ophthalmic Surgery, General Information, pp. 474–475.

Equipment

Suction
Electrosurgical unit
Sitting stools
Power unit for dermatome (optional)

Instrumentation

Limited procedure tray
Basic eye procedures tray
Globe and orbit procedures tray
Dermatome (e.g., Brown) (optional)

Supplies

Basin set
Balanced salt solution (BSS), tear substitute
Electrosurgical pencil
Cotton-tipped applicators or cellulose sponges
Needle magnet or counter
Bone wax
Suction tubing
Packing (e.g., ¼″ gauze)
Antibiotic ophthalmic ointment
Mineral oil (if dermatome is used)

Special Notes

Determine if a skin graft is to be obtained, and prepare the donor site.

CORNEAL TRANSPLANT/KERATOPLASTY

Definition

The grafting of corneal tissue from the eye of one person to another.

Discussion

The indications for corneal transplant are corneal injury or disease resulting in opacification of the cornea. The procedure is performed to improve vision; the retina and optic nerve must be functioning properly.

Types

Lamellar: Replacement of a partial thickness of the cornea

Penetrating: Replacement of a full thickness of the cornea

Total: Replacement of the entire corneal area (limbus to limbus)

Lamellar and total keratoplasty are rarely performed. Penetrating keratoplasty is often performed as an emergency procedure.

Procedure

Penetrating Keratoplasty. The trephine size is chosen, and the donor button is prepared. If the donor button has been prepared by the excision of a cornea with scleral rim, this is placed into a Teflon block, and the button punched from behind (on the endothelial surface). The trephine used for the donor button is 0.5 mm larger than the host trephine. A single nonabsorbable suture is placed through the cut edge of the button. A single suture is placed through the excised button. The excised button is placed epithelial-side down on a moistened (with saline or McCarey-Kaufman medium) gauze pad, and fluid is placed on endothelial surface to prevent drying. The host cornea is now removed by trephining the cornea 0.4 mm deep. The anterior chamber is entered with a sharp knife, and the excision is completed with scissors. Care is taken to remove any adventitious tissue from the host site. Lens extraction, vitrectomy, or any other necessary procedures are performed. The donor button is placed into the host and the previously placed suture is tied at 12 o'clock. The graft is fixed at the 6 o'clock, 3 o'clock, and 9 o'clock positions. The graft is secured with additional sutures. Before the last suture is tied, the anterior chamber is reformed to normal depth with balanced salt solution. Any leaks are repaired. Steroids, as well as antibiotics, may be applied topically.

Preparation of the Patient

The patient is supine; the arm on the side of the operative eye may be tucked in at the patient's side, and the other arm may be extended on an armboard. Tetracaine drops may be instilled. Eyelashes may be clipped. The procedure is performed under general anesthesia. A retrobulbar injection may be administered prior to the skin preparation.

Skin Preparation and Draping

See Ophthalmic Surgery, General Information, pp. 474–475. A drape is needed to cover the microscope.

Equipment

Headrest
Microscope
Sitting stools

Instrumentation

Basic eye procedures tray
Corneal procedures tray

Supplies

Basin set
Cautery (wet field or disposable)
Balanced salt solution (BSS), tear substitute
Cotton-tipped applicators and cellulose sponges
Culture dishes (to store donor corneal button)
Blades (1) No. 15, (1) No. 64 Beaver, (1) superblade 30°
Fluorescein strip (topical stain which temporarily
    stains denuded corneal epithelium)
Antibiotic solution (to wash transplant)
Anti-inflammatory agent (e.g., betamethasone [Celestone Soluspan])

Special Notes

Confirm that the donor cornea is available.

When a portable floor-model microscope is used, it is brought over the patient on the side opposite the operative eye.

A separate sterile table may be requested to cut out donor transplant.

CATARACT EXTRACTION

Definition

Removal of an opaque ocular lens.

Discussion

The ocular lens becomes opacified for a number of reasons including trauma and congenital, drug, and metabolic effects, but it is primarily due to aging. At an appropriate time in the maturation of the cataract, and with sufficient loss of vision, surgery is indicated.

Types

Intracapsular Method. Removal of the opaque lens within its capsule. A cryoprobe is usually applied to the cataract and the lens, and they are removed by gentle pressure.

Extracapsular Method. Removal of an opaque lens by irrigation and expression, leaving the posterior capsule in situ.

Phacoemulsification. A variation of the irrigation-aspiration technique; the contents of the lens capsule are fragmented with ultrasonic energy as the lens material is simultaneously irrigated and aspirated.

An artificial lens is commonly implanted after the cataract has been removed. The surgeon will select a lens prosthesis prior to surgery.

Procedure

Intracapsular. A lid speculum is placed. Traction sutures are placed in the sclera. The conjunctiva is reflected from the corneal superior hemicircumference. Bleeders are cauterized. The anterior chamber is entered. An iridotomy is performed as the cornea is retracted by suture traction. Alphachymotrypsin (Zolyse) is instilled into the anterior chamber (to dissolve the zonules suspending the lens). After 3 minutes a cryoextractor is applied to the lens, which adheres to it, and the lens is withdrawn from the eye. The corneal incision is closed. Traction sutures are removed, and the conjunctival flap is approximated. Ophthalmic ointment may be instilled and an eye pad is applied.

Extracapsular. The lens is opened with a cystotome or capsule forceps. The lens cortex is removed using expression and a lens loop of a coaxial cannula system. Cytoplegic agents may be employed. The corneal incision is closed. The wound is closed as for the intraocular procedure.

An extracapsular intraocular lens may be placed more commonly in the posterior chamber behind the iris. Posterior lenses can be implanted only where the cataract was removed by extracapsular lens extraction. This is the most physiologic position for the artificial lens (composed of polymethyl methacrylate), which has led to a return to extracapsular lens extraction. Anterior chamber lenses are used following intracapsular lens extraction and for secondary lens implants.

Pharmacoemulsification. The anterior lens capsule is excised, the lens nucleus is prolapsed into the anterior chamber, and the ultrasonic probe (with capabilities of irrigation and aspiration as well as delivery of ultrasonic energy) is inserted into the capsule. The remaining lens substance (cortex) in the posterior capsule is "polished" with a moist cellulose sponge (to remove any fragments) or partially excised. Pharmacoemulsification permits a smaller (more cosmetic) wound. The incisions are closed as above. An intraocular lens may be placed.

Preparation of the Patient

The patient is supine; the arm on the side of the affected eye may be tucked in at the patient's side, and the other arm may be extended on an armboard. The head may be supported by a headrest. Prior to the skin preparation, tetracaine drops may be instilled in both eyes followed by the appliction of a Honan intraocular pressure reducer cuff for 10 to 15 minutes. Lashes may be trimmed (infrequently).

Skin Preparation and Draping

See Ophthalmic Surgery, General Information, pp. 474–475.

Equipment

Honan intraocular pressure reducer cuff
Lift sheet for operating table
Headrest (e.g., horseshoe) (optional)
Sitting stools
Microscope
    Intracapsular: Cryoextractor (e.g., Frigitonics)
    Phacoemulsification: Irrigation/aspiration (I/A) unit
      (e.g., Cavitron)

Instrumentation

Basic eye procedures tray
Cataract extraction and lens procedure tray
McIntyre infusion set with connector and coaxial irri-
    gation-aspiration system
Phacoemulsification tray, as indicated by the brand of
    the I/A unit (e.g., Cavitron Phaco Emulsifier unit
    with AVIT handpiece, I/A handpiece, ultrasonic
    handpiece, and irrigation cystotome, available)
Handgrips (or drape) for microscope
Intraocular lens (IOL) implant

Supplies

Basin set
Sterile, plastic adhesive drape
Balanced salt solution (BSS), 500 mL
I/A pack (for phacoemulsification) (available)
Cellulose sponges
Cautery (wet field or disposable)
Beaver blade No. 69
Super blade 30°
Millipore filter (for acetylcholine [Miochol])
Medications (available)

Anesthetic for retrobulbar block (e.g., lidocaine [Xylocaine] 2% with epinephrine or bupivacaine [Marcaine] 0.5% with epinephrine)

Corticosteroid, an anti-inflammatory agent (e.g., betamethasone [Celestone] drops)

Enzyme to increase absorption and dispersion of other drugs (e.g., hyaluronidase [Wydase])

Miotic agent to irrigate and rapidly constrict the pupil (e.g., acetylcholine [Miochol])

Viscoelastic agent acts as a tamponade and a vitreous substitute (e.g., sodium hyaluronate [Healon])

Special Notes

A lift sheet placed on the table will be helpful in transferring the patient to the gurney postoperatively.

A portable (floor-model) microscope, when used, is brought over the patient on the side opposite the affected eye.

Be thoroughly familiar with equipment (i.e., Frigitonics and Cavitron).

Thoroughly check the functioning of the Cavitron unit preoperatively.

When using the Cavitron unit, inform the surgeon as different positions are entered, that is, 1 (on irrigation alone), 2 (on irrigation and aspiration), and 3 (on irrigation, aspiration, and ultrasound). The surgeon is advised by the numbers (e.g., "1, 2, 3, 2, 3").

Follow hospital policy for recording insertion of a lens.

Complete lens manufacturer's forms.

SECONDARY LENS IMPLANT

Definition

Placement of a lens implant in an eye that previously had cataract surgery without a lens implant.

Discussion

Aphakia (absence of a lens) may be corrected with aphakic glasses (only for binocular aphakia) or with corrective (contact) lenses (for monocular aphakia), or preferably by a secondary lens implant.

Procedure

Pupil constricting Pilocarpine drops are instilled. The conjunctiva is exposed at the limbus with a 5 to 6 mm incision into the corneal scleral junction with a keratome. Healon and Miochol are placed in the anterior chamber lens. The implant is slid into position with forceps and/or hook. The cornea wound is closed as in cataract surgery (see pp. 500–501).

Preparation of the Patient

The patient is supine; the arm on the side of the affected eye may be tucked in at the patient's side, and the other arm may be extended on an armboard. The head is supported by a headrest.

Skin Preparation and Draping

See Ophthalmic Surgery, General Information, pp. 473–474.

Equipment

Lift sheet for operating table
Headrest (e.g., horseshoe), (optional)
Sitting stools
Microscope

Instrumentation

See Cataract Extraction, p. 502

Supplies

Basin set
Sterile, plastic adhesive drape
Cellulose sponges
Cautery (wet field or disposable)
Beaver blade, for example, No. 69
Super blade 30°
Millipore filter (for acetylcholine [Miochol])
Balanced salt solution (BSS)
Medications:
    Anesthetic for retrobulbar block (e.g., lidocaine [Xylocaine] 2% with epinephrine or bupivacaine [Marcaine] 0.5% with epinephrine)

Corticosteroid, an anti-inflammatory agent (e.g., betamethasone [Celestone] drops)

Enzyme to increase absorption and dispersion of other drugs (e.g., hyaluronidase [Wydase])

Special Notes

A lift sheet placed on the table will be helpful in transferring the patient postoperatively.

A portable (floor model) microscope, when used, is brought over the patient on the side opposite the affected eye.

Follow hospital policy for recording the insertion of a lens.

Complete lens manufacturer's forms.

EXTRACTION OF AN INTRAOCULAR FOREIGN BODY

Definition

Removal of a foreign body from the eye.

Discussion

Foreign bodies when identified and localized within the eye should be removed, if possible. Particles of iron or copper must be removed to prevent later disorganization of ocular tissues by degenerative changes (siderosis from iron and chalcosis from copper). Particles of glass or porcelain may be tolerated indefinitely and are usually better left alone.

Several different methods may be used to localize intraocular foreign bodies including ultrasonography and coronal CT scan of the orbits. The Berman metal locator, an electronic instrument, is useful in pinpointing an intraocular foreign body. The wand of the instrument can be sterilized and passed over the eye during surgery. The instrument is particularly useful in locating nonmagnetic foreign bodies. The MRI is contraindicated for localization of metallic foreign bodies because it produces a magnetic field during scanning in which magnetic metallic foreign bodies can become high-velocity intraocular projectiles with catastrophic effects.

Procedure

When the foreign body is located anterior to the lens zonules, it is removed through a limbal incision into the anterior chamber at the limbus. If it is located behind the lens and anterior to the equator, it is removed through the area of pars plana nearest to the foreign body (less retinal damage is caused). If the foreign body is located posterior to the equator, it is removed through the pars plana by vitrectomy and intraocular forceps, in order to avoid major choroidal hemorrhages from incisions into the posterior wall of the eyeball. This method is used for both magnetic and nonmagnetic foreign bodies. Special forceps are available for grasping spherical pellets.

Should any area of the retina be damaged, it is treated with diathermy, photocoagulation, or endolaser coagulation to prevent retinal detachment.

Preparation of the Patient, Skin Preparation, and Draping

See Ophthalmic Surgery, General Information, pp. 473–475.

Equipment

Lift sheet for operating table
Headrest
Sitting stools
Loupe or slitlamp
Ophthalmoscope, direct and indirect
Argon laser, available

Instruments

Basic eye procedures tray
Cataract extraction and lens procedure tray
Berman metal locator and wand
Special forceps for grasping spherical pellets
Special magnets (e.g., magnet, electromagnet, rare earth metal magnet)

Supplies

Basin set
Sterile, plastic adhesive drape

Balanced salt solution (BSS)

Cellulose sponges

Cautery (wet field or disposable)

Beaver blade (ask regarding number)

Medications (available)

Anesthetic for retrobulbar block (e.g., lidocaine [Xylocaine] 2% with epinephrine or bupivacaine [Marcaine] 0.5% with epinephrine)

Corticosteroid, an anti-inflammatory agent (e.g., betamethasone [Celestone] drops)

Miotic agent to irrigate and rapidly constrict the pupil (e.g., acetylcholine [Miochol])

Enzyme to increase absorption and dispersion of other drugs (e.g., hyaluronidase [Wydase])

Viscoelastic agent acts as a tamponade and a vitreous substitute (e.g., sodium hyaluronate [Healon])

Antibiotic of choice (drops and/or intravenous)

Special Notes

A lift sheet placed on the table will be helpful in transferring the patient to the gurney postoperatively.

Send foreign body to pathology.

Be prepared to do a vitrectomy, pp. 513–516, if necessary.

Any area of the retina that has been damaged must be treated with diathermy, photodynamic or argon laser coagulation to prevent retinal detachment, see pp. 617–618.

TRABECULECTOMY

Definition

Drainage of the anterior chamber employing a partial-thickness, limbal-based scleral flap.

Discussion

Trabeculectomy is the procedure of choice for primary glaucomas when iridectomy is considered inadequate. Trabeculectomy may also be performed to treat infantile glaucoma and several types of secondary glaucoma.

Procedure

Intraocular pressure is checked; if it is excessively high, measures are taken to bring it into the satisfactory range. A superior rectus bridle suture is placed. A limbal-based conjunctival flap is developed; episcleral tissue is cleaned anteriorly up to and including the corneoscleral sulcus. A caliper is used to measure the width of the flap on the globe. The sclera is outlined with a blade and then incised two-thirds its thickness. Atropine eye drops may be administered to dilate the pupil. The edge of the flap is developed with a Beaver blade; care is taken not to penetrate the base of the flap. The flap is continued to the anterior junction of the conjunctiva and the cornea. A paracentesis track is placed with a sharp-tipped knife into the cornea 1 mm anterior to the limbus. An incision is made through the sclera, through which the iris will prolapse. An iridotomy is performed. The sclera is incised radially. The block of scleral wall is excised. Iridectomy is performed. The scleral flap is sutured in place; after two sutures are placed, the anterior chamber is filled with balanced salt solution or Healon through the paracentesis track as the intraocular pressure is monitored. When filtration is desired postoperatively, a filtering bleb develops as the anterior chamber is shaped. Antibiotic drops or ointment may be instilled and an eye patch is placed.

Preparation of the Patient

The patient is supine; the arm on the side of the operative eye may be tucked in at patient's side and the other arm may be extended on an armboard. A headrest may be used. Tetracaine eyedrops may be instilled. Facial and retrobulbar blocks may be administered. Lashes may be trimmed.

Skin Preparation and Draping

See Ophthalmic Surgery, General Information, pp. 474–475.

Equipment

Headrest (optional)
Sitting stools
Microscope

Instrumentation

Basic eye procedures tray
Glaucoma procedures tray
Handgrips (or drape) for microscope

Supplies

Basin set
Sterile, plastic adhesive drape
Cotton-tipped applicators or cellulose sponges
Blades (e.g., No. 57 Beaver and 15° super blade)
Balanced salt solution (BSS), tear substitute
Cautery (wet field or disposable)
Local and retrobulbar anesthetic (e.g., bupivacaine
  [Marcaine] 0.5%)
Antibiotic ophthalmic drops or ointment

EXCISION OF PTERYGIUM

Definition

Removal of a growth of fibrovascular tissue that extends from the conjunctiva onto the cornea.

Discussion

True pterygia are located in the interpalpabral zone, particularly on the medial aspect of the globe; pterygia often occur bilaterally. All pterygia need not be excised. Indications for removal include an inflamed eye that does not respond to topical medication, growth of a pterygium so that it interferes or is expected to interfere with vision, a change in corneal astigmatism associated with growth of the pterygium, or cosmetic reasons. Several different techniques are advocated.

Procedure

A speculum is inserted. The head of the pterygium may be dissected from the cornea and undermined toward the sclera by superficial stripping (or from sclera to cornea). Alternatively, an incision may be made above or below the pterygium, and a suture is passed under the body of the pterygium. With a sawing motion of the suture, the pterygium is stripped from the cornea as the suture is pulled medially. The corneoscleral limbus is made smooth with a Beaver or No. 15 blade. Hemostasis is achieved with the cautery. With recurrent or large pterygia, every effort is made to carefully excise this tissue to prevent recurrence.

Preparation of the Patient

The patient is supine; the arm on the side of the affected eye may be tucked in at the patient's side, and the other arm may be extended on an armboard. A headrest may be used. The procedure may be performed with a topical anesthetic of cocaine 10%, subconjunctival injection of lidocaine, retrobulbar injection of lidocaine, or a similar agent. See circulator responsibilities regarding local anesthesia, pp. 24–25.

Skin Preparation and Draping

See Ophthalmic Surgery, General Information, pp. 474–475.

Equipment

Headrest (optional)
Sitting stools
Microscope (optional)

Instrumentation

Basic eye procedures tray
Basic eye procedures microscope tray
Handgrips (or drape) for microscope, if used

Supplies

Basin set
Balanced salt solution (BSS), tear substitute
Sterile, plastic adhesive drape
Blades (1) No. 15, and Beaver (1) No. 57 or No. 64
Anesthetic agent
Cotton-tipped applicators or cellulose sponges
Cautery (wet field or disposable)
Anti-inflammatory agent (e.g., hydrocortisone ophthalmic ointment) (optional)

REPAIR OF RETINAL DETACHMENT/SCLERAL BUCKLING

Definition

The sealing of a localized retinal defect by inciting an inflammatory reaction near the defect or by compressing the globe, buckling the sclera to seal a linear defect in the retina.

Discussion

When the neural retinal layer becomes detached from its underlying pigmented layer either because of a defect in the retina or by accumulation of fluid behind the retina, serious visual disturbance results. The inciting events include tumor of the choroid, trauma, and degeneration. Vitreous humor, blood, or tissue may accumulate between the retinal layers and the choroid. Treatment consists of sealing the retinal defect and drainage of the subretinal fluid. Several modalities are employed to effect closure of the defects. Cryoprobe to the sclera overlying the retinal defect creates an inflammatory reaction that seals the defect. Similarly, laser surgery (see Appendix, p. 617) or cryosurgery may be used. To achieve reattachment of the retina, the globe is encircled by suturing a band of silicone to maintain the buckle of the sclera, which decreases the potential space in which unwanted fluids can accumulate.

Procedure

A discrete retinal defect, not surrounded by a detachment, can be sealed by photocoagulation or laser (performed in an "eye laboratory" rather than the operating room). To effect adhesions with a cryoprobe, the preoperatively mapped out section of the globe overlying the defect is exposed. The conjunctiva and Tenon's capsule are incised. The cryoprobe is applied to create adhesions to seal the defect. This maneuver can be controlled by the surgeon viewing through a head-mounted ophthalmoscope as the assistant or surgeon depresses the sclera with the cryoprobe against the defect. An incision can also be made into the subretinal fluid accumulations to evacuate them. The buckling is achieved by incising a groove around the equator of the globe, undermining the edges. A Silastic band is placed in the groove, secured by multiple mattress sutures, which also close the groove. The Silastic band is then tightened around the globe to effect the buckling and maintenance of the retinal layers in apposition. A wedge silicone tire may be used under the band to exert additional pressure and assure the proper degree of buckling. On occasion, one of the extraocular muscles must be retracted (transiently detached) to provide adequate exposure. The conjunctiva is closed. Antibiotic ophthalmic drops and/or ointment may be instilled.

Preparation of the Patient

The patient is supine; the arm on the side of the operative eye may be tucked in at the patient's side, and the other arm may be extended on an armboard. A headrest may be used. General anesthesia is employed.

Skin Preparation and Draping

See Ophthalmic Surgery, General Information, pp. 474–475. Additional drapes may be needed to cover the cryosurgical unit and the microscope.

Equipment

Headrest (optional)
Sitting stools
Cryoprobe
Indirect ophthalmoscope
Cryosurgical unit
Microscope
Laser (optional)

Instrumentation

Basic eye procedures tray
Retinal procedures tray
Tonometer and weights

Cryosurgical retinal probes (curved and straight with
  rubber covering) and cords
Implant

Supplies

Basin set
Sterile, plastic adhesive drape
Balanced salt solution (BSS), tear substitute
Cotton-tipped applicators and cellulose sponges
Cautery (wet field or disposable)
Beaver blade, No. 69 or No. 59
Antibiotic ophthalmic drops and/or ointment (optional)

Special Notes

The surgeon chooses the Silastic band and scleral
sponge prior to the procedure.

Soak the ophthalmoscope lens in aqueous glutaraldehyde (e.g., Cidex).

Have a cryosurgical unit ready.

Implants may be soaked in antibiotic solution after
being flash-autoclaved.

Acetazolamide (Diamox) may be requested (to reduce
intraocular pressure).

The ophthalmoscope may be handled using a sterile
plastic covering for it.

Sterile back vests may be helpful in maintaining
sterility of the field.

If a laser is used, see precautions in Appendix, pp.
619–624.

A culture may be taken prior to closure.

VITRECTOMY

Definition

Removal of vitreous humor.

Discussion

The vitreous body may opacify secondary to retinal
hemorrhage (as in diabetes), endophthalmitis, foreign
bodies and trauma, and preretinal membranes. The

vitreous may also opacify as a result of the formation of bands following anterior chamber surgery (e.g., cataract extraction). Surgery can remove or lyse the bands, restore contour to the globe, and remove organized hemorrhagic areas or foreign matter in order to restore a clear visual pathway to the retina. The argon or the neodymium:yttrium aluminum garnet (Nd:YAG) laser may be used to lyse the bands noninvasively, when applicable. See Appendix, pp. 619–624, for laser precautions.

Procedure

The vitreous is approached by an incision in the pars plana (the anterior attachment of the retina) or via a paralimbal incision. The lens, if not already absent, may be removed. Vitreous, if displaced into the anterior chamber during prior cataract extraction, is removed. A vitrector (e.g., Ocutome), which is a fine, blunt-tipped suction, cutting cannula with the capacity for irrigation (console contolled), is inserted. An additional incision through the pars plana permits endoillumination. The vitreous and its opacities are removed using a combination of cryosurgery, irrigation, and suction. If a retinal tear is present, it is treated by cryopobe, endolaser, and/or a scleral buckle. During the procedure balanced salt solution or sodium hyaluronate (Healon) or a gas such as sulfur hexafluoride or carbon otbfeuroine is infused by catheter to replace vitreous loss and tonicity to the globe. The incisions are closed. Antibiotics and steroids are instilled or injected subconjunctivally, and an eye patch is applied.

Preparation of the Patient

The patient is supine; the arm on the side of the operative eye may be tucked in at the patient's side, and the other arm may be extended on an armboard. The procedure is usually performed under general anesthesia. The table is placed in slight reverse Trendelenburg, the neck is extended, and the head is stabilized with a headrest. Antiembolic hose or elastic bandages may be used. Pressure points are well padded.

Skin Preparation and Draping

See Ophthalmic Surgery, General Information, pp. 474–475. The microscope is draped.

Equipment

Headrest (e.g., doughnut)
Microscope with x-y coupling (allows surgeon to move microscope head over the field)
Endoilluminator light source
Endocoagulator (bipolar, wet field)
Frigitonics unit
Vitrector (e.g., Ocutome II)
Sitting stools

Instrumentation

Basic eye procedures tray
Retinal procedures tray
Forceps (e.g., Lister, curved and straight Pierse-Hoskins, and curved and straight McPherson tying)
Cryoprobe and cord
Endocoagulator handpiece with cord
Endoilluminator handpiece with cord
Vitrectomy instrumentation, vitrectomy handpiece (AVIT) and tubing, scleral plugs (19 or 20 gauge), scleral plug forceps, handheld lens (with irrigator), caliper, special knife and blade, infusion cannula, vitreous scissors, membrane pick, flute needle, foreign body forceps

Supplies

Basin set
Sterile, plastic adhesive drape
Balanced salt solution (BSS), tear substitute
Sodium hyaluronate (Healon), vitreous substitute
Cotton-tipped applicators and cellulose sponges
Acetylcholine (Miochol) and filter to constrict the pupil
Antibiotic and/or steroid ophthalmic drops or injection

Special Notes

Check equipment before beginning the procedure.

The vitrectomy handpiece is attached to sterile tubing, which is connected to the Ocutome unit.

Test suction vacuum, and assess the cutting function of vitrector.

Prime the infusion cannula with solution (surgeon's choice), and remove air bubbles.

Vitrector unit rates are set (infusion, cutting, and aspiration).

Cultures may be taken (from vitreous washings).

REFRACTIVE KERATOPLASTY

Definition

Reshaping of the cornea in order to alter its refractive power.

Discussion

Refractive Keratoplasty refers to a variety of procedures including those performed to correct or improve myopia, astigmatism, hyperopia, aphakia, and keratoconus. In radial keratoplasty, multiple radial incisions are made in the peripheral and paracentral cornea through as much as 90 percent of its depth so that the uncut central cornea may be flattened to correct myopia. For other conditions, as aphakia, a button of cornea from either the patient (keratomileusis) or a donor (keratophakia) is cryolathed by means of a computer-controlled instrument, (re)inserted, and sutured to the cornea. Sophisticated measurements of the corneal shape, thickness, and refractive parameters are performed preoperatively. Following one of these procedures, the patient may see well enough to eliminate the need for glasses.

Procedure

Radial keratotomy requires the patient's cooperation as he or she focuses his or her gaze while being observed through the operating microscope. Employing a micrometer, controlled radial incisions are made in the cornea using a sapphire, diamond, or steel knife, according to preoperative measurements regarding number, depth, and position. Antibiotic ointment and an eye patch may be applied.

Preparation of the Patient

The patient is supine; the arm on the side of the operative eye may be tucked in at the patient's side, and the other arm may be extended on an armboard. A headrest may be employed. Procedure is performed with topical and local anesthesia.

Skin Preparation and Draping

See Ophthalmic Surgery, General Information, pp. 474–475.

Equipment

Headrest (e.g., doughnut)
Microscope (with fixation device attached to the objective lens)
Sitting stools

Instrumentation

Basic eye procedures tray
Cataract extraction lens procedure tray

Supplies

Basin set
Sterile, plastic adhesive drape
Balanced salt solution (BSS), tear substitute
Cotton-tipped applicators and cellulose sponges
Cautery, disposable
Antibiotic ophthalmic ointment (optional)

Special Notes

Surgery is usually performed as an outpatient procedure.

Chapter 20

Pediatric Procedures

PEDIATRIC GENERAL INFORMATION

The surgical care of the infant and small child mandates attention to numerous considerations not ordinarily required for older children or adult surgical patients. The need for appropriately sized smaller instruments, equipment, drapes, supplies, and so on is obvious. Other important factors must be heeded regarding the pediatric patient. It is in this context that the propriety of the phrase the "pediatric patient is not a small adult" is particularly evident. Special precautions for preoperative medication, administration of anesthesia, maintenance of body temperature, accurate fluid balance, and so on, are essential. In addition to the age of the patient, his or her size and weight, nutritional status, degree of hydration, and general medical condition influence care. The operating room is to be prepared prior to transporting the pediatric patient into the room so that specific measures may be instituted immediately upon arrival.

Maintenance of Body Temperature and/or Prevention of Heat Loss Considerations

Transport neonates and small infants in a heated isolette.

Regulate room temperature by adjusting the thermostat:

26° to 27°C (80° to 85°F) infants under 11 kg (25 pounds)

23° to 24°C (75° to 80°F) older children

Use radiant heat lamps (newborns).

Keep warming mattress temperature at approximately 37.7°C (100°F).

Keep head covered (e.g., with stockinette cap).

Cover extremities (e.g., with Webril and plastic wrap or tube stockinette).

Warm intravenous fluids, blood, and so on, to body temperature.

Warm skin preparation solutions.

Do not allow preparation solution to pool under the patient.

Avoid excessive draping.

Warm irrigation fluids to body temperature.

Warm blankets to cover patient postoperatively.

Anesthesia Measures

Pediatric inductions are frequently performed through a mask, after which an intravenous catheter is inserted. Be sure to have available:

Assorted intravenous catheters

Assorted endotracheal tubes:

2.5 to 3.0 mm (8 to 9 Fr) newborn

3.5 to 4.5 mm (10 to 14 Fr) infant

5.0 mm (15 Fr) small child

Pediatric anesthesia circuit

Pediatric rebreathing bag

Small suction catheters

Humidifier

Temperature probe, telethermometer with digital display, for example, axillary, esophageal, rectal (avoid perforation)

Pediatric electrodes for ECG

Restraints

Mummylike wrap (for newborns, small infants, and older children when procedure is performed under local anesthesia)

Soft, padded, nonconstricting extremity restraints

Skin Care Precautions

Avoid pooling of preparation solutions to prevent skin maceration and/or chemical irritation.

Avoid use of direct application of adhesive tape whenever possible.

Use hypoallergenic tape (e.g., Durapore, Transpore, Micropore, Microfoam).

Pad pressure points when positioning patient (e.g., sacrum, elbows, heels, knees and ankles) to avoid skin breakdown and nerve injuries especially in lengthy surgeries.

Positioning Considerations

Avoid hyperextension and hyperflexion to prevent nerve traction injuries (e.g., brachial plexus).

Pad bony prominences to avoid nerve and skin damage, especially in lengthy procedures.

Drop the foot and/or head of the table to facilitate access to the pediatric patient.

Fluid Balance Monitoring

Irrigation solutions accurately measured

Sponges weighed (when significant blood loss anticipated; immediate weighing of sponges reduces evaporation factor)

The surgeon and/or anesthetist may request additional supportive measures. Preferably same will be reviewed prior to transporting the patient into the room.

PEDIATRIC TRACHEOSTOMY

Definition

An opening made into the trachea with the insertion of a cannula to facilitate breathing.

Discussion

The procedure is usually performed under general anesthesia. In infants the trachea is relatively shorter, and the cartilaginous structures are soft and more difficult to palpate than in adults. The thyroid may be situated lower than in the adult, and a pretracheal fat pad may contain substantial blood vessels. In acute respiratory emergencies the cricothyroid membrane may be incised and a trocar and any available hollow tube inserted.

Procedure

The procedure is similar to the procedure for the adult patient (see pp. 459–460), except that segments of the tracheal rings are not excised.

Preparation of the Patient

See Pediatric General Information, pp. 518–520. The patient is supine with the neck extended; a small roll is placed under the shoulders. Small sandbags may be placed at the sides of the head. The extremities are covered and restrained using padded restraints. Apply pediatric electrosurgical dispersive pad.

Skin Preparation

Using warm preparation solutions only, begin cleansing the entire neck extending from the level of the infra-auricular border to the axillae, and down to the table around the shoulders.

Draping

Folded towels and a sheet with a small fenestration

Equipment

Body heat maintenance equipment (e.g., heat lamps, warming mattress)
Small roll and 2 or 3 small sandbags
Covering for extremitites
Electrosurgical unit
Suction

Instrumentation

Tracheostomy tray
Pediatric minor procedures tray

Supplies

Basin set
Blades (2) No. 15, (1) No. 11
Needle magnet or counter
Suction tubing
Tracheostomy tubes, assorted pediatric 2.5 to 5 mm
Umbilical tape
Electrosurgical pencil (with needle tip)

Special Notes

The tracheostomy tube will be held in place with umbilical tapes tied behind the neck.

A gauze dressing split around the tube is applied after the tube is connected to the ventilation equipment.

Tape the obturator to the top of the isolette or crib so that it does not become misplaced while transporting the patient. It will be needed to reinsert the tube if it becomes dislodged.

BRANCHIAL CLEFT SINUSECTOMY

Definition

Excision of a tract resulting from the nonclosure of a branchial cleft.

Discussion

These congenital anomalies are most often noted in later childhood, but they can be treated in infants. Remnants of the first and second branchial clefts are the most common.

The first branchial cleft sinus extends from the auditory canal to just below the midpoint of the mandible.

The second branchial cleft sinus extends from the tonsillar fossae to the lower anterior border of the sternocleidomastoid muscle. The lesion presents as an abscess or a chronically draining sinus.

Procedure

Sinusectomy of First Branchial Cleft. A transverse elliptical incision is made around the external sinus opening (usually in the submandibular or upper neck region). The tract is dissected, and the incision is extended posteriorly toward the angle of the mandible and lower portion of the auditory canal. Care is taken to avoid injury to the mandibular (and other) branches of the facial nerve. The tract is divided at the external auditory canal and ligated. The wound is closed in layers, usually over a small drain secured with a stitch or safety pin.

Preparation of the Patient

See Pediatric General Information, pp. 518–520; the head and extremitites are covered prior to positioning. The patient is supine with the head turned to the side (the affected side is uppermost). A folded sheet may be placed under the shoulders to extend the neck. The extremities are restrained using padded restraints. Apply pediatric electrosurgical dispersive pad.

Skin Preparation

Using warm preparation solutions only, begin by cleansing the entire neck, extending from the infra-auricular border to the nipples, and down to the table at the sides of the neck and shoulders.

Draping

Folded towels and a sheet with a small fenestration

Equipment

Body heat maintenance equipment (e.g., heat lamps, warming mattress)
Covering for head and extremities
Restraints, padded
Suction
Electrosurgical unit

Instrumentation

Pediatric major procedures tray
Weitlaner retractor

Supplies

Basin set
Blades (2) No. 15
Electrosurgical pencil (with needle point)
Suction tubing
Dissectors (e.g., peanut)
Nerve stimulator (locator) (optional)
Drain (e.g., rubber band, ¼″ Penrose)

REPAIR OF CONGENITAL DIAPHRAGMATIC HERNIA

Definition

Repair of an opening in the diaphragm through which the abdominal viscera protrude into the thoracic cavity.

Discussion

Several types of diaphragmatic hernias are seen in the newborn. These hernias require prompt repair to prevent life-threatening cardiorespiratory and obstructive phenomena. The most common of these hernias is through the pleuroperitoneal canal (Bochdaleks hernia). A sac is usually not present; the abdominal viscera enter the pleural space. Hernias through the anterior diaphragm at the sternocostal junction (foramen of Morgagni) are usually small, have a true sac, and are closed by a thoracic or abdominal approach. Eventration of the diaphragm (an attenuation, not a true hernia) is treated by plication of the diaphragm transthoracically. Esophageal hiatal hernia is repaired by a transthoracic approach and is less urgent, the diagnosis often is not suspected in the newborn. Congenital absence of a portion of the diaphragm is rarely encountered; it is repaired by mobilizing the remaining portions or by employing prosthetic sheeting (e.g., Silastic). In all of these patients additional congenital abnormalities may be present.

Procedure

The approach may be abdominal or transthoracic. The abdominal approach is most often employed for

Bochdalek's hernia repair. A paramedian or subcostal incision is made on the side of the hernia. Air is introduced intrapleurally to assist with the delivery of the viscera out of the pleural space. The hernia is repaired with interrupted sutures. Prior to tying the final sutures, air is aspirated from the pleural space as the compressed lung is inflated. If the lung is hypoplastic, an indwelling thoracotomy tube is left in place. Before the abdomen is closed, the viscera are inspected for other abnormalities, especially malrotation, adhesive bands, and intestinal atresia. If the abdomen accommodates the viscera poorly, only skin is closed over the incision in order to avoid respiratory embarrassment because of too tight a closure. Two weeks later, as the abdominal wall stretches, peritoneal and fascial closure may be effected.

Preparation of the Patient

See Pediatric General Information, pp. 518–520; the head and extremities are covered prior to positioning. The patient is supine. Extremities are restrained using padded restraints. Apply a pediatric electrosurgical dispersive pad.

Skin Preparation

Using warm preparation solution only, begin cleansing the abdomen for a paramedian or subcostal incision (same side as the hernia), extending from the suprasternal notch to the pubic symphysis, and down to the table at the sides.

Draping

Folded towels and a pediatric laparotomy sheet

Equipment

Body heat maintenance equipment (e.g., heat lamps, warming mattress)
Covering for head and extremities
Restraints, padded

Suction (with a specimen trap for accurate blood loss measurement)
Electrosurgical unit

Instrumentation

Pediatric major procedures tray
Hemoclip appliers (short, medium)

Supplies

Basin set
Blades (2) No. 15
Needle magnet or counter
Electrosurgical pencil with needle tip
Syringe, 60 mL (for accurate irrigation measurement)
Vessel loops or umbilical tapes, ¼″
Infant chest drainage unit (e.g., Pleurevac) (optional)
Small chest tube (e.g., 10 Fr Argyle) (optional)
Hemoclips (small, medium)
Gastrostomy tube (optional)
Silastic sheeting (for defect repair) (optional)

Special Notes

See Repair of Congenital Atresia of the Esophagus, pp. 534–535.

OMPHALOCELE REPAIR

Definition

Correction of a defect of the umbilicus through which the abdominal viscera protrude outside the abdominal cavity.

Discussion

This congenital defect is evident at birth. The size and extent of an omphalocele is variable from one containing the greater portion of the intra-abdominal viscera including the spleen and liver, to one containing a small loop of intestine. There is no skin covering the defect, but rather amnion or peritoneum, which may rupture at birth, exposing the patient to increased risk of infection. The viscera involved have not undergone the usual rotation and posterior fixation; the blood supply may be under tension and torsion leading to edema and/or circulatory compromise. Additional congenital abnormalities are present in approximately half of these newborns. These considerations and the ability of the abdominal cavity to safely contain the contents of the omphalocele will determine whether a single or a staged repair will be necessary. Hyperalimentation may be required to assure adequate nutrition.

Procedure

Single-Stage Repair. The omphalocele is covered with warm-saline–moistened laparotomy pads. An incision is made separating the skin from the borders of the sac. The umbilical vessels are ligated. The sac and the rim of the defect are excised. A gastrostomy (see Pediatric Gastrostomy, p. 539) may be performed. The viscera are reduced within the abdomen. The abdomen is closed in layers.

Multiple Staged Repair. In the larger omphalocele, when the defect cannot be closed and/or the abdominal cavity is too limited to contain the contents of the sac, an attempt is made to mobilize surrounding skin to cover the protruding viscera. When this, too, is not possible, a synthetic material such as Silastic or silicone mesh or cone is sutured about the periphery over the viscera. As growth permits, in 6 to 24 months complete repair of the defect may be achieved in one or more additional procedures.

Preparation of the Patient

See Pediatric General Information, pp. 518–520; the head and extremities are covered prior to positioning. The patient is supine. Extremities are restrained using padded restraints. Apply a pediatric electrosurgical dispersive pad. A nasogastric tube is passed.

Skin Preparation

The surgeon usually prefers to do skin preparation. If the circulator performs skin preparation, full instructions must be obtained regarding treatment of the omphalocele. Using warm preparation solutions only, cleanse omphalocele according to directions; cleanse the rest of the abdomen extending from the axillae to midthighs, and down to the table at the sides.

Draping

Folded towels and a pediatric laparotomy sheet

Equipment

Body heat maintenance equipment (e.g., heating lamps, warming mattress)
Covering for head and extremities
Padded restraints
Electrosurgical unit
Suction (with specimen trap for accurate blood loss measurement)
Scale (to weigh sponges)

Instrumentation

Pediatric major procedures tray
Hemoclip appliers (short, medium)

Supplies

Basin set
Blades (2) No. 15
Needle magnet or counter
Electrosurgical pencil (with needle tip)
Syringe, 60 mL (for accurate irrigation measurement) (optional)
Hemoclips (small, medium)
Silastic or silicone mesh or cone (for defect repair) (available)

Special Notes

Do not begin the skin preparation without instructions from the surgeon.
    Determine if an intravenous cutdown and/or hyperalimentation line are to be done first.

Accurately measure irrigation fluids.

Weigh sponges immediately to reduce evaporation factor.

Check with the blood bank that blood is available as ordered.

PEDIATRIC UMBILICAL HERNIORRHAPHY

Definition

Repair of an abdominal wall defect at the umbilicus through which viscera protrude.

Discussion

Umbilical hernia is the incomplete closure of the umbilical ring at the fascial level. Skin coverage is intact. Although noted at birth or early infancy, a significant number of these defects close in time. Unless there is a large defect or symptoms present, surgery may be delayed for 18 months or longer. The umbilicus is preserved rather than excised to maintain body image.

Procedure

Usually an infraumbilical hemicircumferential incision is made. The sac is dissected free and the fascial rim of the defect exposed. The dome of the sac is transsected and can be left attached to the undersurface of the umbilical skin. The sac is closed (excess sac is excised) and replaced intra-abdominally. The fascial anterior rectus sheath defect is closed by any of several simple or overlapping layer techniques. The umbilical skin or retained dome of the sac is sutured to the fascia to recreate the umbilical indentation. The skin incision is closed; fine catgut sutures may be used.

Preparation of the Patient

See Pediatric General Information, pp. 518–520. The patient is supine. Extremities are covered and restrained with padded restraints. Apply a pediatric electrosurgical dispersive pad.

Skin Preparation

Using warm preparation solutions only, begin by cleansing the abdomen at the umbilicus, extending from the axillae to the upper thighs, and down to the table at the sides.

Draping

Folded towels and a pediatric laparotomy sheet

Equipment

Body heat maintenance equipment (e.g., heating lamps, warming mattress)
Covering for head and extremities
Restraints, padded
Electrosurgical unit

Instrumentation

Pediatric minor procedures tray

Supplies

Basin set
Electrosurgical pencil (with needle tip)
Blades (2) No. 15
Needle magnet or counter
Dissectors (e.g., peanut)

PEDIATRIC INGUINAL HERNIORRHAPHY

Definition

Ligation of the patent procesus vaginalis through which intra-abdominal viscera have passed into the inguinal canal.

Discussion

Most pediatric inguinal hernias are indirect; correction is accomplished by high ligation of the patent processus vaginalis (sac) without repair of the inguinal floor. In the male, care is taken to avoid injury to the spermatic cord structures. A hydrocele or undescended testis may be associated with the hernia and is corrected at the same time. In females, ovary and fallopian tubes may be encountered within the hernial sac. These hernias are repaired when the diagnosis is made (as an emergency if incarceration occurs). Some surgeons explore the opposite side even if no evidence of contralateral hernia is present preoperatively.

Procedure

A transverse incision is made. The external oblique aponeurosis is exposed and incised. The ilioinguinal nerve is avoided. The contents of the inguinal canal are explored and the sac identified. High ligation is performed; the sac is transsected. If a hydrocele is present, the sac is delivered into the wound and opened to the testis; a portion may be excised. The external oblique aponeurosis is closed, and the skin is closed using a subcuticular suture. In the female, if a sliding component is present (i.e., if part of the sac wall is broad ligament or mesentery), the sac is transsected and ligated, including the round ligament, as close to the sliding portion as possible. Transversalis fascia is closed over the defect prior to closure of the external oblique aponeurosis. The skin is closed.

Preparation of the Patient

See Pediatric General Information, pp. 518–520. The patient is supine. The extremities are covered and restrained using padded restraints. Apply a pediatric electrosurgical dispersive pad.

Skin Preparation

Using warm preparation solutions only, begin cleansing the inguinal area on the affected side extending from nipples to midthighs, and down to the table at the sides.

Draping

Folded towels and a pediatric transverse sheet or sheet with a small fenestration

Equipment, Instrumentation, Supplies, and Special Notes

See Pediatric Inguinal Herniorrhaphy, p. 530.

REPAIR OF CONGENITAL ATRESIA OF THE ESOPHAGUS

Definition

The restoration of esophageal continuity and the repair of the often associated tracheoesophageal fistula.

Discussion

Several types of these anomalies are found. In all there is a lack of a patent esophagus in continuity with the stomach. The stomach either may or may not contain air by virtue of the connection with the trachea. In the most common type the upper esophagus ends blindly, and the lower esophagus communicates with the trachea. The upper and lower esophagus may exhibit muscular continuity but without luminal continuity. Air distends the stomach. The upper esophagus may end blindly, with the lower esophagus extending above the diaphragm for a variable distance but not communicating with the trachea. Here the stomach is empty. Diagnosis is made by the newborns inability to take oral fluids without regurgitation and aspiration; it is confirmed by x-ray studies. Antibiotics are given, and dehydration is corrected. Additional anomalies including those of the cardiovascular and gastrointestinal systems may be encountered.

When air is not present in the stomach, a gastrostomy (see Pediatric Gastrostomy, p. 539) is performed, and tube feedings are begun. Cervical esophagostomy for drainage of secretions and definitive reconstruction is performed in stages. Final restoration may be delayed (even for as long as 2 years). A colonic segment interposition is employed to restore esophageal continuity. If the air-filled stomach compromises respiration and there is reflux of gastric contents into the trachea, gastrostomy is performed immediately, and the definitive surgery is delayed. When the stomach is only moderately distended, definitive single-stage correction may be done, employing a transpleural or extrapleural approach.

Procedure

A transpleural approach may be used. A right postero-lateral incision is made over the fifth rib. The pleura is entered in the fourth intercostal space; the azygous vein is divided. The mediastinal pleura is incised, and the lower esophagus is exposed and mobilized. The tracheoesophageal fistula is transsected and closed. The integrity of the tracheal closure is tested for air leaks by filling the chest with saline. Esophageal continuity is established by any of several one- or two-layer techniques depending on the diameter and muscular wall thickness of the upper and lower segments. A small-gauge feeding tube may be passed transnasally into the esophagus across the anastomotic site into the stomach for postoperative feeding. The connective tissues about the divided azygous vein may be used to reinforce the anastomosis, as is the mediastinal pleura. A chest tube is placed, and the chest is closed.

Preparation of the Patient

See Pediatric General Information, pp. 518–520. The head and the extremities are covered prior to positioning. Following endotracheal intubation the patient is placed in a left lateral position (right side up). A small pillow is placed between the legs. The left leg is straight. The left arm is extended; a small roll may be required just below the axilla to decrease pressure on the brachial plexus. The right arm is positioned on a pillow. The extremities may be restrained with padded restraints. The feet are padded, positioned, and supported as necessary to maintain good body alignment. Apply a pediatric electrosurgical dispersive pad.

Skin Preparation

Using warm preparation solutions only, begin cleansing the chest at the level of the fifth rib extending from the neck to the iliac crest, and down to the table anteriorly and posteriorly.

Draping

Four folded towels, sterile, plastic drape (optional), and
pediatric laparotomy sheet

Equipment

Body heat maintenance equipment (e.g., heat lamps,
warming mattress)
Covering for head and extremities
Restraints, padded
Small pillow
Suction (with specimen trap for accurate blood loss
measurement)
Electrosurgical unit
Scale (to weigh sponges)

Instrumentation

Pediatric major procedures tray
Pediatric thoracotomy tray
Bone cutter, small
Hemoclip appliers (short, medium)
Beaver knife handle (optional)

Supplies

Basin set
Sterile, plastic adhesive drape (optional)
Blades (2) No. 15
Beaver blade (optional)
Suction tubing
Needle magnet or counter
Electrosurgical pencil (with needle tip)
60 mL syringe with cone tip (for accurate irrigation
measurement) (optional)
Vessel loops or ¼" umbilical tape
Infant chest drainage unit (e.g., Pleurevac)
Chest tube (e.g., No. 10 Argyle)
Double cone connector
Hemoclips (small, medium)
Bone wax

Special Notes

Determine if an intravenous cutdown and/or hyperalimentation line are to be done first.

Check with the blood bank that blood is ready and available as ordered.

Weigh used sponges immediately to reduce evaporation factor.

Measure irrigation fluids accurately.

When transferring the patient, keep the closed drainage system below body level.

INSERTION OF CENTRAL VENOUS CATHETER (PEDIATRIC)

Definition

Introduction of Silastic tubing into the subclavian, internal jugular, cephalic, or facial vein in order to administer parenteral nutrition or chemotherapy or to monitor hemodynamics and to replace fluids and blood.

Discussion

A central venous pressure catheter may be inserted on an acute basis for hemodynamic monitoring and for rapid replacement of fluids and blood or for ongoing access for purposes of parenteral nutrition or administration of chemotherapy or any other drug. The main advantage of this technique is to spare the patient frequent venipunctures and to decrease the likelihood of inducing phlebitis if more peripheral veins are used. Several types of Silastic catheters are available.

Procedure

A small incision is made over the external jugular vein in the lateral neck. The catheter is passed into the incised vein (confirmed by the aspiration of blood) to a predetermined length in order to be in the superior vena cava. A subcutaneous tunnel is made from the incision, employing a blunt tunneling instrument, to the anterior chest lateral to the sternum. The catheter exits through the tunnel and is sutured to the skin. The position of the catheter is confirmed by x-ray or fluoroscopy. The catheter is immediately connected by a heparin lock or a three-way stopcock to an appropriate intravenous solution. The venotomy and initial incision are closed.

Preparation of the Patient

See Pediatric General Information, pp. 518–520; the head and extremities may be covered prior to positioning. The patient is supine with the head and neck turned to the left (right side up); a small roll may be used to extend the neck. Cover the extremities, and restrain them using padded restraints. The procedure may be done under local anesthesia with anesthesia standby for newborns and cooperative children; otherwise, general anesthesia is administered. Apply pediatric electrosurgical dispersive pad.

Skin Preparation

Using warm preparation solution only, begin cleansing the supraclavicular area, extending from the infra-auricular border to the umbilicus (including the right shoulder) if the catheter is to exit the anterior thorax. If the catheter is to exit from the epigastrium, extend the preparation to the pubic symphysis. Prepare the skin to the table on the right side and well beyond the midline on the left side.

Draping

Folded towels and a pediatric laparotomy sheet

Equipment

Body heat maintenance equipment (e.g., heating lamps or warming mattress)
Covering for head and extremities
Image intensifier or portable x-ray machine with cassettes
Restraints, padded
Small roll
Electrosurgical unit

Instrumentation

Pediatric major procedures tray
Bulldog clamps, assorted small
Tunneling instrument

Supplies

Basin set
Blades (1) No. 15, (1) No. 11
Needle magnet or counter
Electrosurgical pencil (with needle tip)
Graduate and syringe for heparin solution (optional)
Local anesthetic, for example, lidocaine (Xylocaine) 1%,
    with syringe and needle (local)
Silastic catheter and introducer (e.g., Broviac)
Radiopaque dye (e.g., Hypaque) (optional)
Intravenous tubing
Heparin lock or three-way stopcock
Intravenous solution (e.g., 10% dextrose)

Special Notes

Determine if image intensifier or portable x-ray is to be used, and prepare table accordingly. Notify x-ray department.

Some warming mattresses interfere with fluoroscopy.

Observe x-ray precautions; see p. 21.

PYLOROMYOTOMY FOR CONGENITAL HYPERTROPHIC PYLORIC STENOSIS

Definition

Incision of the hypertrophied muscles of the pylorus in order to relieve pyloric obstruction.

Discussion

This congenital condition usually becomes evident a few weeks after birth with progressive episodes of vomiting caused by pyloric muscular hypertrophy creating a mechanical obstruction. The muscle mass ("olive") can often be palpated transabdominally. A thin solution of barium contrast medium may be necessary to confirm the diagnosis. A Ramstedt-Fredet pyloromyotomy, the procedure of choice, divides the pyloric muscle, leaving the mucosa (and submucosa) intact, relieving the condition.

Procedure

A high right rectus splitting incision is made over the liver; a transverse or oblique incision can also be used. The peritoneum is incised and the pylorus delivered into the wound. The pylorus is incised longitudinally anteriorly from the pyloric vein and pyloroduodenal junction proximally over the extent of the hypertrophic muscle. Using a pyloric spreading forceps, all remaining circular muscle fibers are separated to the level of the submucosa. Any laceration of the gastric or duodenal mucosa is immediately repaired. After hemostasis is obtained, the wound is closed.

Preparation of the Patient

See Pediatric General Information, pp. 518–520; the head and extremities are covered prior to positioning. The patient is supine. Extremities are restrained using padded restraints. Apply a pediatric electrosurgical dispersive pad.

Skin Preparation

Using warm preparation solutions only, begin cleansing over the right upper abdomen, extending from the axillae to the pubic symphysis, and down to the table at the sides.

Draping

Folded towels and a pediatric laparotomy sheet

Equipment

Body heat maintenance equipment (e.g., heating lamps, warming mattress)
Restraints, padded
Electrosurgical unit
Suction (available)

Instrumentation

Pediatric major procedures tray
Pyloric spreader

Supplies

Basin set
Electrosurgical pencil (with needle tip)
Blades (2) No. 15
Needle magnet or counter
Dissectors (e.g., peanut)

PEDIATRIC GASTROSTOMY

Definition

Establishment of an artificial opening into the stomach
exiting onto the skin of the abdominal wall.

Discussion

Gastrostomy is most frequently performed to permit
liquid feedings; it may also be done to permit gastric
drainage or retrograde dilation of an esophageal stricture. Gastrostomy can be an independent procedure or
performed in conjunction with other abdominal surgeries.

Procedure

As an Independent Procedure. A short left upper
quadrant transverse or vertical incision is made. The
greater curvature of the stomach is identified. Two
pursestring sutures are placed in the stomach; a stab
wound is made in the center of the pursestrings, and a
gastrostomy catheter is inserted. The pursestring sutures are then tightened and tied to secure the tube.
The tube is brought out through a stab wound lateral
to the incision. The stomach is sutured to the peritoneum about the stab wound. The tube is sutured to
the skin. The wound is closed.

Preparation of the Patient, Skin
Preparation, Draping, and Equipment

See Pediatric Umbilical Herniorrhaphy, pp. 529–530.

Instrumentation

Pediatric major procedures tray

Supplies

Basin set
Electrosurgical pencil (with needle tip)
Needle magnet
Blades (2) No. 15, (1) No. 11
Gastrostomy catheter (e.g., Pezzer, Malecot, or Foley)

Special Notes

Check with the surgeon regarding the type and size of gastrostomy catheter.

Keep soiled instruments isolated in a basin.

RELIEF OF INTESTINAL OBSTRUCTION (PEDIATRIC)

Definition

Refers to the reestablishment of intestinal patency in any number of conditions that present with blockage of the intestinal tract.

Discussion

Intestinal obstruction in the newborn becomes apparent shortly after birth with symptoms of emesis, abdominal distention, and failure to pass flatus and meconium. Urgent treatment is often mandatory. The conditions responsible for obstruction are numerous including intussusception, esophageal atresia, atresia and stenosis of duodenum, small bowel, and colon, annular pancreas, hypertrophic pyloric stenosis, imperforate anus, congenital malrotation, volvulus, congenital bands, infarction, meconium ileus, aganglionic megacolon, internal hernias, strangulated hernias, and infection. Treatment depends upon the diagnosis; during the course of surgery the search is made for additional abnormalities. Intestinal obstructive symptoms may also be seen in otherwise unrelated conditions such as cerebral injury with persistent emesis and in pulmonary infections.

Procedure

For duodenal atresia a paramedian or transverse incision is made in the upper abdomen. The abdomen is explored, and the site of obstruction and other conditions are identified. Bypass, rather than resection of the obstructed duodenal segment (usually second portion), is performed. An antecolic duodenojejunostomy is usually the procedure of choice. A loop of proximal jejunum is brought anterior to the transverse colon to the side of the distended proximal duodenum. A side-to-side anastomosis is fashioned in one or two layers according to the surgeon's preference and size of the small jejunal lumen. The abdomen is closed in layers.

Preparation of the Patient, Skin Preparation, and Draping

See Pyloromyotomy for Congenital Hypertophic Pyloric Stenosis, p. 538.

Equipment

Body heat maintenance equipment (e.g., heating lamps, warming mattress)
Restraints, padded
Electrosurgical unit
Suction

Instrumentation

Pediatric major procedures tray
Pediatric gastrointestinal tray
Automatic stapling device (optional)

Supplies

Basin set
Electrosurgical pencil (with needle tip)
Blades (2) No. 15
Needle magnet or counter
Dissectors (e.g., peanut)
Staples (optional)

Special Notes

Keep all soiled instruments isolated in a basin.

REDUCTION OF PEDIATRIC INTUSSUSCEPTION

Definition

Reduction of intussusception (in the child) is the correction of a condition in which there is an invagination of a segment of the intestine into an adjacent segment.

Discussion

This entity, typically seen in the older male infant, is characterized by sudden episodes of severe abdominal pain, emesis, and subsequent passage of bloody mucus. The infant seems to feel well shortly thereafter. Additional bouts follow until intestinal obstruction becomes evident. The most common site of intussusception is about the ileocecal valve, in which the terminal ileum (intussusceptum) becomes invaginated into the cecum (intussuscipiens). If not reduced, either spontaneously or by the hydrostatic pressure of a barium enema examination, gangrene will ultimately ensue.

Procedure

A low midline incision is employed. The intussusception is manually reduced. If there is resistance to reduction or compromised bowel is encountered, a resection is done with primary anastomosis, or the ends of the bowel are brought out as stomas through separate incisions. Anastomosis is performed as a secondary procedure. The abdomen is closed.

Preparation of the Patient

See Pediatric General Information, pp. 518–520; the head and extremities are covered prior to positioning patient. The patient is supine. Extremities are restrained using padded restraints. Apply a pediatric electrosurgical dispersive pad.

Skin Preparation

Using warm preparation solutions only, begin cleansing for a low midline incision extending from the nipples to the upper thighs, and down to the table at the sides.

Draping

Folded towels and a pediatric laparotomy sheet

Equipment

Body heat maintenance equipment (e.g., warming mattress, heating lamps)
Restraints, padded
Electrosurgical unit
Suction

Instrumentation

Pediatric major procedures tray
Pediatric gastrointestinal procedures tray
Automatic stapling device (optional)

Supplies

Blades (3) No. 15
Needle magnet or counter
Electrosurgical pencil (with needle tip)
Suction tubing
Vessel loops or umbilical tapes, ¼″
Staples (optional)

Special Notes

If a bowel resection is performed, isolate soiled instruments in a basin.

PEDIATRIC COLOSTOMY

Definition

Formation of an opening into the colon, which is exteriorized onto the anterior abdominal wall as a stoma.

Discussion

Colostomy is performed to bypass an obstructed colonic segment distally or for diversion of the fecal stream to minimize contamination because of perforation or infection and to "protect" a distal anastomosis by eliminating passage of the fecal stream across it. Several types of colostomy may be created; transverse and sigmoid are the most common. Most pediatric colostomies are temporary, but they may be permanent when the rectum is congenitally absent or unable to be reconstructed or in cases of neurologic and neoplastic processes, and so on. Colostomy may be performed as an independent procedure or in conjunction with other abdominal surgery. X-ray studies help to determine the appropriate site. Colostomy may be done as an emergency procedure.

Procedure

For an obstructive process or congenital absence of the distal sigmoid colon or rectum, a sigmoid or descending colon colostomy is made. An oblique incision is made in the left lower abdomen, and the muscles are either separated (as in gridiron incision) or divided. The abdomen is explored to identify any associated abnormalities or obstructive bands. The colon may be brought out as a loop over a rod or bridge to prevent retraction, or it can be divided, the distal end closed, and the proximal end is brought out through the incision or through an adjacent limited incision as an end-colostomy. In either situation, the colon and mesentery are sutured to ensuing layers of abdominal wall to prevent prolapse or herniation. The stoma wall is matured by suturing the full thickness of the stoma to the skin. Tension is avoided in order to prevent retraction or circulatory compromise and to allow for increasing thickness of the abdominal wall, with growth and improved postoperative nutrition. The main incision is closed; additional draping is used to avoid undue contamination. The sequence of closure of the wound and final preparation of the stoma varies with the surgeon. At the completion of the procedure, a colostomy pouch is applied to the stoma.

Preparation of the Patient

See Pediatric General Information, pp. 518–520; the head and extremities are covered prior to positioning.

The patient is supine. Extremities are restrained using padded restraints. Apply a pediatric electrosurgical dispersive pad.

Skin Preparation

Using warm preparation solutions only, begin cleansing the left lower abdomen, extending from the nipples to the upper thighs, and down to the table at the sides.

Draping

Folded towels and a pediatric laparotomy sheet

Equipment

Body heat maintenance equipment (e.g., heating lamps, warming mattress)
Restraints, padded
Electrosurgical unit
Suction (available)

Instrumentation

Pediatric major procedures tray
Pediatric gastrointestinal procedures tray

Supplies

Basin set
Blades (1) No. 10, (2) No. 15
Electrosurgical pencil (with needle tip)
Vessel loops or umbilical tapes ¼″
Dissectors (e.g., peanut)
Suction tubing (optional)
Glass rod and tubing with colostomy pouch (e.g., Karaya Seal or plastic bridge) and loop colostomy set (e.g., Hollister)

Special Notes

Keep soiled instruments isolated in a basin.

PEDIATRIC COLORECTAL RESECTION FOR AGANGLIONIC MEGACOLON/ HIRSCHSPRUNG'S DISEASE

Definition

Removal of the aganglionic portion of the colon and rectum with the anastomosis of the proximal normal colon to the distal rectum or anus.

Discussion

The section of colon removed, which can include a short segment of rectum and/or colon, or less often the entire colon, represents a functional obstruction caused by a lack of ganglion cells in the muscular layer (myenteric plexus) and the inability of this distal segment to relax, permitting passage of feces. The problem may be recognized soon after birth or in later infancy (or if the absence of ganglion cells is partial, diagnosis may be delayed until adulthood). Constipation with abdominal distention, growth failure, anemia, and episodes of paradoxical diarrhea occur. Necrotizing enterocolitis can develop in the neonate and is often fatal if not treated promptly. Barium enema examination and rectal muscle biopsy to demonstrate absence of ganglion cells are diagnostic. Colostomy (see Pediatric Colostomy, pp. 543–545) is indicated in newborns and children who are either ill or not responsive to measures to alleviate constipation and abdominal distention. The site of the colostomy must be proximal to the aganglionic segment, as confirmed by histologic examination. When the infant has regained good health and weight of 13.5 kg (30 pounds), or even until late childhood, surgical correction is undertaken. The aganglionic segment is resected and the proximal colon anastomosed to the distal rectum or anus.

The Swenson "pull-through" procedure is most often employed. The Duhamel procedure in which the distal rectum is not excised but allowed to form a common lumen with a segment of normal proximal colon brought anterior to the rectum by crushing the adjacent bowel walls with clamps has its advocates. In the Soave procedure the distal rectum is preserved but denuded of mucosa, forming a sleeve through which a normal colonic segment is passed to the anus with local anastomosis. These latter procedures avoid dissection in the pelvis, sparing possible injury to genital nerves but do not necessarily give better results than the Swenson procedure or its several modifications.

Procedure

A left paramedian incision is made. The colostomy, if present, is excised. The sigmoid colon is mobilized, and superior hemorrhoidal vessels are divided, taking care not to injure the ureters. Frozen section of colon muscle biopsies may be done at the level of the division of the bowel to make certain of the presence of ganglia. The pelvis is entered, the lateral rectal ligaments are cut, and the rectum is further mobilized, staying close to the bowel to avoid injury to the autonomic nerves. A ring clamp or long Babcock forceps is inserted transanally, and a segment of dissected colon is seized from within; with counterpressure from the pelvis, the colon is everted and "pulled through" the anus. The coats of the everted bowel are circumferentially incised, suturing the rim of the retained portion of colon to the anal canal in a single or double layer. The specimen is thereby amputated and the anastomosis completed. The anastomotic ring is then inverted, replacing it within the anal canal. The abdominal incision is closed.

Preparation of the Patient

See Pediatric General Information, pp. 518–520; the head and extremities are covered prior to positioning. Following the induction of anesthesia, the patient is positioned in a modified lithotomy or supine position with the knees bent in a modified frog-leg position. A folded towel is placed under the buttocks. The legs may be held in position using adominal dressing pads and adhesive tape. Padded restraints are used on the upper extremities. Apply a pediatric electrosurgical dispersive pad. Check with the surgeon regarding insertion of a Foley catheter and irrigation of the rectum with warm saline.

Skin Preparation

Use warm preparation solutions only. For a *combined approach:* Begin cleansing for a left paramedian incision extending from the nipples to the knees, and down to the table at the sides. Cleanse inner thighs, genitalia, exposed buttocks, perineum, and anus (discarding each sponge after prepping anus).

For *separate approaches: perineal:* Begin at the pubic symphysis, cleanse inner thighs, genitalia, exposed buttocks, perineum, and anus (discarding each sponge after prepping anus). *Abdominal:* Begin cleansing for a left paramedian incision, extending from the nipples to the midthighs, and down to the table at the sides.

Draping

The patient may be draped all at once for both the abdominal and perineal approaches, or the patient may be reprepared and redraped for the perineal approach.

For the *combined approach,* tuck in a drape sheet under the patient's buttocks. Drape the abdomen and perineal area with folded towels. Towels may be secured by a sterile, plastic adhesive drape, staples, or with sutures. A pediatric laparotomy sheet covers the field.

For the *perineal approach,* the abdominal wound is covered, and a hole is cut in the laparatomy sheet in the perineal area. If the patient is to be reprepared and redraped: Tuck a drape sheet under the patient's buttocks; drape the perineum with folded towels and a pediatric laparotomy sheet.

For the *abdominal approach,* gowns and gloves are changed, the patient is reprepared and redraped, and the instruments are changed. The patient is draped with folded towels on the abdomen and a pediatric laparotomy sheet.

Equipment

Body heat maintenance equipment (e.g., heating lamps, warming mattress)
Covering for the head and extremities
Pediatric stirrups (modified lithotomy)

Suction (with specimen trap for accurate blood loss measurement)
Electrosurgical unit
Scale (to weigh sponges)
Mayo stand (additional) and/or back table for perineal approach

Instrumentation

Abdominal Approach
Pediatric major procedures tray
Pediatric Balfour retractor
Brain/ribbon/malleable retractor (small)
Hemoclip appliers (short, medium)
Hegar dilators (small)
Automatic stapling device (optional)

Perineal Approach
Pediatric major procedures tray
Ruler

Supplies

Basin set
Electrosurgical pencil (with needle tip)
Bulb syringe
Hemoclips (small, medium)
Suction tubing
Sterile, plastic adhesive drape (optional)
Needle magnet or counter
Blades (1) No. 10, (4) No. 15
Foley catheter (e.g., No. 8 for bladder)
Dissectors (e.g., peanut)
Staples (optional)

Special Notes

In positioning the patient, do not allow adhesive tape to come in direct contact with the skin. Protect skin with tincture of benzoin.

Check with the blood bank to determine that blood is available as ordered.

Weigh used sponges immediately to reduce evaporation factor.

Measure irrigation fluids accurately.

Be prepared for multiple bowel tissue biopsies.

REPAIR OF IMPERFORATE ANUS

Definition

Establishment of colorectal continuity where there is an absence of an anal opening.

Discussion

There are four classes of imperforate anus:

Types

I   Stenosis at the anus or distal rectum

II   Membranous barrier at the anus

III   Rectum ending in a blind pouch above the perineum

IV   Anus and distal rectum ending in a blind pouch proximally, and the more proximal rectum ending in a blind pouch above the distal segment

Type I may be treated by dilation, ultimately if stricture persists, a plastic procedure will be necessary.

In *Type II* a simple anal membrane needs only to be incised and dilated. The mucosa can be sutured to the skin.

Type III is often associated with various fistulae (rectovesical, rectourethral, rectovaginal, rectoperineal) that may allow the passage of the fecal stream by way of the genitourinary tract. Correction of these conditions depend upon the presentation.

Type IV, which is rare, is treated by preliminary colostomy with definitive repair several months later by direct anastomosis, or "pull-through," procedure. Type III with its variety of fistulae is initially treated by colostomy, especially if other abnormalities are present and the infant is in otherwise ill health or premature. Definitive repair can be performed after 3 months of age.

Procedure

In the male type III procedure without fistula, the procedure is done by the *perineal approach* only if x-ray confirms the blind pouch is less than 1.5 cm from the anal dimple. A catheter (8 or 10 Fr) is passed into the bladder. The location of the anal sphincter is determined by a nerve stimulator. A small vertical incision is made within the anal dimple. The rectal pouch is dissected free from surrounding stricture so that it can be brought to skin level without tension. The bowel is opened and meconium aspirated. The full thickness of the rectal wall is sutured to the skin.

When the rectal pouch is greater than 1.5 cm above the sphincter, a combined *abdominoperineal approach* is used. The bladder is catheterized with the patient in modified lithotomy position. (This gives simultaneous access to the abdomen and perineum.) An incision is made within the anal dimple as above, and the sphincter is dilated. A left lower oblique or a left paramedial abdominal incision is made. The sigmoid colon and rectum are mobilized, taking care not to injure the ureters. Meconium is aspirated from the distal portion of the colon with a large-bore needle and the puncture site sutured closed. Dissection continues until the rectum can reach the perineal floor without tension. Care is taken to preserve vascular arcades. The end of the bowel is passed through a tunnel within the levator muscles, made via the perineal incision. The pelvic peritoneum is closed. The abdominal wound is closed. The full thickness of the rectum is sutured to the skin about the sphincter as above.

Preparation of the Patient

See Pediatric General Information, pp. 518–520; the head and extremities are covered prior to positioning. Following the induction of anesthesia, the patient is positioned in a modified lithotomy or supine position with the knees bent in a modified frog-leg position. A folded towel is placed under the buttocks. The legs may be held in position using abdominal dressing pads and adhesive tape. Padded restraints are used on the upper extremities. Apply a pediatric electrosurgical dispersive pad. Check with the surgeon regarding insertion of a Foley catheter.

Skin Preparation

Use warm preparation solutions only. See Pediatric Colorectal Resection, p. 548. For an extensive procedure, follow the preparation for a combined approach; for a limited procedure, follow the preparation for a perineal approach.

Draping

See Pediatric Colorectal Resection, p. 548. For an extensive procedure, drape as for a combined approach; for a limited procedure, drape as for a perineal approach.

Equipment

Covering for head and extremities
Body heat maintenance equipment (e.g., heat lamp, warming mattress)
Electrosurgical unit
Suction (with specimen trap for accurate blood loss measurement)
Scale (to weigh sponges for an extensive procedure)

Instrumentation

Pediatric major procedures tray
Hegar dilators, probes
    For extensive procedures, see Pediatric Colorectal Resection, p. 549.

Supplies

Basin set
Blades (2) No. 15
Needle magnet or counter
Suction tubing
Bulb syringe
Electrosurgical pencil (with needle tip)
Nerve stimulator (locator)
    For extensive procedures, see Pediatric Colorectal Resection, p. 549.

Special Notes

In positioning the patient, do not allow adhesive tape to come in direct contact with the skin. Protect the skin with tincture of benzoin.

For extensive procedures, see Pediatric Colorectal Resection, pp. 549–550.

Isolate soiled instruments in a basin.

PEDIATRIC LIMITED ACCESS PROCEDURES

At present, pediatric laparoscopy and thoracoscopy have not had the wide application as practiced in the adult; one reason is that the physical size of smaller children is a limiting factor in certain procedures with currently available instrumentation. The cost of endoscopic surgeries must be considered. An overriding principle of any limited access procedure is that it must be promptly converted to an open procedure when the endoscopic approach is deemed unfeasible or the patient's safety is compromised.

PEDIATRIC LAPAROSCOPY

This modality has been applied to a number of conditions including gastroesophageal reflux (fundoplication), hematologic entities as spherocytosis, idiopathic thrombocytopenic purpura, and so on, splenectomy, sickle cell disease, cholelithiasis (cholecystectomy), and acute appendicitis (appendectomy). Less common indications include identification of contralateral patent processus vaginalis in performance of inguinal herniorrhalphy whereby a scope can be inserted intraperitoneally through the hernia sac on the ipsilateral side, search for nonpalpable intra-abdominal testis, which if abnormal, can be excised or can be mobilized for later replacement into the scrotum, and assistance in mobilizing the colon as in a pull-through procedure for Hirschsprung's disease. Diagnostic evaluation of tumors, including retroperitoneal node biopsy, and so on, may be performed.

Pneumoperitoneum is established with a Verres needle or by direct puncture under direct vision utilizing a limited cutdown. During needle insertion the abdominal wall is pulled up manually or by the use of tissue hooks or stay sutures. The usual pediatric preparatory precautions are observed as previously noted (see pp. 518–520).

Under development are shortened modifications of certain adult endoscopic instruments. Currently available are shortened graspers, scissors, dissectors, and 5 mm trocars. Several commonly employed instruments as right-angle clamps, Babcock clamps, clip appliers, and linear staplers inherently require adult size 10 mm trocar parts as well as adequate room intraperitoneally to permit full excursion of the working parts of these instruments.

PEDIATRIC LAPAROSCOPIC APPENDECTOMY

Definition

Excision of the appendix through a laparoscope.

Discussion

Indications for laparoscopic pediatric laparoscopy are similar to the standard approach, but it should not be attempted when the disease has reached an advanced stage or when peritonitis is present. An additional use of the laparoscopic approach is the ability to identify other causes of the acute abdomen as ovarian pathology, congenital abnormalities (e.g., Meckel's diverticulum), and numerous abdominal infections. Many pediatric surgeons prefer in the smaller child and the thin male to perform an open procedure regardless, as the abdominal portal incision may be longer than the standard incision.

Procedure

The umbilical portal is made using a 12 mm trocar following the establishment of pneumoperitoneum. If early appendicitis is identified, two additional 5 mm portals are established at the right anterior axillary line and in the left lower quadrant. The appendix is placed in traction with the endoloop or grasping forceps; the mesoappendix is either clipped or stapled and the appendix ligated, also with either endoloop or staples, and the speimen is delivered (using a specimen bag, if desired). If the appendix is perforated or covered by purulent exudate, the use of a specimen bag is mandatory in order to avoid contamination. The abdomen may be irrigated and a drain placed as indicated. The portals are removed and the incisions closed.

PEDIATRIC LAPROSCOPIC FUNDOPLICATION/NISSEN PROCEDURE

Definition

Endoscopic wrapping of the gastric fundus about the cardia to correct esophageal reflux.

Discussion

This procedure is employed to prevent gastroesophageal reflux. The laparoscopic approach is particularly beneficial in children with chronic cough (e.g., cystic fibrosis) in that postoperative pain is minimized with easier pulmonary toilet.

Procedure

After pneumoperitoneum is established, four portals are placed: umbilical, mid-upper rectus, and left and right paraumbilical. A 30° laparoscope is used. The triangular ligament of the liver is incised, and the phrenicoesophageal ligament is divided. A dilator is passed into the esophagus. The esophagus is dissected, protecting the vegas nerves. The crura are dissected, and the dilator is removed. The gastric fundus is mobilized dividing short gastric muscles as necessary. A Nissen wrap (or partial wrap) is accomplished with two or three nonabsorbable sutures (sometimes reinforced by staples). The fundus can then be stapled to the right crus.

If a gastrostomy is indicated, the stomach is inflated with carbon dioxide through a nasogastric tube. Four T-fasteners are inserted into the stomach percutaneously with a special slotted needle, and a catheter (e.g., Foley) is passed into the center of the square of fasteners. The T-fasteners are tied over stents.

If gastric emptying is a problem, pyloromyotomy or

pyloroplasty may be performed, laparoscopically mobilizing the pylorus, which may be delivered onto the abdominal wall through an enlarged port, and the definitive procedure performed. The pneumoperitoneum is released, and the ports are closed in the routine manner.

PEDIATRIC THORACOSCOPY

Definition

The endoscopic approach to the thorax.

Discussion

Indications include identification and biopsy of solitary peripheral lesions, lysis of empyema cavity in the early stages, identification of mediastinal masses, and so on. This procedure is contraindicated for larger lesions, small children (less than 6 months old), established pleural symphysis, and for patients on whom mechanical ventilation must be maintained. It should be noted that a limited biopsy through a small opening incision is efficient and less costly, especially when diffuse disease is present.

Technical Considerations

Local anesthesia may be employed. Using pediatric laparoscopic 5 mm trocars for simple biopsies, a cup biopsy forceps is employed. (Note that direct leaks are rare following biopsies.) For more involved procedures, selective intubation is necessary so that the ipsilateral lung is well collapsed. On occasion a Fogarty catheter can be placed to obstruct the ipsilateral bronchus. Low pressure CO_2 insufflation, 4 to 6 mm, can further assist in collapsing the operative side (in which case laparoscopy ports must be used).

Portal placement and position of the patient depend upon preoperative localization of the lesion (e.g., if the lesion is posterior, lean the patient forward). The initial portal is made in the fifth or sixth intercostal space on the midaxillary line. After exploration other ports are placed accordingly. Endoscopic staplers are helpful in sealing the wound edges following excision of tissues excised; note however, that in small patients an endo-gastrointestinal stapler must be introduced as far from the operative site as possible to allow 5 mm clearance to operate the instrument. Certain lesions such as a posterior mediastinal neuroblastoma can be excised employing cautery or a laser. A larger specimen can be morcellated in a specimen bag to facilitate its extraction.

After lysis of empyema cavities prior to the fibrotho-rax stage, urokinase (an enzyme) may be instilled into the pleural space: 100,000 to 200,000 units of uroki-nase in 30 mL of saline.

A chest tube is usually not employed postoperatively unless the patient requires assisted ventilation. The use of staplers permits removal of the chest tube prior to the patient's leaving the operating room.

PEDIATRIC LAPAROSCOPIC SPLENECTOMY

Definition

The endoscopic excision of the spleen.

Discussion

Primary indications for this procedure are hematologic. If cholecystectomy is likewise indicated, laparoscopic cholecystectomy similar to that performed in the adult can be done. Intraoperative cholangiogram to identify the small biliary ductal structures is done through the gallbladder or cystic duct. A colonic preparation is nec-essary.

Procedure

With the patient in the supine position, pneumoperi-toneum is established. Three or four portals in the mid-line or left of the midline are placed. The short gastric vessels are divided. The patient may then be placed in the left lateral position. The splenocolic ligament is di-vided, employing electrosurgery or an endoscopic lin-ear stapler; attachments to the diaphragm and perinephric tissues are divided. The remaining short gastric vessels are also divided. The linear stapler is placed across the splenic hilum avoiding the tail of the pancreas. The patient may then be returned to the supine position and the specimen delivered in a specimen retrieval bag with morcellation of the spleen as necessary. Accessory spleens, if present, are excised. The pneumoperitoneum is released, and the ports are closed.

PART IV

INSTRUMENT TRAYS

The chapters on instrument trays complement the instrumentation section of each procedure. The instruments included are meant to be representatives of particular types used for specific functions. Substitutions for instruments that can be similarly used can be made according to the preference of the surgeons at each institution.

Today there is an ever-increasing number and variety of surgical instruments. Many traditionally used instruments have been discarded or modified. Some instruments are known by more than one name or by various colloquial names even within the same institution. The composition of the trays appearing in this guide, therefore, will be familiar to most readers, though perhaps not precisely what might be encountered at their own surgical facility.

These trays are based upon anatomic regions or frequently performed specific procedures. To simplify the listings of the tray components certain liberties have been taken to avoid excessive terminology and subsections. Therefore, the category of forceps refers only to "thumb" forceps; the category of clamps includes hemostatic forceps, grasping forceps, towel clips, and needle holders. The "Miscellaneous" subheading is an all-inclusive category for all instruments that do not fit under any of the main categories.

Chapter 21

General Surgery Trays

MAJOR PROCEDURES TRAY

Retractors

2 Ribbon/malleable (1) 1½", (1) 2½"
3 Richardson (1) small, (1) medium, (1) large
2 Goulet
2 Army-Navy
3 Deaver (1) narrow, (1) medium, (1) wide

Forceps

2 Tissue without teeth (1) 5½", (1) 10"
3 Tissue with teeth (1) 5½", (1) 8", (1) 10"
2 Russian (1) 7", (1) 10"
6 DeBakey (2) 6", (2) 7¾", (2) 9"
2 Adson with teeth

Scissors

2 Straight Mayo 6¼"
1 Curved Mayo 6¼"
1 Metzenbaum 7"
1 Wire cutter

Clamps

10 Towel clip 5½"
18 Curved Crile 5½"
6 Straight Crile 5½"

6 Straight Kocher 6¼"
6 Allis 6"
4 Babcock 6"
12 Curved Pean (6) 6¼", (6) 8"
4 Tonsil (Schnidt) 7½"
2 Right-angle 8"
6 Needle holder (2) 6", (2) 7", (2) 8"
4 Sponge forceps 10"
2 Carmalt 8"

Suction Tubes or Tips

1 Poole
1 Yankauer 10⅜"

Miscellaneous

3 Knife handles (2) No. 3, (1) No. 7
1 Probe, malleable
1 Grooved director

BASIC/MINOR PROCEDURES TRAY

Retractors

2 Goulet
2 Army-Navy
1 Weitlaner, sharp 6½"
1 Ribbon/malleable 1"
1 Deaver, narrow
1 Richardson, small
2 Senn, sharp

Forceps

2 Tissue without teeth 5½"
2 Tisssue with teeth 5½"
1 Adson without teeth
2 Adson with teeth
1 Russian 7"
4 DeBakey (2) 6", (2) 7¾"

Scissors

1 Curved Mayo 6¼"
2 Straight Mayo 6¼"

3 Metzenbaum (1) 5¼", (1) 6", (1) 7"
1 Stevens tenotomy
1 Straight iris
1 Curved iris

Clamps

10 Towel clip (6) 3½", (4) 5½"
12 Curved mosquito 5¼"
2 Straight mosquito 5¼"
12 Curved Crile 5½"
2 Babcock 6"
4 Allis 6"
4 Straight Kocher 6¼"
2 Webster needle holder
4 Needle holder (2) 6", (2) 7"
2 Sponge forceps 7"

Suction Tubes or Tips

1 Yankauer 10⅜"
1 Poole
1 Frazier No. 10

Miscellaneous

3 Knife handles (2) No. 3, (1) No. 7
1 Probe, malleable
1 Grooved director
2 Medicine cups

LIMITED PROCEDURE TRAY

Retractors

2 Joseph skin hook
2 Senn, sharp

Forceps

1 Tissue with teeth 5½"
2 Adson with teeth
1 Adson without teeth
1 Adson-Brown

Scissors

1 Straight Mayo 6¼"
2 Metzenbaum (1) 5¼", (1) 6"
1 Stevens tenotomy
1 Curved iris
1 Straight iris

Clamps

4 Curved Crile 5½"
2 Straight Crile 5½"
4 Curved mosquito 5¼"
2 Needle holder 6"
8 Towel clip (4) 3½", (4) 5½"

Suction Tubes or Tips

1 Frazier No. 10

Miscellaneous

2 Knife handles No. 3
2 Medicine cups

THYROID TRAY

Retractors

2 Senn (sharp)
1 Mahorner
2 Greene
2 Cushing vein
2 Gelpi
1 Weitlaner, sharp 5½"
2 Lahey

Forceps

2 Tissue without teeth 5½"
2 Tissue with teeth 5½"
2 Adson with teeth
2 DeBakey 6"

Scissors

2 Straight Mayo (1) 5¼", (1) 6¼"
2 Metzenbaum (1) 5¼", (1) 6"
1 Straight Metzenbaum 5¼"

Clamps

12 Curved mosquito 5¼"
6 Curved Crile 5½"
2 Curved Pean 6¼"
6 Allis 6"
2 Right-angle, fine
2 Right-angle 6¼"
2 Straight Kocher 6"
2 Lahey
2 Needle holder 6"
12 Towel clip 3½"

Suction Tubes or Tips

1 Frazier No. 8
1 Andrews 9½"

Miscellaneous

2 Knife handles No. 3

LONG INSTRUMENTS TRAY

Forceps

1 Tissue without teeth 10"
1 Tissue with teeth 10"

Scissors

1 Metzenbaum 9"

Clamps

4 Collier 10½"
3 Right-angle 11"
6 Pean 10"
4 Allis 10"
2 Babcock 10"
2 Needle holder 10"

Miscellaneous

1 Knife handle No. 3L, 8"

BILIARY TRACT PROCEDURES TRAY

Forceps

4 Randall stone (¼ curved length through 1 full curved length)

Scissors

1 Metzenbaum 9″

Scoops

3 Ferguson gallstone scoops (1) small, (1) medium, (1) large

Miscellaneous

9 Bakes common duct dilators (sizes 3 to 11)
1 Knife handle No. 3L
1 Spoon
1 Medicine cup
1 Probe, malleable
1 Alcock conical catheter adaptor
1 Ochsner gallbladder trocar

CHOLEDOCHOSCOPY TRAY

1 Choledochoscope
1 Light adaptor (for scope)
1 Fiberoptic cord
1 Biopsy forceps, flexible
1 Biopsy forceps, rigid
1 Foreign body forceps, flexible
1 Instrument guide
1 Stone crusher
1 Stopcock
1 Rubber washer
2 Rubber caps

BASIC RIGID SIGMOIDOSCOPY TRAY

1 Sigmoidoscope with obturator (steel) or 1 disposable sigmoidoscope with obturator
1 Illuminator head unit (for disposable scope only)
1 Sigmoidoscopy light cord

1 Insufflation bulb
1 Anoscope (e.g., Hirschmann, medium)

Special Notes

Standard sigmoidoscope is 25 × 1.9 cm.
   Disposable sigmoidoscopes are preferred over metal ones.

GASTROINTESTINAL PROCEDURES TRAY

Clamps

12 Pean (8) 6¼″, (4) 10″
4 Babcock 10″
4 Kocher (Ochsner) 9″
2 Straight Doyen intestinal 9¼″
2 Curved Doyen intestinal 9¼″
Assorted variety, additional pairs of noncrushing bowel
   clamps, straight or right angle such as:
      Glassman intestinal
      DeBakey vascular
      Bainbridge intestinal
      Wertheim

Miscellaneous

8 Latex tubing pieces 6″ × ³⁄₁₆″ (for Doyen)

RECTAL PROCEDURES TRAY

Retractors

1 Parks or 1 Pratt rectal speculum (with set screw)
3 Sawyer (1) small, (1) medium, (1) large

Forceps

1 Tissue without teeth 5½″
1 Tissue with teeth 5½″
1 Adson-Brown

Scissors

1 Straight Mayo 6¼″
1 Curved Mayo 6¼″
1 Metzenbaum 7″

Clamps

6 Curved Crile 5½"
6 Allis 6"
4 Towel clip 5½"
4 Pennington 5½"
2 Needle holder 6"

Suction Tubes or Tips

1 Yankauer 10⅜"

Miscellaneous

2 Knife handles No. 3
1 Probe, malleable
1 Grooved director
1 Crypt hook

Chapter 22

Gynecologic and Obstetric Trays

DILATATION AND CURETTAGE (D & C) TRAY

Retractors

1 Auvard vaginal speculum, weighted

Forceps

1 Tissue without teeth 10″
1 Tissue with teeth 10″

Scissors

1 Straight Mayo 6¼″

Clamps

1 Straight Crile 5½″
2 Towel clip 5½″
1 Needle holder 8″

Tenaculums

1 Schroeder single-toothed
1 Jacobs

Dilators

8 Hegar (Nos. 3 to 4 through 17 to 18)
1 Goodell

Curettes

3 Sims sharp (1) small, (1) medium, (1) large
1 Thomas blunt (1) medium
1 Heaney endometrial

Miscellaneous

1 Biopsy punch
1 Randall stone forceps (¼ curved length)
1 Bozeman packing forceps
1 Sponge forceps 10″
1 Uterine sound

CERVICAL CONE TRAY

Retractors

2 Heaney

Forceps

1 Tissue without teeth 10″
2 Tissue with teeth (1) 5½″, (1) 10″

Scissors

1 Straight Mayo 6¼″
1 Curved Mayo 6¼″
1 Metzenbaum 7″

Clamps

6 Curved Crile 5½″
2 Straight Kocher 6¼″
6 Allis 6″
2 Towel clip 5½″
1 Needle holder 7″

Miscellaneous

2 Knife handles (1) No. 3, (1) No. 7

VAGINAL HYSTERECTOMY TRAY

Retractors

1 Auvard vaginal speculum, weighted
1 Glennor, weighted
1 Deaver, narrow
2 Jackson, short
2 Heaney

Forceps

3 Tissue without teeth (1) 5½″, (1) 8½″, (1) 10″
3 Tissue with teeth (1) 5½″, (1) 8½″, (1) 10″
1 Russian 7″

Scissors

1 Curved Mayo 6½″
2 Straight Mayo 6½″
1 Metzenbaum 7″

Clamps

8 Straight Crile 5½″
8 Curved Crile 5½″
8 Allis 6″
4 Curved Pean 6¼″
12 Straight Kocher (Ochsner) (8) 6¼″, (4) 8″
4 Curved Kocher (Ochsner) 8″
4 Heaney 8¼″
2 Babcock 10″
4 Sponge forceps 10″
4 Needle holder (2) 6″, (2) 7″
2 Heaney needle holder
6 Towel clip 5½″

Suctions

1 Yankauer 10⅜″
1 Poole

Tenaculums

1 Jacobs
1 Schroeder single-toothed
1 Schroeder double-toothed

Miscellaneous

1 Bozeman packing forceps
1 Uterine sound
3 Knife handles (1) No. 3, (1) No. 3L 10″, (1) No. 7

ABDOMINAL HYSTERECTOMY TRAY

Forceps

1 Tissue with teeth 10″

Scissors

1 Curved Mayo 6¼″

Clamps

2 Lahey
5 Heany 8¼″
6 Straight Kocher (Ochsner) 8″
6 Curved Kocher (Ochsner) 8″
6 Curved Phaneuf 8¼″
6 Long Allis 10″

Tenaculums

1 Jacobs
1 Schroeder single-toothed
1 Schroeder double-toothed

CESAREAN SECTION TRAY

Retractors

2 Richardson (1) small, (1) medium
1 Deaver, extra wide 3″
2 Goulet
1 DeLee universal

Forceps

2 Tissue with teeth 5½″
2 Adson with teeth
1 Russian 7″

Scissors

2 Straight Mayo 6¼"
1 Curved Mayo 6¼"
1 Metzenbaum 7"
1 Umbilical
1 Lister bandage

Clamps

4 Towel clip 5½"
12 Curved Crile 5½"
4 Straight Crile 5½"
2 Babcock 6"
6 Allis 6‴
6 Straight Kocher 6¼"
6 Pean 6¼"
4 Sponge forceps 7"
4 Pennington
4 Needle holder (2) 7", (2) 8"

Suction Tubes or Tips

1 Poole
1 Yankauer 10⅜"

Miscellaneous

3 Knife handles (2) No. 3, (1) No. 4

Chapter 23

Genitourinary Trays

VASECTOMY TRAY

Retractors

2 Joseph skin hook
2 Senn, sharp

Forceps

1 Tissue without teeth 5½″
1 Tissue with teeth 5½″
1 Adson with teeth

Scissors

1 Metzenbaum 5¼″
1 Straight Mayo 6¼″

Clamps

2 Curved Crile 5½″
2 Curved mosquito 5¼″
2 Allis 6″
2 Towel clip 5½″
1 Needle holder 6″

Miscellaneous

1 Knife handle No. 3

ABDOMINAL PROSTATECTOMY TRAY

Retractors

1 Judd-Mason

Clamps

6 Allis 10″
6 Babcock 10″
4 Lahey
1 Stratte needle holder 9″

Scissors

1 Metzenbaum 9″
1 Jorgenson 9″

KIDNEY TRAY

Forceps

4 Randall Stone (¼ curved length through 1 full curved length)

Scissors

1 Metzenbaum 9″

Clamps

4 Babcock 9″
2 Herrick kidney pedicle 9½″
1 Pean vessel 10″

Chapter 24

Thoracic Trays

MEDIASTINOSCOPY TRAY

Retractors

2 Senn, sharp
2 Army-Navy
2 Carlen introducer
1 Weitlaner, blunt 5½″

Forceps

1 Tissue with teeth 5½″
1 Adson with teeth
1 DeBakey 6″

Scissors

1 Straight Mayo 6¼″
1 Metzenbaum 7″

Clamps

1 Straight Crile 5½″
4 Curved Crile 5½″
4 Towel clip 5½″
2 Needle holder, fine 6″

Suction Tubes or Tips

1 Frazier No. 10
2 Suction-electrocoagulator and cords

Miscellaneous

1 Fiberoptic mediastinoscope
1 Fiberoptic light cord
3 Biopsy forceps, assorted
1 Circular biopsy
1 Electrosurgical cord
2 Staimey needles
1 Knife handle No. 3
1 Aspirating tube
1 Syringe, Luer-lok, 5 mL

THORACOTOMY TRAY

Retractors

1 Finochietto rib (with 4 blades) adult size, total opening 10″
1 Finochietto rib (with 4 blades) child size, total opening 6″

Forceps

1 Russian 10″

Scissors

1 Metzenbaum 11″
1 Nelson 8″

Clamps

2 Duval-Crile lung
2 Mixter 9″
2 Right-angle 11″
4 Babcock 10″
1 Needle holder, fine 10½″

Rib Elevators

2 Doyen elevator and raspatory, (1) left, (1) right
1 Matson stripper and elevator
1 Alexander costal periosteotome
1 Langenbeck periosteal elevator
1 Alexander rib raspatory

Rib Shears

1 Bethune
2 Gluck (1) narrow, (1) wide
1 Sauerbruck double-action rongeur
1 Stille

Miscellaneous

2 Bailey rib contractors

PACEMAKER TRAY

Retractors

2 Senn, blunt
2 Weitlaner (1) 5½″, (1) 7½″
2 Rake, blunt (4 prong)
2 Army-Navy

Forceps

1 Tissue without teeth 5½″
1 Tissue with teeth 5½″
1 Adson without teeth
2 Adson with teeth
1 DeBakey 6″

Scissors

1 Metzenbaum 7″
1 Straight Mayo 6¼″
1 Stevens tenotomy
1 Curved iris
1 Straight iris
1 Potts

Clamps

2 Right-angle 8″
2 Tonsil (Schnidt)
8 Curved Crile 5½″
6 Curved mosquito 5¼″
2 DeBakey, multipurpose 6″ (1) 30°, (1) 60°
1 Needle holder 6″

1 Ryder needle holder 6″
4 Towel clip 5½″
2 Sponge forceps 10″

Suction Tubes or Tips

1 Frazier No. 10
1 Andrews 9½″

Miscellaneous

2 Knife handles No. 3
1 Medicine cup
1 Bozeman packing forceps

Chapter 25

Cardiovascular Trays

VASCULAR PROCEDURES TRAY

Forceps

6 DeBakey (2) 6″, (2) 8″, (2) 9½″

Scissors

1 Potts

Clamps

2 DeBakey multipurpose (1) 9¾″, (1) 12″
1 DeBakey curved aorta aneurysm 11¼″
5 DeBakey tangential occlusion 7½″, 9¾″, 10″, 10¼″, 10⅝″
1 Hufnagel ascending aorta
2 Angled DeBakey 90° 10″
1 DeBakey Aorta 10½″
1 Medium curved Crawford auricle 9¼″
1 Glover coarctation, straight 8¾″
1 Glover coarctation, angled 8¾″
1 Glover patent ductus, straight 8″
1 Glover patent ductus, angled 8″
1 Straight Glover 6¾″
2 Curved Glover (1) 6¾″, (1) 8¼″
1 Cooley multipurpose, angled 6¼″
2 Cooley multipurpose, straight 7″
1 Curved Cooley 6¾″
6 Cardiovascular needle holder (2) 7″, (2) 8″, (2) 9″

VASCULAR SHUNT TRAY

Retractors

2 Army-Navy
2 Goulet
2 Senn, blunt
2 Rake, blunt (4 prong)
2 Cushing vein
2 Straight Weitlaner, blunt 6½"
1 Curved Weitlaner, blunt 6½"
2 Alm, blunt

Forceps

1 Tissue without teeth 5½"
1 Tissue with teeth 5½"
1 Russian 6"
2 Adson without teeth
1 Adson with teeth
1 Adson-Brown
2 DeBakey 6"

Scissors

2 Straight Mayo 6¼"
3 Metzenbaum (1) 5", (1) 5¾", (1)7"
1 Straight Metzenbaum 5"
1 Stevens tenotomy
1 Straight iris
1 Curved iris

Clamps

6 Straight Crile 5½"
6 Curved Crile 5½"
3 Straight mosquito 5¼"
3 Curved mosquito 5¼"
3 Curved Pean 6¼"
3 Tonsil (Schnidt) 7½"
5 Right-angle (2) 5¼", (3) 7"
12 Towel clip 3½"
2 Sponge forceps 7"

2 Shunt
1 Needle holder (fine) 6″
4 Ryder needle holder (2) 6″, (2) 7″
1 Castroviejo needle holder

Suction Tubes or Tips

1 Andrews 9½″

Miscellaneous

1 Probe (malleable)
2 Knife handles No. 3
8 Rubber tubing pieces 2″
Various vascular clamps (e.g., DeBakey peripheral, De-
    Bakey multipurpose, patent ductus, and coarctation)

CARDIAC PROCEDURES TRAY*

Retractors

1 Richardson, small
3 Army-Navy
2 Cushing vein
2 Senn, sharp
2 Rake (3 prong), sharp
2 Adson self-retaining, straight
2 Himmelstein sternal (with hinged arms)
2 Lamina spreader (1) small, (1) large

Forceps

4 Tissue with teeth 5½″
3 Adson with teeth
2 Russian 10″
10 DeBakey (1) 7¾″, (8) 9½″ (1) 12″

---

*A wide variety of instruments have been developed for car-
diovascular surgery. Similar instruments with minor modifications are available. The selection and nomenclature of similar clamps vary between institutions and sections of the
country.

Scissors

4 Straight Mayo 6¼″
1 Curved Mayo 6¼″
5 Metzenbaum 7″
3 Potts (1) 25°, (1) 45°, (1) 60°
2 Wire cutter

Clamps

6 Curved mosquito 5¼″
18 Curved Crile 5½″
2 Curved Pean 6¼″
2 Herrick kidney 9½″
2 Straight Kocher (Ochsner) 8″
2 Right-angle 8″
2 Tonsil (Schnidt) 7½″
6 Tube occluding
3 Derra (1) small, (1) medium, (1) large
2 DeBakey coarctation (1) 8½″, (1) 8⅜″
2 Crafoord aortic aneurysm 9½″
2 DeBakey tangential occlusion (1) 9¾″, (1) 10″
2 Satinsky 9½″
1 DeBakey patent ductus, straight 7½″
1 DeBakey patent ductus, angular 7½″
12 Needle holder (6) 6″, (6) 8″
16 Vascular needle holder, variety
4 Sternal needle holder
2 Sponge forceps 10″
26 Towel clip 5½″

Suction Tubes or Tips

2 Yankauer 10⅜″

Miscellaneous

4 Knife handles (1) No. 3, (2) No. 7, (1) No. 3L
2 Beaver knife handles
1 Lebsche sternal knife
1 Aortic punch
2 Awls
1 Ruler
2 Aortic dilators

10 Vessel dilators
1 Toomey adaptor
3 Heparin needles
3 Olive-tipped heparin needles
1 Mallet
1 Pliers, needlenose
2 DeBakey bulldog clamps, curved
4 DeBakey bulldog clamps, straight
1 Pituitary rongeur, straight

For Valves Add

4 Allis clamps (2) 6″, (2) 10″
4 Babcock clamps 10″
4 Richardson retractors (2) 9½″ with ¾″ × 1″ blade, (2) 9½″ with 1″ × 1¼″ blade
Valve retractor
1 Atrial retractor
1 Valve dilator
1 Smithwick hook

Chapter 26

Orthopedic Trays

BASIC ORTHOPEDIC PROCEDURES TRAY

Retractors

2 Rake (4 prong) sharp
2 Rake (6 prong) sharp
1 Weitlaner, sharp
2 Army-Navy

Forceps

2 Tissue with teeth 5½″
2 Adson with teeth

Scissors

2 Straight Mayo 6¼″
1 Curved Mayo 6¼″
2 Metzenbaum (1) 6″, (1) 7″
1 Bandage 8″
1 Wire cutter
1 Pin cutter

Clamps

2 Curved Pean 6¼″
2 Kocher-Lovelace
5 Curved Crile 5½″
2 Needle holder 7″

8 Towel clip 5½″
1 Sponge forceps

Suction Tubes or Tips

1 Yankauer 10⅜″

Miscellaneous

3 Knife handles (2) No. 3, (1) No. 7
2 Pliers (1) regular, (1) needlenose
2 Screwdrivers (1) Phillips, (1) blade
1 Mallet
1 Ruler
1 Depth gauge
3 Guide wires
1 Drill bit ⁷⁄₆₄″
1 Rasp
1 Hand drill with chuck
3 Bone cutters
1 Langenbeck elevator
1 Joker
1 Freer dissector
6 Currettes Nos. 0 to 5
1 Lewin bone holding forceps
1 Duckbill ronguer
1 Straight double action rongeur
1 Rongeur (Stille-Luer)
1 Blunt nerve hook
1 Gigli saw with 2 handles
5 Osteotomes, various sizes

MINOR ORTHOPEDIC PROCEDURES TRAY

Retractors

2 Weitlaner, sharp 5½″
2 Senn (sharp)
2 Joseph skin hook
2 Volkmann rake, 2 prong

Forceps

1 Tissue without teeth 5½″
1 Tissue with teeth 5½″

1 Adson without teeth
2 Adson with teeth
1 Adson-Brown

Scissors

2 Straight Mayo 6¼″
3 Metzenbaum (1) 5¼″, (1) 6″, (1) 7″
1 Stevens tenotomy
1 Curved iris
1 Straight iris
1 Wire cutter

Clamps

4 Curved Crile 5½″
2 Straight Crile 5½″
4 Curved mosquito 5¼″
2 Straight mosquito 5¼″
2 Allis 6″
6 Kocher (Ochsner) (4) 6″, (2) 10″
1 Needle holder 6″
1 Scissors needle holder
1 Webster needle holder 5″
8 Towel clip (4) 3½″, (4) 5½″

Suction Tubes or Tips

1 Frazier No. 10

Miscellaneous

2 Knife handles No. 3
1 Langenbeck elevator
1 Small rasp
1 Small double-action rongeur (Ruskin)
1 Small bone cutter (Ruskin-Lister)
1 Small mallet
1 Small chisel
1 Freer elevator dissector
1 Short blunt nerve hook
1 Straight Key elevator ½″
1 Curved Key elevator ¼″
3 Curettes 000 to 0
1 Ruler
5 Osteotomes

BONE HOLDING INSTRUMENTS TRAY

2 Lane retractors
2 Lowman clamps
5 Verbrugge forceps (1 large, 1 medium, 1 small, 2 very small)
2 Lewin bone clamps
2 Bishop clamps

HIP RETRACTORS TRAY

2 Bennett
2 Hibbs
3 Israel
2 Meyerding
3 Cobra
4 Hohmann

KNEE ARTHROTOMY TRAY

Retractors

6 Grey
1 Blount
1 Doane

Scissors

1 Cartilage

Clamps

1 Cartilage (modified Martin)
2 Lahey

Miscellaneous

1 Semilunar cartilage knife
3 Smilie cartilage knives (1) right, (1) left, (1) neutral
1 Meniscotome
1 Beaver knife handle
1 O'Donahue suture passer
1 Adson blunt hook

Chapter 27

Neurologic Procedures Trays

CRANIOTOMY TRAY

Retractors

1 Mastoid
2 Weitlaner (1) 5½", (1) 6½"
1 Curved Weitlaner 6½"
1 Adson cerebellar
2 Brain spoons
8 Malleable brain spatulas, double-ended (Davis) (¼" to 1½")
2 Nerve hooks (1) sharp, (1) blunt
2 Nerve root
2 Hoen dura separators (1) 45°, (1) 90°
2 Dura hooks

Forceps

2 Adson with teeth
2 Adson cup
4 Cushing with teeth (2) 7", (2) 8"
2 Cushing without teeth 8"
2 Bayonet 8"

Scissors

2 Straight Mayo 6¼"
1 Curved Mayo 6¼"

2 Metzenbaum (1) 6″, (1) 7″
1 Wire cutter

Clamps

2 Curved Pean 6¼″
10 Curved Crile 5½″
6 Curved Mosquito 5¼″
36 Hemostatic scalp (Dandy)
2 Allis 6″
2 Tonsil (Schnidt) 7½″
2 Needle holder, fine 6″
2 Needle holder, heavy 7¼″
12 Towel clip (4) 3½″, 2″, (8) 5½″

Suction Tubes or Tips

4 Frazier No. 7, No. 9, No. 10, No. 12

Miscellaneous

3 Knife handles (2) No. 3, (1) No. 7
1 Langenbeck periosteal elevator
1 Freer
5 Penfield dissectors Nos. 1 to 5
2 Short Kerrison rongeur, up
1 Flat Kerrison rongeur
1 Kerrison rongeur 30° up
1 Leksell double-action rongeur
1 Small double-action rongeur
1 Straight pituitary forceps
1 Angled pituitary forceps, up
3 Blunt ventricular needles, (1) No. 11, (1) No. 14, (1) No. 16
1 Sharp ventricular needle
4 Stylets
4 Syringes, Luer-Lok (control) 10 mL
3 Pituitary spoons (1) small, (1) medium, (1) large
1 Perforator (Raney, Hudson)
2 Scalp clip appliers (Raney, Michel)
4 Hemoclip appliers (2) small, (2) medium
1 Hand drill with key
1 Set drill bits
2 Gigli saws with (2) handles

1 Saw guide (Bailey)
1 Hudson brace
1 Basin (tiny)
4 Medicine cups
10 Rubber bands
1 Bayonet bipolar electrocoagulating forceps and cord
1 Neurosurgical sponge tray (pattie plate)
Prongs for skull clamp (e.g., Yasargil, Gardner, May-field)

LAMINECTOMY TRAY

Retractors

1 Downing (with 6 blades) (2) small, (2) medium, (2) large
4 Taylor (2) small, (2) large
2 Beckman (sharp)
2 Gelpi
2 Straight Weitlaner, blunt
2 Curved Weitlaner, sharp
2 Angled nerve root
2 Goulet
2 Army-Navy
1 Laminar spreader
4 Love root (4) 45°, (2) 90°
2 Straight Love root

Forceps

2 Tissue with teeth 5½"
1 Adson with teeth
2 Cushing without teeth
3 Bayonet without teeth

Scissors

1 Straight Mayo 6¼"
1 Curved Mayo 6¼"
1 Metzenbaum 7"

Clamps

18 Curved Crile 5½"
6 Curved mosquito 5¼"

2 Curved Pean 6¼"
2 Short Kocher (Ochsner) 6¼"
2 Kocher-Lovelace
4 Needle holder (2) 6", (2) 7"

Suction Tubes or Tips

1 Frazier No. 10

Miscellaneous

4 Knife handles (2) No. 3, (2) No. 7
1 Long Beaver handle
1 Probe, malleable
1 Grooved director
1 Blunt nerve hook (Hoen)
1 Ruler
2 Jokers
2 Freer dissectors
1 Freer chisel
1 Langenbeck periosteal elevator $^{11}/_{16}$"
2 Penfield dissectors
2 Medicine cups
4 Long curettes 0 to 3
2 Ring curettes (1) small, (1) medium
3 Cobb elevators (1) small, (1) medium, (1) large
2 Key elevators (1) ¾", (1) 1"
1 Leksell double-action ronguer
1 Stille-Luer double-action ronguer (gooseneck)
1 Neurosurgical sponge tray (pattie plate)

KERRISON RONGEURS AND PITUITARY FORCEPS TRAY

Pituitary Forceps

2 Straight (1) 2 × 10 mm, (1) 4 × 10 mm
2 Angled, up (1) 2 × 10 mm, (1) 4 × 10 mm
2 Angled, down (1) 2 × 10 mm, (1) 4 × 10 mm

Clamps

1 Ligamenta flava forceps

Kerrison Rongeurs

2 Straight (1) 3 mm, (1) 5 mm
2 Angled, up (1) 3 mm, (1) 5 mm
2 Angled, down (1) 3 mm, (1) 5 mm

Chapter 28

Plastic Procedures Tray

BASIC PLASTIC PROCEDURES TRAY

Retractors

2 Joseph skin hook, single
2 Joseph skin hook, double
2 Army-Navy
2 Senn, blunt
2 Cushing vein
2 Rake, blunt (four prong)
2 S-shaped
5 Malleable brain (1) ⅜″, (1) ½″, (1) ⅝″, (1) ¾″, (1) 1″

Forceps

1 Tissue without teeth 5½″
1 Tissue with teeth 5½″
1 Adson-Brown
1 Adson without teeth
2 Adson with teeth
2 Bayonet

Scissors

1 Straight Mayo 6¼″
3 Metzenbaum (1) 5¼″, (1) 6″, (1) 7″
1 Straight Metzenbaum 5¼″
1 Straight iris

1 Curved iris
1 Stevens tenotomy

Clamps

10 Towel clip 3½"
4 Curved Crile 5½"
2 Straight Crile 5½"
12 Curved mosquito 5¼"
4 Straight mosquito 5¼"
2 Allis 6"
2 Kocher 6"
2 Needle holder 6"
2 Brown needle holder
2 Webster needle holder

Suction Tubes or Tips

3 Frazier (with stylets) (1) No. 7, (1) No. 9, (1) No. 11
1 Andrews 9½"

Miscellaneous

3 Knife handles (2) No. 3 (1) No. 7
1 Probe, malleable
1 Ruler
1 Freer septal elevator
1 Caliper

Chapter 29

Otorhinolaryngologic (ENT) Trays

EAR PROCEDURES TRAY

Retractors

2 Joseph skin hook
2 Senn, sharp
2 Army-Navy
1 Richardson, small
2 Wullstein-Weitlaner
2 Mastoid
1 Shea speculum holder (with 4 specula)
6 Ear specula 1 to 6

Forceps

2 Adson with teeth
1 Adson-Brown
1 Bayonet, short (Jansen)

Scissors

1 Straight Mayo
2 Metzenbaum (1) 5¼″, (1) 7″
1 Strabismus
3 House-Bellucci alligator (1) straight, (1) left, (1) right

Clamps

4 Straight mosquito 5¼"
6 Curved mosquito 5¼"
2 Curved Crile 5½"
2 Curved Pean 6¼"
2 Allis 6"
2 Webster needle holder 5"
10 Towel clip (6) 3½", (4) 5½"

Suction Tubes or Tips

2 Frazier with stylets (1) No. 5, (1) No. 7
4 Baron (2) No. 5, (2) No. 7
2 House
4 Rosen

Miscellaneous

1 Knife handle No. 3
1 Ruler
1 House elevator
1 Endaural speculum
1 Malleus nipper
1 House-Dieter malleus nipper
3 Cup forceps (1) small, (1) medium, (1) large
2 Alligator forceps (1) small, (1) large
1 Hartman forceps
2 Mastoid gouges (1) 2 mm, (1) 4 mm
2 House curettes (double-ended)
3 Mastoid curettes (1) size 000, (1) size 00, (1) size 0
1 House Gelfoam pressure forceps

Middle Ear Sharp Instruments (Usually in Protective Rack)

1 Duckbill knife-elevator
1 Right-angle elevator
1 Oval curette
1 Excavator
1 Heavy needle
2 Pick (1) 45°, (1) 90°
1 Rosen needle
1 Attic dissector

1 Strut caliper
1 Straight chisel
1 Canal knife
1 Sickle knife (House)
1 Drum scraper
1 Oval window rasp
1 Incal stapedial knife
1 Hough hoe
2 Footplate hooks
1 House alligator crimper forceps

NASAL PROCEDURES TRAY

Retractors

2 Nasal specula (Killian) (1) 3″, (1) 2″
1 Nasal speculum, short
2 Aufricht nasal (1) long, (1) short

Forceps

1 Jansen bayonet without teeth
1 Cottle columella

Scissors

1 Fomon dorsal angular
1 Fomon lower lateral
1 Cottle bulldog
1 Knight nasal

Clamp

1 Bayonet needle holder (Jacobson)

Suction Tip

1 Antrum

Miscellaneous

1 Asch septal forceps
1 Mallet, small
2 Long metal applicators
1 Cartilage knife
2 Joseph knives (1) sharp, (1) blunt

1 Joseph button-end-knife
1 McKenty knife
1 Ballenger swivel knife
1 Freer septum knife
1 Freer septum elevator
1 Joseph periosteal elevator
1 Takahashi nasal forceps
1 Ferris-Smith fragment forceps
3 Knight polyp forceps (1) small, (1) medium, (1) large
1 Septal cutting forceps
1 Kazanjian nasal hump forceps
1 Double-action nasal rongeur
3 Kerrison rongeurs (1) 2 mm, (1) 4 mm, (1) 6 mm
1 Nerve hook
1 Reamer
1 Antrum trocar and stylet
3 Nasal rasps, assorted
2 Nasal saws, (1) right, (1) left
2 Chisels, curved, guarded (1) right, (1) left
2 Gouges (1) 2 mm, (1) 4 mm
2 Osteotomes (1) 2 mm, (1) 4 mm
6 Nasal curettes, angles (Coakley) assorted

MYRINGOTOMY TRAY

Retractors

3 Aural specula, plastic (1) small, (1) medium, (1) large
4 Aural specula, metal (assorted)

Forceps

1 Bayonet 5½″

Scissors

1 Straight iris

Suction Tubes or Tips

3 Frazier (with stylets), (1) No. 5, (1) No. 7, (1) No. 9

Miscellaneous

1 Smooth alligator
2 Curettes (1) small, (1) medium

1 Folding myringotomy Deaver knife
1 Medicine cup

TONSILLECTOMY AND ADENOIDECTOMY TRAY

Retractors

1 Fulton mouth gag
3 Jennings mouth gags (1) 4″, (1) 4½″, (1) 6″
1 Love uvula
1 Hurd dissector and pillar retractor
2 Tongue blades (1) large, (1) small

Scissors

1 Metzenbaum 7″
1 Straight Mayo 6¼″

Clamps

2 Tonsil (Schnidt) 7½″
2 Allis 6″
1 Curved Allis 10″
1 Straight sponge forceps 10″
2 Curved sponge forceps 7″
2 Towel clip 3½″
1 Needle holder 7″

Suction Tubes or Tips

1 Yankauer 10⅜″

Miscellaneous

1 Knife handle No. 7
1 Beck-Schenck tonsil snare with wire (and 2 extra wires)
1 Adenoid punch
1 Fisher tonsil knife
3 Barnhill adenoid curettes (1) No. l, (1) No. 2, (1) No. 3
3 La Force adenotomes (1) small, (1) medium, (1) large
2 Medicine cups

TRACHEOSTOMY TRAY

Retractors

2 Army-Navy
2 Senn, blunt

Forceps

1 Tissue with teeth 5½″
1 Adson with teeth

Scissors

1 Metzenbaum 7″
1 Curved Mayo 6¼″
1 Straight Mayo 6¼″

Clamps

4 Curved Crile 5½″
4 Curved mosquito 5¼″
2 Allis 6″
1 Needle holder 6″
4 Towel clip 3½″

Suction Tubes or Tips

1 Yankauer 10⅜″
1 Andrews 9½″
1 Frazier No. 10

Miscellaneous

2 Knife handles No. 3
2 Knife blades (1) No. 11, (1) No. 15
1 Syringe 5 mL, Luer-Lok control
2 Needles (1) 20 gauge 1″, (1) 25 gauge 1″
1 Tracheostomy dilator
1 Tracheostomy hook
10 Sponges 4″ × 4″
1 Preparation cup

Chapter 30

Ophthalmic Trays

BASIC EYE PROCEDURES TRAY

Scissors

1 Blunt (Stevens)
1 Curved iris
1 Stevens tenotomy
1 Suture

Clamps

2 Halsted straight mosquito 5¼″
1 Halsted curved mosquito 5¼″
4 Towel clip 3½″

Miscellaneous

1 Irrigating tip No. 21
1 Knife handle No. 9
6 Medicine cups
Needles:
    (1) 23 gauge 1″, (1) 25 gauge ⅝″
    (2) 23 gauge retrobulbar
    (2) 25 gauge retrobulbar
Syringes:
    (2) 5 mL Luer-Lok
    (5) 2 mL Luer-Lok
1 Eye pad

2 Eye shields (1) metal, (1) plastic
2 Serrefine clamps

Special Notes

Labeling syringes and medicine cups avoids confusion.
Leave eye pads in wrapper when sterilizing the tray.

EYELID AND CONJUNCTIVAL PROCEDURES TRAY

Retractors

1 Eye speculum (Barraquer, Lancaster)
1 Lacrimal sac
1 Chalazion clamp (Des Marres)
2 Senn
2 Skin hook
2 Skin hook, double-prong
5 Des Marres (2) No. 1, (1) No. 2, (2) No. 3
2 von Graefe muscle hook (1) No. 1, (1) No. 3

Forceps

2 Fixation (e.g., Lester)
2 Bishop-Harmon suturing
1 Castroviejo suturing
1 Conjunctival, with teeth
1 Conjunctival, serrated
1 Dressing
1 Tying (e.g., Castroviejo)
1 Lid (Green)
1 Chalazion
1 Entropion (Snellen)

Scissors

1 Wescott tenotomy
1 Vannas iridocapsulotomy

Clamps

1 Kalt needle holder
1 Castroviejo needle holder

Miscellaneous

1 Corneal knife (Gill)
1 Beaver knife handle
1 Castroviejo caliper
3 Chalazion curettes

BASIC EYE MUSCLE PROCEDURES TRAY

Retractors

1 Eye speculum (Lancaster, Barraquer)
1 Lacrimal sac (self-retaining)
2 Muscle hook (Stevens)
4 Muscle hook (von Graefe) (2) No. 1, (2) No. 3

Forceps

1 Fixation (Lester)
1 Recession
2 Suturing (Bishop-Harmon) (1) heavy, (1) fine
2 Suturing (Castroviejo 0.5 mm)
2 Muscle (Jameson, Berens)

Scissors

1 Straight Wescott tenotomy
1 Curved Wescott tenotomy
1 Suture (Troutman)

Clamps

2 Needle holder (Kalt, Barraquer)

Miscellaneous

1 Caliper (Castroviejo)

DACRYOCYSTORHINOSTOMY TRAY

Retractors

2 Lacrimal sac, 4 prong (Knapp)
1 Lacrimal sac, self-retaining (Agricola)
2 Nasal specula (1) short, (1) medium

Forceps

2 Bayonet

Clamps

2 Webster needle holder

Suction Tubes or Tips

2 Frazier with stylets (1) No. 5, (1) No. 7

Miscellaneous

1 Lacrimal irrigating cannula
1 Lacrimal trephine (Arruga)
3 Lacrimal dilators
2 Lacrimal cannulas (1) straight, (1) bulbous tip
2 Lid everter (Berens)
6 Lacrimal probes (0000 to 000 to sizes 7 to 8)
1 Worst pigtail probe
2 Lacrimal chisels (1) 2 mm, (1) 4 mm
2 Lacrimal gouges (1) 2 mm, (1) 4 mm
2 Lacrimal osteotomes (1) 2 mm, (1) 4 mm
1 Small mallet
2 Kerrison rongeurs (1) 2 mm, (1) 4 mm
1 Takahashi straight nasal forceps
1 Lempert rongeur, delicate curved
1 Freer elevator
1 Joseph periosteal elevator

GLOBE AND ORBIT PROCEDURES TRAY

Retractors

1 Eye speculum (Guyton-Park, Lancaster)
1 Lacrimal sac (Fink)
4 von Graefe muscle hook (2) No. 1, (2) No. 3
1 Arruga orbital/elevator
1 Schepens orbital
1 Converse alar, double-ended

Forceps

2 Tissue (Bishop-Harmon)
2 Fixation (Lester, von Graefe)

2 Suturing (Castroviejo)
1 Recession (Jameson)

Scissors

1 Suture (Stevens)
2 Wescott (1) left, (1) right
1 Straight tenotomy (Stevens)
1 Curved tenotomy (Stevens)
1 Enucleation

Clamps

1 Curved mosquito 5¼″
4 Straight mosquito 5¼″
1 Straight Crile 5½″
1 Right-angle (Mixter)
2 Tonsil (Schnidt)
2 Needle holder (Barraquer, Alabama-Green)

Miscellaneous

2 Kerrison mastoid rongeurs (1) up, (1) down
1 Lacrimal sac chisel
1 Freer periosteal elevator
1 Cottle septum elevator
1 Enucleation snare
1 Evisceration spoon
1 Enucleation spoon
1 Sphere introducer
1 Small mallet
1 Bone cutter
1 Rongeur, single-action (Lempert)
1 Blade breaker and holder

CORNEAL PROCEDURES TRAY

Retractors

1 Eye speculum (Lancaster, Barraquer)
2 Muscle hook (Green, O'Connor, Jameson, von Graefe)

Forceps

2 Tissue (Bishop-Harmon)
1 Corneal (Colibri 0.12 mm)

2 Suturing (Castroviejo)
1 Corneal-scleral
1 Straight tying (McPherson)
1 Curved tying (McPherson)

Scissors

1 Curved suture
2 Troutman-Castroviejo (1) right, (1) left
1 Straight Castroviejo
1 Straight iris (Barraquer-DeWecker)

Clamps

2 Straight micro needle holder (Castroviejo, Barraquer)

Miscellaneous

1 Iris spatula
1 Paton spatula
1 Castroviejo spatula
1 Corneal knife (Gill)
1 Corneal dissector (Troutman)
1 Air cannula, 27 gauge
1 Castroviejo caliper
2 Corneal markers
2 Trephine handles (Weck)
3 Trephine blades 7.5 mm, 8.0 mm, 8.5 mm
1 Teflon block
1 Corneal punch (Troutman), 2 parts
1 Base plate with corneal block

CATARACT EXTRACTION AND LENS PROCEDURE TRAY

Retractors

1 Eye speculum (Barraquer, child size)
1 Muscle hook (von Graefe) No. 1
1 Muscle hook (Green)

Forceps

1 Curved iris (von Graefe)
1 Capsulotomy (Arruga)

1 Corneal (Colibri 0.12 mm)
1 Straight tying (McPherson)
1 Curved tying (McPherson)
2 Suturing (Castroviejo [1] 0.12 mm, [1] 0.5 mm)
1 Lens holding (Shepard)
1 Bonn 0.12 mm

Scissors

1 Tenotomy (Wescott)
1 Straight iris (Barraquer-DeWecker)
1 Capsulotomy (Vannas)
1 Iridotocapsulotomy
2 Corneal (Troutman) (1) left, (1) right
1 Barraquer-DeWecker

Clamps

1 Castroviejo needle holder
1 Barraquer needle holder

Miscellaneous

1 Beaver knife handle
1 Lens loop (Knapp)
1 Olive tip irrigator
1 Iris spatula (Wheeler)
1 Castroviejo cyclodialysis spatula
1 Irrigating vectis loop
1 Corneal knife (Gill)
1 Air or Healon cannula
1 Lacrimal irrigator
1 Blade breaker
1 Castroviejo caliper
Irrigation and aspiration set
1 Micro lens hook (Sinsky)
1 Lens manipulator (Kugler)
1 Iris hook (Bonn)
1 Lens hook (Fenzl)

GLAUCOMA PROCEDURES TRAY

Retractors

1 Eye speculum (Barraquer, Lancaster)

Forceps

1 Corneal (Colibri 0.12 mm)
1 Suturing (Castroviejo 0.12 mm)
1 Bonn 0.1 mm
2 Tissue (Bishop-Harmon)

Scissors

1 Wescott (blunt tipped)
1 Suture (Troutman)
1 Iris (Barraquer-DeWecker)
1 Strabismus (Knapp)
1 Iridocapsulotomy (Vannas)
1 Tenotomy (Wescott)

Clamps

1 Kalt needle holder
1 Barraquer needle holder (curved, nonlocking)

Miscellaneous

1 Tonometer (Schiotz)
1 Irrigating tip No. 27
1 Corneal dissector (Troutman)
1 Castroviejo caliper
1 Castroviejo cyclodialysis spatula
1 Iris spatula (Wheeler)
1 Blade breaker (Castroviejo, Barraquer)
1 Beaver knife handle
1 Corneal knife (Gill)
1 Iris hook (Bonn)
1 Air cannula
1 Scleral punch (Holth)

BASIC EYE PROCEDURES MICROSCOPE TRAY

Retractors

1 Eye speculum (Barraquer, Lancaster)
5 Lid (Des Marres) (2) No. 1, (1) No. 2, (2) No. 3
2 Muscle hook

Forceps

2 Castroviejo suturing (0.12 mm, 0.5 mm)
1 Bishop-Harmon suturing
1 Fixation (Lester, von Graefe)
1 Corneal (Colibri 0.12 mm)
1 Curved tying (McPherson)
1 Straight tying (McPherson)
2 Straight suture tying (Castroviejo)

Scissors

2 Corneal (Castroviejo) (1) left, (1) right
1 Suture (Troutman)
1 Suture iris (Barraquer-DeWecker)
1 Iridocapsulotomy (Vannas)

Clamps

1 Nonlocking needle holder (Barraquer)
2 Needle holder (Kalt, Troutman-Barraquer)

Miscellaneous

1 Knife handle No. 9
1 Beaver knife handle
1 Iris spatula (Barraquer)
1 Corneal knife (Gill)

RETINAL PROCEDURES TRAY

Retractors

1 Eye speculum (Lancaster, Guyton-Park)
1 Muscle hook (von Graefe) No. 1
1 Muscle hook (Jameson)
1 Retinal detachment hook (Gass)
1 Des Marres lid No. 2
1 Arruga
1 Schepens

Forceps

1 Castroviejo suturing (0.12 mm)
2 Suturing (Bishop-Harmon) (1) heavy, (1) fine

2 Tying (McCollough, Alabama)
1 Fixation (Lester, von Graefe, Elshnig)
1 Recession (Jameson)

Scissors

1 Tenotomy (Wescott)
1 Suture
1 Straight Stevens
1 Curved Stevens
1 Iris

Clamps

1 Curved Castroviejo needle holder
1 Barraquer needle holder
1 Kalt needle holder

Miscellaneous

2 Beaver knife handles
1 Corneal knife (Gill)
1 Castroviejo caliper
2 Air cannulas (1) 27 gauge, (1) 30 gauge
1 Tonometer (Schiotz)
1 Scleral depressor (Schepens)
3 Diathermy tips
1 Straight retinal probe
1 Curved retinal probe
1 Retinal probe sleeve

Chapter 31

Pediatric Trays

PEDIATRIC MAJOR PROCEDURES TRAY

Retractors

2 Senn, blunt
4 Gans (2) No. 1, (2) No. 2
5 Malleable brain (spatulas) (1) ⅜″, (1) ½″, (1) ⅝″, (1) ¾″, (1) 1″
1 Small Balfour (total opening 3¾″)
1 Heiss self-retaining
2 Richardson (1) ½″ × 1″, (1) 1″ × 1″

Forceps

1 Tissue with teeth 5½″
2 Adson without teeth
2 Adson with teeth
1 Cushing without teeth 7″
1 Cushing with teeth 7″
4 DeBakey (fine) (2) 6″, (2) 7¾″

Scissors

2 Straight Mayo 6¼″
1 Curved Mayo 5½″
3 Metzenbaum (1) 5¼″, (1) 6″, (1) 7″
1 Straight Metzenbaum 6″
1 Potts

1 Stevens tenotomy
1 Curved iris
1 Straight iris

Clamps

4 Straight Crile 5½″
6 Curved Crile 5½″
4 Straight mosquito 5¼″
10 Curved mosquito 5¼″
6 Curved Pean 5½″
4 Curved Kocher 5½″
6 Straight Kocher 5½″
2 Kocher-Lovelace
4 Babcock 5¾″
4 Allis 6″
6 Allis (fine) 5¾″
6 Right-angle (2) 5½″, (2) 7″, (2) 7½″
2 Tonsil (Schnidt) 7½″
2 Needle holder 6″
2 Needle holder, fine 7½″
6 Towel clip 3½″
4 Sponge forceps 7″

Suction Tubes or Tips

1 Poole 9¼″
1 Andrews 9½″
1 Frazier No. 7

Miscellaneous

4 Knife handles (2) No. 3, (1) No. 7, (1) No. 9
1 Ballinger elevator
1 Elevator dissector
1 Elevator probe

PEDIATRIC MINOR PROCEDURES TRAY

Retractors

2 Gans No. 1
2 Senn, blunt

Forceps

2 Tissue without teeth
2 Adson without teeth
2 Adson with teeth
2 DeBakey 6″

Scissors

1 Straight Mayo 6¼″
2 Metzenbaum (1) 5½″, (1) 6″
1 Straight Metzenbaum 5¼″
1 Stevens tenotomy
1 Curved iris
1 Straight iris

Clamps

2 Curved Crile 5½″
2 Straight mosquito 5¼″
6 Curved mosquito 5¼″
2 Babcock 5¾″
2 Needle holder 6″
4 Towel clip 3½″

Miscellaneous

2 Knife handles No. 3
1 Medicine cup

PEDIATRIC GASTROINTESTINAL PROCEDURES TRAY

Clamps

2 Curved pediatric Doyen 7½″
2 Straight pediatric Doyen 7½″
2 Curved pediatric Bainbridge 7½″
2 Straight pediatric Bainbridge 7½″

Miscellaneous

8 Robinson catheter No. 18 Fr, pieces 2″

PEDIATRIC THORACOTOMY TRAY

Retractors

1 Finochietto rib (4 blades) child size, total opening 6″
2 Finochietto rib, infant size, total opening (1) 2½″, (1) 3½″

Miscellaneous

2 Langenbeck periosteal elevators (1) ¼″, (1) ¹¹⁄₁₆″
1 Beyer double-action rongeur 7″
1 Bailey rib contractor 6¾″

Appendix

LASER TECHNOLOGY

Definition

The *laser* (an acronym for *light amplification by stimulated emission of radiation*) is an energy source derived from light.

Discussion

The laser emits light energy produced by stimulating the electrons of various media (solid, liquid, tunable dye, or gas) with electricity (or xenon flash lamp or another laser) to reach a high-energy state, releasing this energy in the form of photons. The photons collide within the laser chamber between mirrors, creating more energy that then escapes in a controlled manner as the laser beam. This beam is collimated, maintaining a constant diameter for great distances (unlike an ordinary light beam, which expands). This beam is monochromatic and of a single optical frequency, and the energy particles (photons) travel in a coordinated fashion, in phase with each other (coherent). These properties allow the laser beam to travel over great distances with extremely concentrated energy. Each individually stimulated substance emits energy of a different wavelength, which influences the absorption of this energy in a selective manner. The laser does not, however, produce ionizing radiation and is not hazardous in that sense, as are radioactive substances or x-rays.

Body tissues are affected by the laser beam as the light energy is converted to heat (or acoustical energy), resulting in the vaporization, fragmentation, cutting,

616

coagulation (or "welding") of these tissues. The level of the power setting (wattage), the duration of the contact time with the target tissues, the use of continuous or pulsed mode, and the cooling action of the local blood flow, and pigmentation and translucency of the target and adjacent tissues determine the effect of the laser beam on tissues.

Several lasers of different wavelengths measured in nanometers (nm) and clinical capabilities are in common usage in the operating room. The CO_2 (carbon dioxide) 10,600 nm laser is used in a noncontact mode for cutting and vaporization of tissues (and welding of certain tissues, for example, vascular anastamoses). Previously, because of its longer wavelength, the CO_2 laser beam could not be transmitted through lengthy fiber delivery systems. A recent adaptation of a flexible hollow wave guide lined with metal ribbons and dielectric (electrically nonconducting) coating increases the CO_2 laser's ability to treat previously inaccessible areas, but with loss of laser energy. The Nd:YAG (neodymium yttrium aluminum garnet) 1064 nm laser is used for deeper-tissue effect or can be transmitted by a flexible probe (fiber) through an endoscope for destruction of gastrointestinal, urinary, and respiratory tract lesions. With the use of a sapphire tip, the Nd:YAG laser can be used in a contact mode. The argon 488 to 515 nm (blue-green) laser energy is absorbed by melanim and hemoglobin and is used in ophthalmology (photo coagulation of retinal tests and bleeding points) and in plastic surgery to ablate hemangiomata. The KTP 532 nm laser is a variant of the Nd:YAG wherein the beam is passed through a potassium-titanyl-phosphate crystal, doubling its frequency (halving its wavelength), giving this laser properties similar to the argon laser but with increased tissue destructive capability. Pulsed dye lasers are of various frequencies depending upon the particular liquid dye medium and a pulsed light source. For example, this laser (with a frequency of 504 nm), as conducted through a fine quartz fiber, can be passed through a urethroscope in direct application to a calculus in order to shatter it. A 530 nm wavelength yellow dye laser will also disrupt urinary tract calculi. A flash lamp laser (Candela, 585 nm) is used for similar urologic purposes, or it can be used to ablate colored skin lesions as hemangiomata. The ruby laser (694 nm) is used for tattoo removal. The excimer (excited dimeric medium) laser utilizes an inert gas-halide system (including argon-fluoride 193 nm, krypton-fluoride 248 nm, xenon-chloride 308 nm, and xenon-fluoride 351 nm), which can be incorporated in a fine catheter that includes a video system and irrigating mechanism used to open occluded coronary arteries (pulsed 308 nm) by direct contact destruction of intimal plaque. An additional excimer laser use is in optical contouring of the cornea.

An additional modality is photodynamic therapy, which involves the systemic injection of a photosensitive dye (e.g., modified porphyrin), which is selectively retained by malignant tissues. These tissues (e.g., urinary bladder, breast, retina, maxillary sinus) are exposed to a laser light of appropriate wavelength to produce a photochemical reaction, resulting in tumor destruction. Thus a tunable dye laser adjusted (tuned) by prism to emit, for example, red light (argon laser energy source for rhodamine B laser 630 nm) produces the photochemical effect in conjunction with the administration of hematoporphyrin to ablate certain superficial lesions as carcinoma-in-situ and transitional cell bladder tumors.

Newer lasers whose clinical role is yet to be defined include Ho:YAG (Holmium), Er:YAG (Erbium), and CO (carbon monoxide). Diode lasers, 75 to 950 nm (e.g., Gallium arsenide, 840 to 910 nm), a more compact system for photocoagulation in ophthalmologic use, delivered directly by fiber or introduced through a slit lamp, have been developed. Newly designed delivery fibers with a rotary mirror (metallic) to orient the beam are available, as are units that can deliver a selection of lasers of different wavelengths.

As CO_2 and Nd:YAG laser beams are colorless, an accompanying neon-helium beam that emits a red light is used for "aiming."

Adapted to use with the operating microscope, the laser is invaluable in microlaryngeal and ophthalmologic procedures. Many laser procedures can be performed in outpatient surgery or special-procedure units (e.g., eye laboratory) with reduced operating room and anesthesia time. In many of its applications the laser permits minimal tissue trauma with reduced injury to adjacent structures and a relatively dry field with reduced blood loss. Direct tissue contact is often not necessary, and otherwise inaccessible areas may be treated. Faster wound healing with less pain, edema (due to sealing of nerve endings and lymphatics), scarring, and so on, are often attributed to laser surgery (though not necessarily realized in various applications, e.g., "laser" hemorrhoidectomy). However, the laser and its obligate special equipment, complex maintenance, and evolving technological advances with continuously upgraded instrumentation make laser surgery costly. More significant is that laser procedures are potentially hazardous to patients and operating room personnel.

Safety Precautions

Any time a laser procedure is performed, a scrub nurse, circulating nurse, and laser nurse should be present.

Table of Commonly Used Lasers

	CO_2	Argon	Nd:YAG
Laser wavelength	10,600 nm	488–515 nm	1064 nm
Depth of tissue destruction	0.1 mm	0.5 mm	4–5 mm
Effect dependent upon tissue pigment	None	Yes	Minimal
Contact	Noncontact	Contact and noncontact	Contact and noncontact
Delivery by fiberoptics	Developmental	Yes	Yes
Beam delivery mode	Focus	Quartz fiber or focus	Quartz fiber or focus
Eye protection	Yes Clear	Yes Tinted	Yes Tinted
Lens filters on endoscope/microscope	None	Tinted	Tinted

Strict safety precautions must be enforced. Signs posted on the operating room doors warn of laser use. All equipment must be checked prior to the procedure, including but not limited to testing the beam focus, electrical connections, suction apparatus, and so on. Only personnel trained in laser safety and technique should participate. A master key enabling operation of the laser must be obtained and then returned at the completion of the procedure. The laser is set at "standby" or "stop" mode during significant interruptions in its use.

Eye protection for patients and all personnel is mandatory. For the CO_2 laser, clear glasses with side wings are used by everyone, including the patient if he or she is awake. Under general anesthesia the patient's eyes are taped shut and covered with wet pads, and the face is covered with a wet towel (unless of course the procedure involves this area). The Nd:YAG laser requires blue-green safety goggles, and the argon laser, orange goggles.

Fire is a realistic potential hazard, particularly when the CO_2 laser is used near the airway (as in laryngeal procedures). Only nonflammable anesthetics are used. Conventional endotracheal tubes must be wrapped with aluminum foil tape. Flexible metallic and insulated silicone endotracheal tubes are available. A protocol for endotracheal tube fire must be rehearsed to minimize any untoward effects. A variety of instruments to protect the tissue surrounding the laser target have been devised (e.g., Donnez "backstop"), some with plume suction incorporated. Similarly, nonreflective instruments (with anodized or ebonized finishes, etc.) that defocus and disperse the laser energy are used. Wet towels or sponges surround the operating field, but precautions are taken to prevent strikethrough contamination. A saline-filled irrigating syringe is available to cool local tissues or extinguish a flash fire about the operative field, and special fire extinguishers (e.g., Halon) can be used for a flash fire in any portion of the laser system apparatus without significant damage to the expensive and delicate components. The skin preparation solution must contain no combustible agents (i.e., no alcohol or ether).

The laser should be in the standby mode when not in use. The laser activation switch or pedal must be controlled only by the surgeon; other controls (e.g., for the electrosurgical unit) may be delegated to the assistant. When a laser fiber is passed through a scope or tube, the laser must not be activated until the laser tip is beyond the tip of the scope or tube to avoid heating and other damage. A satisfactory smoke evacuator to remove noxious smoke (plume) is necessary. Plume smoke evacuate filters should be changed as recommended. Laser masks that filter out particles of finer size than do ordinary masks are employed. Movement of the patient is limited by restraints if the patient is awake, and for delicate microscopic surgery, general anesthesia with muscle paralysis is used.

The circulator enforces these precautions, provides support to the patient, explains the need for protective eye covering, and documents the procedure. The scrub person keeps the immediate field surrounded by wet towels or sponges while guarding against contamination, assists in suctioning the plume, and anticipates the need for special instruments or supplies. The laser nurse, working in conjunction with the surgeon, tests to see that the laser equipment is functioning properly. The laser nurse also sees that all rules and regulations and precautions regarding the use of the laser are maintained by all personnel and maintains an individual patient record in the laser log book for each patient. An example of an OR Laser Log Sheet is on pp. 622–623.

Care standards and competency standards for use of the different types of lasers have been established (with ongoing revisions) by several agencies including the Food and Drug Administration (FDA), Occupational Safety and Health Administration (OSHA), American Society for Laser Medicine in Surgery (ASLMS), Association of Operating Room Nurses (AORN), and the American National Standards Institute (ANSI). Indeed, the Joint Commission on Accreditation of Health Care Organizations (JCAHO) mandates that physicians employing the laser are credentialed, that operating room personnel are instructed in laser use and safety including hands-on

LASER OPERATIVE PROCEDURE REPORT

DATE:	O.R. NO.:	CASE NO.:	CLEAN □ CONTAMINATED □ IP □ BURN □ MAJOR □	
			CLEAN CONT. □ DIRTY □ OP □ CENTER □ MINOR □	VIDEO EQUIP USED □

Pre-operative Diagnosis: (VIDEO TAPE USED □, LAMINAR AIR FLOW USED □)

Operative Procedure:

Post Operative Diagnosis: SAME AS PRE-OP □ PENDING PATH □ Other:

Surgeon(s): MD Circ Nurse(s): RN IN OUT

Assistant(s): MD Laser Nurse/Tech: RN IN OUT RN □ ST □ RN □ ST □

MD Scrub Nurse(s): MD RN □ ST □ IN OUT

Anesthesiologist: MD Intubated □ Oral □ Nasal □ LTA Kit □ Monitors On □

Anesthesia: Gen □ Spinal □ Epidural □ MAC □ Local □ Bier Block □ Other □

Anesthetic Agent: Pentothal □ Diprivan □ Brevital □ O_2 □ N_2O_2 □ Forane □ Ethrane □ Halothane □

Local Agents & Dose:

Entered O.R.: Entered O.R. VIA: Guerney □ Bed □ Nurses Arms □ Walking □ Crib □

Anesthesia Start: Position: SUPINE □ LITHOTOMY □ PRONE □ LATERAL □ FROGGED □ LEGS UP TOGETHER □ LEGS DOWN TOGETHER □

Operation Start: Other:

Operation End: Prep: Shave □ By: Surgeon □ RN □ RN Initial: ( )

Anesthesia End: Exit O.R.: Prep Agents: Bet S&P □ Bet Paint Only □ Hibiclens □ Phisohex □ None □ ( ) INIT

Cautery: BI-POLAR □ UNI-POLAR □ SERIAL NO. GROUND PLATE LOT NO. GROUND CONTACT INTACT □ Location: ANT. THIGH □ OTHER: ANT. THIGH □ ( ) INIT

Ground Pad/site: CLEAN □ DRY □ CLEAR/INTACT □ GOOD CONTACT APPARENT □ Post-Op Pad site: INTACT □ CLEAR □ OTHER:

Tourniquet □ mmHg: Location: RA □ LA □ RL □ LL □ By: Surgeon □ RN □ RN Initial ( ) TOTAL TIME:

Prothesis □ SEE SEPARATE IMPLANT SHEET Lab Studies Sent: CBC/H & H □ LITES/K □ PT/PTT □ T & X □ ABG's □ OTHER:

Irrigants/Solutions: Saline 1000cc (x); Sterile H_2O 1000cc (x); Double Antibiotic 1000cc (x)

Medications & Times:

						HEMOSTATIC AGENTS							XYLO USED
Pre-Op Invasive Lines	Solutions	Size Angio	Site	Site Clear	DC/ED	Intra-Op Invasive Lines	Solutions	Size Angio	Site	Site Clear	By Initial		
Peripheral ☐			☐	☐	☐	Peripheral ☐	1000 L.R. ☐			☐			☐

					NO. 2		NO. 3		NO. 4	

LASER ☐ CO2 ☐ KTP ☐ YAG ☐
- ☐ SIGNS POSTED
- ☐ SAFETY GLASSES
- ☐ WINDOWS COVERED
- ☐ PATIENT PROTECTED

- ☐ FOOT PEDAL TO SURGEON
- ☐ "STANDBY" MODE ON
- ☐ NO DYSFUNCTION LIGHTS ON
- ☐ LASER TEST FIRED

- ☐ SMOKE EVACUATOR USED
- ☐ OPERATIVE SITE DRAPED WITH WET TOWELS
- ☐ FIRE EXTINGUISHER IN ROOM
- ☐ LASER E.T. TUBE USED
- ☐ EYE/WEAR INSPECTION

SETTINGS:
WATTS:
CW: PULSE:

- ☐ HAND PIECE
- ☐ MICRO MANIPULATOR
- ☐ LASER GUIDE
- ☐ FIBER

X-Rays In O.R. ☐   Fluro ☐   Cell Saver ☐   No. of Units _____

BLOOD & ASSOCIATED PRODUCTS

AUTOLOGOUS	DIRECTED	RED CROSS	F.F. PLASMA
UNIT NO.	UNIT NO.	UNIT NO.	UNIT NO.

Admission Drains/Caths/Packing: Foley ☐   Salem Sump ☐   Other: _____

Discharge Drains/Caths: Foley ☐ Size ( )   Penrose ☐ Size ( )   Flat Jc/JP ☐ Size ( )

Round ie Hemovac ☐ Size ( )   Chest ☐   Size ( )   Other

URINE OUTPUT:

Discharge Packing: _____

Additional Supplies: _____

ALBUMIN 250 cc (x)	PLASMANATE 250 cc (x)	PLASMANATE 250 cc (x)	PLASMANATE 500 cc (x)

Dressing: Telfa ☐ 4 x 4's ☐ Adaptic ☐ Xeroform ☐ Abd ☐ (x) Ace ☐ (x) Kling ☐ (x) Kerlix ☐ (x)   Periped ☐ T-Binder ☐ Steristrip ☐ Other:

Specimens and/or Number: _____   Pathologist In Room ☐   Frozen Section ☐   Cultures ☐   Site:

Complications and/or additional nursing intervention not addressed above or on intraoperative Patient Care Plan:

PATIENT PLATE

Sponge & Needle Count: Opening by ( )   Closing #1 by ( )   Closing #2 by ( )
Instrument Count ☐   Correct ☐   Correct ☐

DISCHARGED TO: PACU ☐ SDS ☐ NURSING UNIT ☐ NICU ☐ ICU ☐ VAG QUERNEY ☐ BED ☐ INCUBATOR ☐
AIRWAY: NATURAL ☐ ORAL ☐ NASAL ☐ ENDOTUBE ☐ CRIB ☐
REPORT TO: RN   CRNI   SIGNATURE: RN

training, and that quality maintenance of equipment is observed. Documentation of laser procedures becomes part of the patient's operating room record. Data include type of procedure, type of laser, duration of use, wattage settings, and documentation that the safety protocol was observed, and if necessary, documentation of untoward occurrences and measures taken to minimize them.

ARGON BEAM COAGULATOR

The argon beam coagulator allows a jet of argon gas to carry electrons from a unipolar electrode through space to impact on tissue in a grounded patient to deliver electrosurgical energy in a way similar to a standard unipolar cautery. However, inherent is a no-touch technique, and the plume of argon gas, as it conducts the electrical energy, simultaneously has a "blast" effect on the target tissues momentarily blowing away blood, fluid, and debris for more efficient coagulation. The flow of gas (e.g., 4 L/min), power (40 to 50 W), and spot diameter of the beam can be adjusted. The coagulation effect is good on solid organ surfaces such as the spleen, liver, and myometrium and broad oozing surfaces such as in enterolysis. Smoke is minimal as argon gas surrounds the target site.

Laparoscopic adaptation is evolving with 10 and 5 mm diameter disposable probes. Excess gas then must be evacuated as not to unduly increase intraperitoneal pressure. A suction irrigation probe is therefore placed near the argon beam coagulator probe when it is activated.

Recently the argon beam coagulator has been used to obliterate endometrial implants and to perform presacral neurectomy through laparotomy or laparoscopy.

Whereas the electrical generator is less costly than a laser, the electrode tips are relatively expensive, requiring frequent replacement; however, the efficacy of the argon beam coagulator with potential reduction of operating room time and with efficient achievement of otherwise tedious hemostasis may negate these expenses.

RADIOFREQUENCY ENDOMETRIAL ABLATION

Currently being investigated is radiofrequency endometrial ablation for dysfunctional uterine bleeding in patients who do not desire further pregnancy. The goal of therapy is to create endometrial fibrosis or stenosis of the uterine cavity. The system does not depend upon a distensive medium (as for hysteroscopy) and is less expensive than laser equipment. The endometrial tissues are heated to 62° to 65°C for approximately 15 minutes. Uterine blood flow, thermal nonconductivity of the myometrium, and the geometrically proportional fall-off of the heating effect combine to protect surrounding organs.

The cervix is dilated to Hegar size 10 and the uterus sounded. A probe length appropriate to avoid heating the endocervical canal is selected. The probe is then passed into the uterine cavity through an insulated vaginal sleeve (which also affords protection to the bladder). Thermal monitoring probes and a special grounding belt are employed. Care is taken to be certain that the patient is not in contact with any metal surfaces. During the procedure the thermal probe may be rotated to achieve more uniform tissue destruction.

A thermotherapeutic modality for prostatic disease is available, but results of this treatment do not appear to be reliable enough to replace the standard transurethral resection of the prostate (TURP).

Bibliography

Adams, GL, Lawrence, RB, and Paparella, MM: Boies' Fundamentals of Otolaryngology: A Text of Ear, Nose, and Throat Diseases, ed 5. WB Saunders, Philadelphia, 1978.

Aimino, PA: Perioperative nursing documentation: Developing the record and using care plans. AORN J 46:73, 1987.

Anderson, BA: Endoscopic carpal tunnel release. AORN J 57:413, 1993.

Aronoff, BL: The star wars revolution: Lasers in cancer surgery. Bull Am Coll Surg 72:8, 1987.

Atkinson, LJ, and Kohn, ML: Berry and Kohns Introduction to Operating Room Technique, ed 6. McGraw-Hill, New York, 1986.

Ball, KA: Controlling smoke evacuation and odor during laser surgery. Today's OR Nurse 8:4, 1986.

Ball, KA: Developing a laser program. Today's OR Nurse 8:16, 1986.

Ball, KA: Laser safety. Today's OR Nurse 8:10, 1986.

Ballenger, JJ: Diseases of the Nose, Throat and Ear, ed 12. Lea and Febiger, Philadelphia, 1977.

Beck, CF: Malignant hyperthermia. AORN J 59:2, 1994.

Bendick, PJ: Laser safety in the operating room. Bull Am Coll Surg 71:10, 1987.

Bennett, CN (ed): Lasers. Humana Technos 1:1, 1982.

Benson, CD, et al: Pediatric Surgery. Year Book Medical Publishers, Chicago, 1962.

Bigos, DM, and Davis, JL: Idiopathic radial tunnel syndrome: Surgical treatment and nursing care. AORN J 46:255, 1987.

Braunwald, E: Heart Disease: A Textbook of Cardiovascular Medicine, ed 4. WB Saunders, Philadelphia, 1992.

Brooks, SM: Instrumentation for the Operating Room, ed 2. CV Mosby, St. Louis, 1983.

Campbell, AD, and Ferrara, BE: Toupet partial fundoplication. AORN J 57:671, 1993.

Canala, L: Advancements in internal surgical stapling. Today's OR Nurse 8:11, 1986.

Churchill-Davidson, H: Wylie and Churchill-Davidson's A Practice of Anesthesia. Year Book Publishers, Chicago, 1984.

Coltharp, WH, et al: Videothorascoscopy: Improved technique and expanded indications. Ann Thorac Surg 53:776–779, 1992.

Corman, ML: Colon and Rectal Surgery, ed 3. JB Lippincott, Philadelphia, 1993.

Cowden, JW, et al: Repeated radial keratotomy in the prospective evaluation of radial keratotomy study. Am J Ophthalmol 103:423, 1987.

Crenshaw, AH (ed): Campbell's Operative Orthopedics, ed 7. CV Mosby, St. Louis, 1987.

Crenshaw, AH (ed): Campbell's Operative Orthopedics, ed 8, vol 4, 2226–2237. Mosby Year Book, St. Louis, 1992.

Danforth, DN (ed): Obstetrics and Gynecology, ed 4. Harper and Row, Philadelphia, 1982.

Deitz, MR, Sanders, R, and Raanan, MG: A consecutive series of radial keratotomies performed with a diamond blade. Am J Ophthalmol 103:417, 1987.

Devita, VT (ed), et al: Cancer Principals and Practice of Oncology, ed 4, Vol 2, pp 1695–1706. JB Lippincott, Philadelphia, 1993.

De Weese, DD, and Saunders, WH: Otolaryngology, ed 5. CV Mosby, St. Louis, 1977.

Dienno, ME: Esophageal atresia: Corrective procedures and nursing care. AORN J 45:1356, 1987.

Dixon, JA: Surgical Application of Lasers. Year Book Medical Publishers, Chicago, 1983.

Donnelly, J, and Livacz, L: New instruments in ophthalmic surgery. Today's OR Nurse 8:8, 1986.

Dornier Medical Systems, Inc.: Instructional films, and personal communication. Marietta, Georgia, 1987.

Drucker, MD: Arthroscopic surgery of the knee joint. AORN J 36:585, 1982.

Durtschi, MB: Use of thoracoscopy in clinical practice. Am J Surg 165:5, 1993.

Feldman, ST, and Brown, SI: Reduction of astigmatism after keratoplasty. Am J Surg 103:477, 1987.

Ferkel, RD, et al: An Illustrated Guide to Small Joint Arthroscopy. Smith & Nephew Dyonics, 1991.

Ferson, PF, et al: Thorascopic wedge resection of the lung. Surgical Rounds. 16:5, 1993.

Fezer, SJ: Cricoid pressure: How, when, and why. AORN J 45:1374, 1987.

Friel, JP (ed): Dorlands Illustrated Medical Dictionary, ed 26. WB Saunders, Philadelphia, 1981.

Fuller, JR: Surgical Technology Principles and Practice. WB Saunders, Philadelphia, 1986.

Gadacz, T: Video-assisted transthoracic hiatal hernioplasty using stapled, uncut gastroplasty and fundoplication. Surgical Rounds 17:7, 1994.

Glenn, JF (ed): Urologic Surgery, ed 4. JB Lippincott, Philadelphia, 1991.

Goldberg, SM, Gordon, P, and Nivatavongs, S: Essentials of Anorectal Surgery. JB Lippincott, Philadelphia, 1980.

Greene, VW, Klapes, NA, and Langholz, AC: Interhospital transportation: Monitoring sterility of instrument packs. AORN J 45:1420, 1987.

Gruendemann, BJ, and Meeker, MH: Alexander's Care of the Patient in Surgery, ed 8. CV Mosby, St. Louis, 1987.

Hirvela, ER, et al: General surgery. JAMA 271:21, 1994.

Huff, BB (ed): Physicians' Desk Reference, ed 41. Medical Economics, Oradell, NJ, 1987.

Jackson, EW (ed): Caring for Surgical Patients. Intermed Communications, Springhouse, PA, 1982.

Johns, ME, et al: Otolaryngology—Head and neck surgery. JAMA 271:21, 1994.

Kaufman, HE: Refractive surgery (editorial). Am J Ophthalmol 103:355, 1987.

Krumeich, JH, and Swinger, C: Non freeze epikeratophakia for the correction of myopia. Am J Ophthalmol 103:397, 1987.

Kuhn, PA: Operating Room Procedure Manual. Reston Publishing, Reston, VA, 1981.

Lach, J: OR Nursing: Preoperative Care and Draping Technique. Kendall, Chicago, 1974.

Lambrix, K: Epikeratophakia: Correcting visual deficits with corneal tissue. AORN J 46:218, 1987.

Laskin, RS, and Varrichio, DM: Total knee replacement. AORN J 36:577, 1982.

Le Maitre, G, and Finnegan, J: The Patient in Surgery, ed 4. WB Saunders, Philadelphia, 1980.

Linberg, JV: Oculoplastic and Orbital Emergencies. Appleton and Lange, Norwalk, CT, 1990.

LoCicero, J, Quebbeman, E, and Nichols, R: Health hazards in the operating room: An update. Bull Am Coll Surgeons 72(9):4, 1987.

Lore, JM: Atlas of Head and Neck Surgery, ed 2. WB Saunders, Philadelphia, 1973.

Mack, MJ, et al: Video thoracoscopy in thoracic surgery. Surgical Rounds 16:11, 1993.

Madden, JL: Atlas of Techniques in Surgery, ed 2. Appleton-Century-Crofts, New York, 1964.

Magovern, GJ, et al: Cardiothoracic surgery. JAMA 271:21, 1994.

Marshall, JG, and Ross, JL: Hydrocephalus: Ventriculoperitoneal shunting in infants and children. AORN J 40:842, 1984.

Mattingly, RF, and Thompson, JD: Te Linde's Operative Gynecology, ed 6. JB Lippincott, Philadelphia, 1985.

McCord, CD Jr (ed), et al: Occuloplastic Surgery, ed 3. Raven Press, New York, 1995.

Miner, D: Patient positioning: Applying the nursing process. AORN J 45:1117, 1987.

Moore, DC: Regional Block, ed 3. Charles C Thomas, Springfield, IL, 1962.

Nicholson, C, et al: Are you ready for video thoracoscopy? Am J Nurs 93:3, 1993.

Noguchi, M, et al: Mastectomy with and without immediate breast reconstruction using a musculocutaneous flap. Am J Surg 166:279, 1993.

Noone, J, et al: A six year experience with immediate reconstruction after mastectomy for cancer. Plast Reconstr Surg 76:258, 1985.

Pack, GT, and Oropeza, R: A technique for superficial and deep groin dissection. Surgical Procedures 3:2, 1966.

Partain, N: Laparoscopic Surgery and the OR Nurse. Ethicon, Somerville, NJ, 1991.

Pellegrini, CA: Thorascopic management of achalasia of the esophagus. Techniques in General Surgery 1:2, 1992.

Perez, RP, and Wood, RE: Update on pediatric flexible bronchoscopy. Pediatr Clin North Am 41:385, 1994.

Pernoll, ML (ed): Obstetrics and Gynecologic Diagnosis and Treatment, ed 7. Appleton and Lange, Norwalk, CT, 1991.

Peyman, GA, and Schulman, JA: Intravitreal surgery principles and practice. Appleton-Century-Crofts, New York, 1986.

Podrasky, P, and Rudzinski, HM: Percutaneous endoscopic gastrostomy: An alternative to laparotomy. AORN J 45:1403, 1987.

Quattro, LS: Spinal instrumentation: An introduction to Cotrel-DuBousset instrumentation. AORN J 46:54, 1987.

Quilici, PJ: New developments in laparoscopy. Auto Suture Co, 1992.

Raffensperger, JG: Swensons Pediatric Surgery, ed 4. Appleton-Century-Crofts, New York, 1980.

Reddick, EJ: Atlas of Laparoscopic Surgery. Raven Press, New York, 1993.

Richert, M: Laparoscopic instruments. AORN J 57:637, 1993.

Sabiston, D (ed): (Christopher's) Textbook of Surgery, ed 13. WB Saunders, Philadelphia, 1986.

Schuessler, W, and Vancaillie, TG: Laparoscopic Lymphadenectomy. Ethicon, Somerville, NJ, 1991.

Semm, K: Morcellment and suturing using pelviscopy—not a problem anymore. Geburtshilfe Frauenheilkd 51:843, 1991.

Smith, RR: Essentials of Neurosurgery. JB Lippincott, Philadelphia, 1980.

Smith, SR: Gasless laparoscopy: The next phase of laparoscopic surgery? Contemporary Surgery 45:171, 1994.

Snyder, SL, and Karzel, RP: The Orthopedic Clinics of North America. WB Saunders, Philadelphia, 1993.

Solomon, RP, and Koch, FA: The new tracking implant regulations. AORN J 58:6, 1993.

Spaeth, GL: Ophthalmic Surgery. WB Saunders, Philadelphia, 1982.

Spaeth, GL: Ophthalmic Surgery: Principles and Practice, ed 2. WB Saunders, Philadelphia, 1990.

Sutton, C, and Diamond, MP (eds): Endoscopic Surgery for Gynecologists. WB Saunders, Philadelphia, 1993.

Takeda, M, et al: Laparoscopic adrenalectomy for primary aldosteronism: Report of initial ten cases. Surgery 115:5, 1994.

Tampinco-Golos, I: Endoscopic thoracotomy. AORN J 55:1167, 1992.

Tanagho, EA, and McAninch, JW: Smith's General Urology, ed 13. Appleton and Lange, Norwalk, CT, 1992.

Te Linde: Operative Gynecology, ed 7. JB Lippincott, 1991.

Thomas, CL (ed.): Taber's Cyclopedic Medical Dictionary, ed 17. FA Davis, Philadelphia, 1989.

Torresyap, PM: Esophagogastrectomy for carcinoma of the esophagus. Today's OR Nurse 9:10, 1987.

Tupa, B: Alleviating the fears of pediatric patients. Today's OR Nurse 9:33, 1987.

Turek, S: Orthopaedics, ed 4, vol 2. JB Lippincott, Philadelphia, 1984.

Vaiden, RE, and White, WR: Arteriovenous malformations of the brain. AORN J 46:37, 1987.

Vaughn, D, and Ashbury, T: General Ophthalmology, ed 10. Lange Medical Publications, Los Altos, CA, 1983.

Vaughn, DG, et al: General Ophthalmolgy, ed 13, pp 187–189, 366–367. Appleton and Lange, Norwalk, CT, 1992.

Voyles, RC, et al: Trocar/cannula systems in laparoscopic surgery. Surgical Rounds 15:9, 1992.

Walker, WS, et al: Video assisted thoracoscopic pneumonectomy. Br J Surg 81:1, 1994.

Walsh, PC, Gittes, RF, and Perlmutter, AD (eds): Campbell's Urology, ed 5. WB Saunders, Philadelphia, 1986.

Watson, DS: The use of the benzodiazepine antagonist flumazenil. AORN J 57:497, 1993.

Waughman, WR, Jordan, LM, and Norris, JL: Nurse anesthetist: Patient-centered nursing. Today's OR Nurse 8:16, 1986.

White, RA, and Klein, SR (eds): Endoscopic Surgery. Mosby Year Book, St. Louis, 1991.

Wiklund, RA, and Barash, PG: Anesthesiology. JAMA 271:21, 1994.

Wilkins, RH: Neurological surgery. JAMA 271:21, 1994.

Wilson, JR, Beeacham, CT, and Carrington, ER: Obstetrics and Gynecology. CV Mosby, St. Louis, 1971.

Youmans, JR (ed): Neurological Surgery. WB Saunders, Philadelphia, 1982.

Zook, EG: Plastic surgery. JAMA 271:21, 1994.

Zucker, KA (ed): Surgical laparoscopy. Quality Medical Publishing, St. Louis, 1991.

Index

A "t" following a page number indicates a table.

Abdominal aortic endarterectomy, 274–278
Abdominal aortic neurysmectomy, 274–278
Abdominal aortic procedures, 274–278
Abdominal extraintestinal surgery, 60–94
  abdominal herniorrhaphy, 66–71
  abdominal laparoscopy, 62–66
  abdominal laparotomy, 60–62
  cholecystectomy, 71–79
  drainage of abscess in region of liver, 84–86
  drainage of pancreatic cyst (pseudocyst), 79–81
  hepatic resection, 86–88
  pancreatectomy, 83–84
  pancreaticoduodenectomy (Whipple procedure), 81–83
  splenectomy, 89–94
Abdominal herniorrhaphy, 66–71

Abdominal hysterectomy, total, 170–172
Abdominal hysterectomy tray, 572
Abdominal laparoscopy, 62–66
Abdominal laparotomy, 60–62
Abdominal lipectomy/abdominoplasty, 430–432
Abdominal prostatectomy tray, 575
Abdominoperineal resection of rectum, 135–138
  laparoscopic-assisted, 142
Abdominoplasty/abdominal lipectomy, 430–432
Abortion, therapeutic, by suction curettage, 5, 160–161
Abscess(es), liver region, drainage of, 84–86
Acoustic neuroma, 368–369
Acquired immunodeficiency syndrome (AIDS), 11, 22

Adenoidectomy and tonsillectomy, 454–456

Admission procedure, 5

Adrenalectomy, 230–233

Aganglionic megacolon, colorectal resection for, pediatric, 546–550

AIDS. *See* Acquired immunodeficiency syndrome (AIDS)

Amputation of lower extremity, 5, 363–366

Anesthesia
  conduction anesthesia, 27
    commonly used, 33t–34t
    local, 34–35
    nerve blocks, 32
    regional, local, topical, 42–44
    spinal, epidural, caudal, 40–42
    topical, 35–36
  general, anesthesia, 27, 29–30, 30t, 31, 31t, 37–39
  general information, 27–36
  ophthalmic surgery and, 473–474
  pediatric measures, 519

Aneurysm, intracranial, 368

Ankle and foot, arthroscopy of, 350–353

Ankle joint replacement, total, 354–356

Ankle, open reduction of, 348–350

Ankle, triple arthrodesis of, 353–354

Anterior and/or posterior colporrhaphy, 166–167

Anterior dislocation of shoulder, recurrent, repair of, 310–312

Anterior resection of sigmoid colon and rectum, 134

Antrostomy, intranasal/intranasal fenestration of the nasoantral wall, 444–447

Antrum of the maxillary sinuses, radical drainage of (Caldwell-Luc procedure), 447–448

Aortic valve replacement, 288, 291, 293

Aortoiliac graft, 274–278

Appendectomy, 122–123
  laparoscopic, 123–126
  pediatric, 554–555

Argon beam coagulator, 624

Arteriovenous fistula/arteriovenous shunt, 286–288

Arteriovenous malformation, 368

Arteriovenous shunt/arteriovenous fistula, 286–288

Arthrodesis, triple, of ankle, 353–354

Arthroscopic carpal tunnel release, 301

Arthroscopy of the ankle and foot, 350–353

Arthroscopy of the elbow, 318–321

Arthroscopy of the knee, 336–341

Arthroscopy of the shoulder, 312–316

Arthroscopy of the wrist, 307–310

Arthrotomy of the knee, 332–336
  tray for, 588

Atresia of the esophagus, congenital, repair of, 532–535

Augmentation mammoplasty, 428–430

Augmentation mentoplasty, 409–410

Baker's (popliteal) cyst, excision of, 341–343
Bankart procedure, 310
Bartholin's duct cyst, marsupialization of, 161–163
Basic/minor procedures tray, 562–563
Basic rigid sigmoidoscopy tray, 566–567
Biliary tract procedures tray, 566
Bladder or bladder neck, transurethral resection of (TURB), 215–217
Blepharoplasty, 410–412
Blepharoptosis repair, 483–484
Body mechanics for operating room personnel, 20–21
Bone fracture(s)
  "Blowout," 404
  internal fixation of hip, 321–323
  open reduction
    of ankle, 348–350
    of carpal, 296–298
    of femoral condyle, 333
    of femoral shaft, 330–332
    of humeral head, 316–318
    of humerus, 301–303
    of olecranon process, 305–307
    of orbital floor, 404–406
    of patella, 334
    of radius and/or ulna, 303–305
    of tibial plateau, 333
    of tibial shaft, 346–348
  reduction
    of a mandibular, 399–402
    of a nasal, 397–399
    of a zygomatic, 402–404
Bone holding instruments tray, 588

Branchial cleft sinusectomy, pediatric, 522–524
Breast biopsy, 53–55
Breast procedures, 53–59
Bristow procedure, 310
Bronchoscopy, 246–249
Bunionectomy, 356–358
Burr hole(s), 367
Bypass, femoropopliteal, 278–281
Byron-Smith procedure, 481

Caldwell-Luc procedure, 447–448
Canthorrhaphy/tarsorraphy, 478–480
Canthotomy, 477–478
Carbon dioxide laser, 617–618, 619t
Cardiac procedures, 288–295
Cardiac procedures tray, 582–584
Cardiopulmonary bypass, 288 290, 292 293
Cardiopulmonary resuscitation (CPR), 18–19
Cardiovascular surgery
  abdominal aortic endarterectomy, 274–278
  abdominal aortic neurysmectomy, 274–278
  abdominal aortic procedures, 274–278
  aortoiliac graft, 274–278
  arteriovenous shunt/arteriovenous fistula, 286–288
  cardiac procedures, 288–295
  carotid endarterectomy, 272–274
  femoropopliteal bypass, 278–281
  greater saphenous vein ligation and stripping, 281–283

Cardiovascular surgery—
Continued
portasystemic shunt, 283–
285
Cardiovascular trays
cardiac procedures tray,
582–584
vascular procedures tray,
580
vascular shunt tray, 581–
582
Carotid endarterectomy,
272–274
Carpal bone fracture, open
reduction of, 296–298
Carpal tunnel release, 300–
301
Cataract extraction, 500–503
Cataract extraction and lens
procedure tray, 607–
608
Caudal, spinal, epidural
anesthesia, 40–42
Centers for Disease Control
and Prevention, 22
Central venous catheter, pediatric, insertion of,
535–537
Cerebrospinal fluid otorrhea
or rhinorrhea, 368
Cervical cone tray, 570
Cervical intervertebral disc,
excision of with fusion,
390–392
Cervix
conization of, 158–159
curettage of, 156–158
Cesarean section, 190–193
Cesarean section tray, 572–
573
Chalazion, excision of, 476–
477
Chemical hazards, 22–23
Chevron procedure, 357
Cholangiogram, 72–73, 75
Cholecystectomy, 71–74
Cholecystotomy, 71

Choledochoscopy, 71–73, 75–
76
Choledochoscopy tray, 567
Choledochotomy, 71–72
Cidex, 18
Circulator
abdominal extraintestinal
surgery and, 66, 78–
79, 94
anesthesia and, 28–29, 32,
34–35, 39, 41, 43
breast surgery and, 54–55,
58
cardiovascular surgery
and, 294
gastrointestinal surgery
and, 106, 112, 144
genitourinary surgery and,
238
gynecologic and obstetric
surgery and, 161,
192
orthopedic surgery and,
340
protection of patient and,
5, 13–15
psychological support of
the patient and, 4
thoracic surgery and, 267
Circumcision, 197–198
Classic radical mastectomy,
55, 57
Cleft lip repair, 393–395
Cleft palate repair, 395–397
Closure of colostomy, 128–
130
Closure of a perforated peptic
ulcer, 113
laparoscopic (with vagot-
omy), 113–114
Colectomy
anterior resection of the
sigmoid colon and rec-
tum, 134
right hemicolectomy, 130–
132
transverse, 132–133

Collateral or cruciate ligament repair, 333–334
Colon resection, laparoscopic-assisted, 138–144
Colonoscopy, 98
Colorectal resection for aganglionic megacolon/Hirschsprung's disease, pediatric, 546–550
Colostomy, 126–128
    closure of, 128–130
    pediatric, 543–545
Colporrhaphy, anterior and/or posterior, 166–167
Colpotomy, posterior, 174–176
Conduction anesthesia, 27
    commonly used, 33t–34t
    local, 34–35
    nerve blocks, 32
    regional, local, topical, 42–44
    spinal, epidural, caudal, 40–42
    topical, 35–36
Congenital abnormalities, neurologic, 369
Congenital atresia of esophagus, repair of, 532–535
Congenital diaphragmatic hernia, repair of, 524–526
Congenital hypertrophic pyloric stenosis, pyloromyotomy for, 537–539
Conization of uterine cervix, 158–159
Consent form(s), 4–5
Cordotomy, 385
Corneal procedures tray, 606–607
Corneal transplantation/keratoplasty, 497–500
Coronary artery bypass graft, 288, 292–293

Correction of hammer toe deformity with interphalangeal fusion, 359
Correction of ectropion, 480–482
Correction of entropion, 482–483
Correction of pectus excavation, 259–260
Correction of scoliosis, 360–363
Correction of strabismus, 490–492
Counting procedure, 14–16
CPR. See Cardiopulmonary resuscitation (CPR)
Craniectomy, 367
Craniopharyngioma, 368
Cranioplasty, 375–378
Craniotomy, 367–375
Craniotomy tray, 589–591
Cruciate or collateral ligament repair, 333–334
Culdoscopy, 163
Cutaneous ileostomy, 120–122
Cutaneous ureterostomy, 227–228
Cutaneous vasostomy, 206
Cyst, Popliteal (Baker's), excision of, 341–343
Cystectomy, 212–215
    pilonidal and sinusectomy, 149–151
Cystoscopy, 208–210
Cystotomy, 210–212

D & C, 156–158
D & C tray, 569–570
Dacryocystorhinostomy, 488–490
Dacryocystorhinostomy tray, 604–605
Death, 19
Decortication of lung, 256
Dermabrasion, 414–416

Diaphragmatic hernia, congenital, repair of, 524–526

Digital flexor tendon repair, 420–422

Dilatation and curettage (D & C) tray, 569–570

Dilatation of cervix and curettage of uterus (D & C), 156–158

Dislocation of shoulder, anterior, recurrent, repair of, 310–312

Drainage of antrum of the maxillary sinuses (Caldwell-Luc procedure), 447–448

Drainage of abscess(es) in the region of the liver, 84–86

Drainage of frontal sinus, 449–451

Drainage of pancreatic cyst (pseudocyst), 79–81

Ear procedures tray, 596–598

Ectropion, correction of, 480–482

Elbow, arthroscopy of, 318–321

Electrical and fire hazards, 12

Electrohydraulic lithotripsy, 243–245

Electrosurgery, 12–13

Emergencies and disasters in the operating room, 18–19

Endarterectomy, abdominal aortic, 274–278

Endarterectomy, carotid, 272–274

Endocardial pacemaker, insertion of transvenous, 256–258

Endometrial ablation, radiofrequency, 625

Endoscopic microsurgery, transanal, 144–147

Endoscopy, sinus, 451–454

ENT surgery. See Otorhinolaryngologic surgery

ENT trays. See Otorhinolaryngologic trays

Entropion, correction of, 482–483

Enucleation of globe, 494–495

Environmental controls, 10–12

Epidural, spinal, caudal anesthesia, 40–42

Epidural hematoma, 368

Epigastric herniorrhaphy, 67–68

Epispadias repair, 196–197

Esophageal atresia repair, congenital, 532–535

Esophageal hiatal herniorrhaphy, 102–103

Esophagogastromyotomy, video-assisted thoracoscopic, 270–271

Esophagoscopy, 95–97

ESWL. See Extracorporeal shock wave lithtripsy (ESWL)

Evisceration of eye, 492–494

Excision(s)

cervical intervertebral disc, with fusion, 390–392

chalazion, 476–477

eyelid lesions, 485–487

ganglion, 298–300

oral cavity lesions, 469–472

popliteal (Baker's) cyst, 341–343

pterygium, 509–510

submaxillary (submandibular) gland, 461–462

Exenteration, orbital, 495–497

Exenteration, pelvic, 186–189

Extended radical mastectomy, 55

External levator resection, 483–484

Extracapsular cataract extraction, 500–501

Extracorporal shockwave lithotripsy without water bath, 239–242

Extracorporeal shock wave lithtripsy (ESWL), 233–238

Extraction of an intraocular foreign body, 505–507

Eye, evisceration of, 492–494

Eye muscle procedures tray, 604

Eye procedures, basic, tray, 602–603

Eye procedures microscope tray, 609–610

Eyelid and conjunctival procedures tray, 603–604

Eyelid laceration repair, 487–488

Eyelid lesions, excision of, 485–487

Fallopian tubes, tuboplasty of, 183–186

Fasciectomy, palmar, 425–426

Fatigue factors for operating room personnel, 21

Femoral condyle and tibial plateau fractures, open reduction, 333

Femoral condyle, open reduction of, 333

Femoral head prosthetic replacement, 323–326

Femoral herniorraphy, 66–67

Femoral shaft, open reduction of, 330–332

Femoropopliteal bypass, 278–281

Fire and electrical hazards, 12

Fistula, arteriovenous/arteriovenous shunt, 286–288

Fixation, internal, hip, 321–323

Flash sterilizer, 16–17

Flexible sigmoidoscopy, 99, 101

Foot and ankle, arthroscopy of, 350–353

Fracture(s). See Bone fracture(s)

Frontal sinus, drainage of, 449–451

Fundoplication, laparoscopic (Nissen procedure), 103–106
  pediatric, 555–556

Gamma knife, 369

Ganglion, excision of, 298–300

Gas chemical sterilization, 16–18

Gastrectomy, 116–119

Gastrointestinal procedures tray, 567
  pediatric, 614

Gastrointestinal surgery, 95–155
  abdominoperineal resection of rectum, 135–138
  anterior resection of sigmoid colon and rectum, 134
  appendectomy, 122–123
  closure of colostomy, 128–130
  closure of a perforated peptic ulcer, 113
  colonoscopy, 98

Gastrointestinal surgery—
Continued
  colostomy, 126–128
  cutaneous ileostomy, 120–
      122
  esophageal hiatal hernior-
      rhaphy, 102–103
  esophagoscopy, 95–97
  gastrectomy, 116–119
  gastroscopy, 97–98
  gastrostomy, 114–116
  hemorrhoidectomy, 147–
      149
  laparoscopic appendec-
      tomy, 123–126
  laparoscopic-assisted colon
      resection, 138–144
  laparoscopic closure of a
      perforated ulcer (with
      vagotomy), 113–114
  laparoscopic fundoplication
      (Nissen procedure),
      103–106
  laparoscopic vagotomy,
      108–112
  perineal resection of the
      rectum for complete
      rectal prolapse (proci-
      dentia), 154–155
  pilonidal cystectomy and
      sinusectomy, 149–151
  right hemicolectomy, 130–
      132
  Ripstein procedure (presac-
      ral rectopexy), 153–154
  sigmoidoscopy, 98–101
  small-bowel resection, 119–
      120
  Thiersch procedure, 151–
      152
  transanal endoscopic mi-
      crosurgery, 144–147
  transverse colectomy, 132–
      133
  vagotomy and pyloroplasty,
      106–108
Gastroscopy, 97–98

Gastrostomy, 114–116
  pediatric, 539–540
General anesthesia, 27, 29–
    30, 30t, 31, 31t, 37–39
General surgery trays
  basic rigid sigmoidoscopy
      tray, 566–567
  basic/minor procedures
      tray, 562–563
  biliary tract procedures
      tray, 566
  choledochoscopy tray, 566
  gastrointestinal procedures
      tray, 567
  limited procedures tray,
      563–564
  long instrument tray, 565
  major procedures tray,
      561–562
  minor/basic procedures
      tray, 562–563
  rectal procedures tray,
      567–568
  thyroid tray, 564–565
Genitourinary surgery
  adrenalectomy, 230–233
  circumcision, 197–198
  cutaneous ureterostomy,
      227–228
  cutaneous vasotomy, 206
  cystectomy, 212–215
  cystoscopy, 208–210
  cystostomy, 210–212
  electrohydraulic
      lithotripsy, 243–245
  epispadias repair, 196–197
  extracorporal shock wave
      lithotripsy without wa-
      ter bath, 239–242
  extracorporeal shock wave
      lithotripsy (ESWL),
      233–238
  hydrocelectomy, 202–203
  hypospadias repair, 194–
      196
  ileal conduit, 228–230
  lesions of the bladder or

bladder neck (TURB), 215–217
Marshall-Marchetti-Krantz procedure, 200–202
nephrectomy, 221–224
nephrolithotomy, 225–227
open prostatectomy, 217–221
orchiectomy, 207–208
penile implant, 198–200
pyelolithotomy, 225–227
spermatocelectomy, 206–207
transurethral resection of lesions of bladder or bladder neck (TURB), 215–217
transurethral resection of the prostate (TURP), 215–217
ultrasonic lithotripsy, 242–243
upper tract urolithotomy, 225–227
ureterolithotomy, 225–227
vasectomy, 203–205
vasovasotomoy, 205–206
Genitourinary trays
abdominal prostatectomy tray, 575
kidney tray, 575
vasectomy tray, 574
Glaucoma procedures tray, 608–609
Globe and orbit procedures tray, 605–606
Globe, enucleation of, 494–495
Glossectomy, partial, with marginal resection of mandible, 469–472
Graft, aortoiliac, 274–278
Greater saphenous vein ligation and stripping, 281–283
Gynecologic and obstetric surgery

anterior and/or posterior colporrhaphy, 166–167
cesarean section, 190–193
conization of uterine cervix, 158–159
culdoscopy, 163
dilation of cervix and curettage of uterus (D & C), 156–158
hysteroscopy, 180–183
laparoscopic hysterectomy and laparoscopic-assisted vaginal hysterectomy with or without salpingo-oophorectomy, 176–180
marsupialization of Bartholin's duct cyst, 161–163
pelvic extenteration, 186–189
pelvic laparoscopy/pelviscopy, 167–170
salpingo-oophorectomy, 172–174
Shirodkar procedure, 189–190
therapeutic abortion by suction curettage, 160–161
total abdominal hysterectomy, 170–172
tubal sterilization, 174–176
tuboplasty of fallopian tubes, 183–186
vaginal hysterectomy, 163–165
Gynecologic and obstetric trays
abdominal hysterectomy tray, 572
cervical cone tray, 570
cesarean section tray, 572–573
dilatation and curettage (D & C) tray, 569–570

Gynecologic and obstetric trays—Continued
vaginal hysterectomy tray, 571–572

Hammer toe deformity, correction of, with interphalangeal fusion, 359
Harrington rod, 361
Hartmann's procedure, 141–142
Hematoma, subdural or epidural, 368
Hemicolectomy, left, laparoscopic-assisted, 140, 142
Hemicolectomy, right, 130–132
laparoscopic-assisted, 139–140, 142
Hemorrhoidectomy, 147–149
Hepatic resection, 86–88
Hepatitis B virus (HBV), 11, 22
Hernia, congenital diaphragmatic, 524–526
Herniorrhaphy
abdominal, 66–71
epigastric, 67–68
esophageal hiatal, 102–103
femoral, 66–67
incisional, 67–68
inguinal, 66–67
pediatric, 530–532
laparoscopic groin, 68–71
pediatric umbilical, 529–530
Hip
internal fixation of, 321–323
total replacement of, 326–330
Hip retractors tray, 588
Hirschsprung's disease, pediatric colorectal resection for, 546–550

Human immunodeficiency virus (HIV), 11, 22
Humeral head, open reduction of fracture of including prosthesis, 316–318
Humerus, open reduction of, 301–303
Hydrocelectomy, 202–203
Hydrocephalus, 369, 382–383
Hydrodissection, 177
Hyperthermia, malignant, 19
Hypophysectomy, transphenoidal, 378
Hypospadias repair, 194–196
Hysterectomy
laparoscopic, with or without salpingo-oophorectomy, 176–180
total abdominal, 170–172
tray for, 572
vaginal, 163–165
tray for, 571–572
Hysteroscopy, 180–183

Ileal conduit, 228–230
Ileostomy, cutaneous, 120–122
Imperforate anus, repair of, 550–553
Implant, secondary lens, 503–505
Incident report(s), 19
Incisional (Ventral) herniorrhaphy, 67–68
Infection control, 22
Informed consent, 4–5
Inguinal herniorrhaphy (direct, indirect), 66–67
pediatric, 530–532
Injury, prevention of, 5, 10
body mechanics for, 20–21
Insertion of transvenous endocardial pacemaker, 256–258
In-service education for operating room personnel, 20

Instrument count(s), 16
Instrument trays, 559
  cardiovascular trays, 580–584
  general surgery trays, 561–568
  genitourinary trays, 574–575
  gynecologic and obstetric tray, 569–573
  neurologic procedures trays, 589–593
  ophthalmic trays, 602–611
  orthopedic trays, 585–588
  otorhinolaryngologic (ENT) trays, 596–601
  pediatric trays, 612–615
  plastic procedures tray, 594–595
  thoracic trays, 576–579
Internal fixation of the hip, 321–323
Internal tarsal-obicularis resection, 482–483
Interphalangeal fusion, correction of hammer toe deformity with, 359
Intestinal obstruction, pediatric, relief of, 540–541
Intra-aortic balloon catheter, 290–291
Intracapsular cataract extraction, 500–501
Intracranial aneurysm, 368
Intracranial vessel, occluded, 368
Intraocular foreign body extraction, 505–507
Intraocular lens implant (IOL), 500–501, 503–505
Intranasal antrostomy/intranasal fenestration of nasoantral wall, 44–447

Intussusception, pediatric, reduction of, 542–543
Iridectomy, 507

Jackknife position, 100
Joint Commission on Accreditation of Healthcare Organizations (JCAHO), 13–14
Joint replacement, total ankle, 354–356

Keller procedure, 357–358
Keratoplasty, refractive, 516–517
Keratoplasty/corneal transplant, 497–500
Kerrison rongeurs and pituitary forceps tray, 592–593
Kidney tray, 575
Knee
  arthroscopy of, 336–341
  arthrotomy of, 332–336
  synovectomy of, 333–334
  total replacement of, 343–346
Knee arthrotomy tray, 588

Laceration repair, eyelid, 487–488
Lacrimal duct probing, 484–485
Laminectomy, 385–390
Laminectomy tray, 591–592
Laparoscopic appendectomy, 123–126
  pediatric, 554–555
Laparoscopic cholecystectomy, 74–79
Laparoscopic fundoplication (Nissen procedure), 103–106
  pediatric, 555–556

Laparoscopic groin hernior-
    rhaphy, 68–71
Laparoscopic hysterectomy
    and laparoscopic-as-
    sisted vaginal hyster-
    ectomy with or with-
    out salpingo-
    oophorectomy, 176–
    180
Laparoscopic splenectomy,
    91–94
  pediatric, 557–558
Laparoscopic vagotomy, 108–
    112
Laparoscopic-assisted abdom-
    inal perineal resection
    of the rectum, 142
Laparoscopic-assisted colon
    resection, 138–144
Laparoscopy, pediatric, 553–
    554
Laparotomy, abdominal, 60–
    62
Laparotomy, suprapubic, 212
Laryngectomy, 464–467
Laryngoscopy, 456–459
Laser technology, 616–625
  argon beam coagulator,
    624
  commonly used laser, 619t
  radiofrequency endome-
    trial ablation, 625
  safety precautions, 619–
    622, 624
    operative procedure re-
      port, 622f–623f
Left hemicolectomy, laparo-
    scopic-assisted, 140,
    142
Lens implant, secondary,
    503–505
Lens procedure and cataract
    extraction tray, 607–
    608
Lesion excision(s)
  eyelid, 485–487
  oral cavity, 469–472

Lifting, body mechanics of,
    20–21
Ligament repair, collateral or
    cruciate, 333–334
Ligation and stripping,
    greater saphenous
    vein, 281–283
Limited access procedures,
    pediatric, 553
Limited procedure tray, 563–
    564
Lipectomy, abdominal/abdom-
    inoplasty, 430–432
Liposuction, 432–434
Liquid chemical sterilization,
    18
Lithotomy position, 100
Lithotripsy, electrohydraulic,
    243–245
Lithotripsy, extracorporal
    shock wave without
    water bath, 239–242
Lithotripsy, extracorporeal
    shock wave (ESWL),
    233–238
Lithotripsy, ultrasonic, 242–
    243
Liver, drainage of abscess in
    region of, 84–86
Lobectomy, pulmonary,
    254
Local anesthesia, 34–35, 42–
    43
Long instruments tray, 565
Low anterior resection, laparo-
    scopic-assisted, 140–
    141
Lower extremity, amputation
    of, 5, 363–366
Lumpectomy, 55
Lung
  decortication of, 256
  resection of, 251–253
  wedge resection of, 253–
    254
    thoracoscopic, 268–
      269

Major procedures tray, 561–562
  pediatric, 612–613
Malignant hyperthermia, 19
Mammoplasty, augmentation, 428–430
Mammoplasty, reduction, 426–428
Mandible, partial resection of with partial glossectomy, 469–472
Mandibular fracture, reduction of, 399–402
Marshall-Marchetti-Krantz procedure, 200–202
Marsupialization of Bartholin's duct cyst, 161–163
Mastectomy, 55–59
Mastoidectomy, 437–440
Maxillary sinuses, radical drainage of, 447–448
McDonald procedure, 189
Mediastinoscopy, 249–250
Mediastinoscopy tray, 576–577
Meniscectomy, 333–334
Mentoplasty augmentation, 409–410
Metatarsal head resection, 359–360
Microlaryngoscopy, 458
Minilaparotomy, 174–176
Minor/basic procedures tray, 562–563
  pediatric, 613–614
Mitral valve replacement, 288, 291, 293
Modified Lateral/Sims' position, 100
Modified radical mastectomy, 55, 57
Myringotomy, 435–437
Myringotomy tray, 599–600

Nasal fracture, reduction of, 397–399

Nasal polypectomy, 448–449
Nasal procedures tray, 598–599
Nasal septum, submucous resection of, 443–444
Nasoantral wall, intranasal antrostomy/intranasal fenestration of, 444–447
National Institute of Occupational Safety and Health (NIOSH), 22
Neck, radical dissection of, 467–469
Neck surgery, 48–52
Neodymium/YAG laser, 617–618, 619t
Nephrectomy, 221–224
Nephrolithotomy, 224–227
Nerve block(s), 32
Nerve repair, peripheral, 422–425
Neurologic disorders, 369
Neurologic procedures trays
  craniotomy tray, 589–591
  Kerrison Rongeurs and pituitary forceps tray, 592–593
  laminectomy tray, 591–592
Neuroma, 368–369
Neurosurgical surgery
  cranioplasty, 375–378
  craniotomy, 367–375
  excision of cervical intervertebral disc with fusion, anterior approach, 390–392
  laminectomy, 385–390
  transsphenoidal hypophysectomy, 378–381
  ventricular shunts, 381–385
Neurysmectomy, abdominal aortic, 274–278
NIOSH. See National Institute of Occupational Safety and Health (NIOSH)

Nissen procedure (laparo-
        scopic fundoplication),
        103–106
    pediatric, 555–556

Occluded intracranial vessel,
        368
Olecranon process fracture,
        open reduction of,
        305–307
Omphalocele repair, 526–528
Oophorectomy,
Open prostatectomy, 217–221
Open reduction(s)
    ankle, 348–350
    carpal bone fracture, 296–
        298
    femoral condyle, 333
    femoral shaft, 330–332
    humeral head, 316–318
    humerus, 301–303
    olecranon process, 305–307
    patella, 334
    radius and/or ulna, 303–305
    tibial plateau, 333
    tibial shaft, 346–348
Operative record, 8–9t, 13–14
Ophthalmic surgery, 34, 473–
        476
    blepharoptosis repair, 483–
        484
    canthorrhaphy/tarsorra-
        phy, 478–480
    canthotomy, 477–478
    cataract extraction, 500–
        503
    corneal transplant/kerato-
        plasty, 497–500
    correction of ectropion,
        480–482
    correction of entropion,
        482–483
    correction of strabismus,
        490–492
    dacryocystorhinostomy,
        488–490

    enucleation of globe, 494–
        495
    evisceration of eye, 492–
        494
    excision of chalazion, 476–
        477
    excision of eyelid lesions,
        485–487
    excision of pterygium, 509–
        510
    extraction of an intraocular
        foreign body, 505–507
    eyelid laceration repair,
        487–488
    iridectomy, 507
    keratoplasty/corneal trans-
        plant, 497–500
    lacrimal duct probing, 484–
        485
    orbital exenteration, 495–
        497
    refractive keratoplasty,
        516–517
    repair of retinal detach-
        ment/scleral buckling,
        511–513
    secondary lens implant,
        503–505
    tarsorrhaphy/canthorrha-
        phy, 478–480
    trabeculectomy, 507–509
    vitrectomy, 513–516
Ophthalmic trays
    basic eye muscle proce-
        dures tray, 604
    basic eye procedures micro-
        scope tray, 609–610
    basic eye procedures tray,
        602–603
    cataract extraction and
        lens procedure tray,
        607–608
    corneal procedures tray,
        606–607
    dacryocystorhinostomy
        tray, 604–605
    eyelid and conjunctival

procedures tray, 603–604

glaucoma procedures tray, 608–609

globe and orbit procedures tray, 605–606

retinal procedures tray, 610–611

Optic glioma, 368

Oral cavity, excision of lesions, 469–472

Orbit and globe procedures tray, 605–606

Orbital exenteration, 495–497

Orbital floor fracture, open reduction of, 404–406

Orchiectomy, 207–208

Orientation (teaching) session, psychological support of the patient and, 3

Orthopedic surgery

amputation of lower extremity, 363–366

arthroscopy of the ankle and foot, 350–353

arthroscopy of elbow, 318–321

arthroscopy of knee, 336–341

arthroscopy of shoulder, 312–316

arthroscopy of wrist, 307–310

arthrotomy of knee, 332–336

bunionectomy, 356–358

carpal tunnel release, 300–301

correction of hammer to deformity with interphalangeal fusion, 359

excision of ganglion, 298–300

excision of popliteal (Baker's) cyst, 341–343

femoral head prosthetic replacement, 323–326

humeral head prosthesis, 316–318

internal fixation of hip, 321–323

metatarsal head resection, 359–360

open reduction of ankle, 348–350

open reduction of carpal bone fracture, 296–298

open reduction of femoral shaft, 330–332

open reduction of fracture of humeral head (including humeral head prosthesis), 316–318

open reduction of humerus, 301–303

open reduction of olecranon process fracture, 305–307

open reduction of radius and/or ulna, 303–305

open reduction of tibial shaft, 346–348

procedure for correction of scoliosis, 360–363

repair of recurrent anterior dislocation of shoulder, 310–312

total ankle joint replacement, 354–356

total hip replacement, 326–330

total knee replacement, 343–346

triple arthrodesis of ankle, 353–354

Orthopedic trays

basic orthopedic procedures tray, 585–586

bone holding instruments tray, 588

hip retractors tray, 588

knee arthrotomy tray, 588

Orthopedic trays—Continued
  minor orthopedic proce-
    dures tray, 586–587
Otoplasty, 416–418
Otorhinolaryngologic (ENT)
    surgery
  Caldwell-Luc procedure,
    447–448
  drainage of frontal sinus,
    449–451
  excision of lesions of oral
    cavity, 469–472
  excision of the submaxil-
    lary (submandibular)
    gland, 461–462
  intranasal antrostomy/
    intranasal fenestration
    of nasoantral wall,
    444–447
  laryngectomy, 464–467
  laryngoscopy, 456–459
  mastoidectomy, 437–440
  myringotomy, 435–437
  nasal polypectomy, 448–
    449
  parotidectomy, 462–464
  partial glossectomy with
    marginal resection of
    mandible, 469–472
  radical drainage of antrum
    of maxillary sinuses,
    447–448
  radical neck dissection,
    467–469
  sinus endoscopy, 451–
    454
  stapedectomy, 442–443
  submucous resection of
    nasal septum (SMR),
    443–444
  tonsillectomy and adenoid-
    ectomy (T & A), 454–
    456
  tracheostomy, 459–461
  tympanoplasty, 440–442
Otorhinolaryngologic (ENT)
    trays

  basic ear procedures tray,
    596–598
  myringotomy tray, 599–
    600
  nasal procedures tray,
    598–599
  tonsillectomy and ade-
    noidectomy (T & A)
    tray, 600–60
  tracheostomy tray, 601
Otorrhea, cerebrospinal fluid,
    368

Pacemaker, transvenous en-
    docardial, insertion of,
    256–258
Pacemaker tray, 578–579
Palmar fasciectomy, 425–
    426
Pancreatectomy, 83–84
Pancreatic cyst, drainage of,
    79–81
Pancreaticoduodenectomy
    (Whipple procedure),
    81–83
Parkinson's disease, 369
Parasellar tumor, 368
Parathyroidectomy, 50–51
Parotidectomy, 462–464
Partial gastrectomy, 116
Partial glossectomy with
    marginal resection of
    mandible, 469–472
Partial mastectomy, 55–56
Partial pancreatectomy, 83–
    84
Patient
  anesthesia and, 27–29
    conduction, 32, 34–35,
      40–44
    general, 29, 37–39
  identification of, 4–5
  lifting of, 20–21
  preparation for surgery in
    abdominal extraintesti-
    nal surgery, 61, 64, 67,

70, 72, 76, 80, 82, 85, 87, 89, 92
breast surgery, 54, 57
cardiovascular surgery, 273, 276, 279, 282, 285–286, 292
gastrointestinal surgery, 96, 99–100, 104, 107, 110, 115, 117, 120–121, 123, 125, 127, 129, 131–134, 136, 142, 146, 150–151, 153
genitourinary surgery and, 195, 199, 201–202, 204, 209, 211, 214, 216, 219, 222–223, 226–227, 229, 231–232, 235, 240
gynecologic and obstetric surgery and, 157–159, 161–162, 164, 167, 169, 171, 173, 175, 178–179, 184, 187, 189–191
neck surgery, 49, 52
neurosurgical surgery, 371–372, 370, 979–380, 383, 385–388, 391
ophthalmic surgery and, 476–478, 481, 484–486, 488–489, 491–493, 495–497, 499, 501–502, 504, 508, 510, 512, 514, 517
orthopedic surgery, 297, 300, 302, 304, 306, 308, 311, 314, 317, 319–320, 324–325, 331, 335, 338, 341–342, 344–345, 347, 349, 351–352, 357, 362, 364
otorhinolaryngologic (ENT) surgery, 435–436, 438, 445, 447, 450, 452–453, 455, 457, 460–463, 465–466, 468, 470
pediatric patient, 518–520, 523, 525, 527, 529, 531, 533, 536, 538, 542, 544–545, 547, 551
plastic surgery, 394, 396, 398, 400, 403, 405, 407, 409, 411, 413–416, 418–419, 421, 424, 427, 429, 431–433
thoracic surgery, 247, 250 252, 257, 261, 265
protection of in surgery, 5–19
psychological support of, 3–4
Patellectomy, 333
Pectus excavatum, correction of, 259–260
Pediatric procedures, 518–520
branchial cleft sinusectomy, tracheostomy, 522–524
colorectal resection for aganglionic mega-colon/Hirschsprung's disease, 546–550
colostomy, 543–545
gastrostomy, 539–540
inguinal herniorrhaphy, 530–532
insertion of a central venous catheter, 532–535
laparoscopic appendectomy, 554–555
laparoscopic fundoplication/Nissen procedure, 555–556
laparoscopy, 553–554
limited access, 553
omphalocele repair, 526–528

Pediatric procedures—
  Continued
pyloromyomotomy for con-
    genital hypertrophic
    pyloric stenosis, 537–
    539
  reduction of pediatric in-
    tussusception, 542–
    543
  relief of intestinal obstruc-
    tion, 540–541
  repair of congenital atresia
    of the esophagus, 532–
    535
  repair of congenital dia-
    phragmatic hernia,
    524–526
  repair of imperforate anus,
    550–553
  splenectomy, laparoscopic,
    557–558
  thoracoscopy, 556–557
  tracheostomy, 520–522
  umbilical herniorrhaphy,
    529–530
Pediatric trays
  gastrointestinal procedures
    tray, 614
  major procedures tray,
    612–613
  minor procedures tray,
    613–614
  thoracotomy tray, 615
Pelvic exenteration, 186–189
Pelvic laparoscopy/pelvi-
    scopy, 167–170
Penetrating keratoplasty,
    498–499
Penile implant, 198–200
Perforated ulcer, closure of,
    113
  laparoscopic (with vagot-
    omy), 113–114
Perineal resection of the rec-
    tum for complete rec-
    tal prolapse (prociden-
    tia), 154–155

Perioperative considerations
  protection of the patient in
    surgery, 5–19, 29
  psychological support of the
    surgical patient, 3–4
  safety for operating room
    personnel, 20–23
Peripheral nerve repair, 422–
    425
Permanent colostomy, 126–
    127
Phacoemulsification, 500
Pilonidal cystectomy and
    sinusectomy, 149–151
Pituitary forceps and Kerri-
    son Rongeurs tray,
    592–593
Pituitary, tumors near the,
    368
Plasma scalpel, 88
Plastic procedures tray, ba-
    sic, 594–595
Plastic surgery, 34
  abdominoplasty/abdominal
    lipectomy, 430–432
  augmentation mammo-
    plasty, 428–430
  blepharoplasty, 410–412
  cleft lip repair, 393–395
  cleft palate repair, 395–397
  dermabrasion, 414–416
  digital flexor tendon repair,
    420–422
  liposuction, 432–434
  mentoplasty augmenta-
    tion, 409–410
  open reduction of orbital
    floor fracture, 404–406
  otoplasty, 416–418
  palmar fasciectomy, 425–
    426
  peripheral nerve repair,
    422–425
  reduction mammoplasty,
    426–428
  reduction of mandibular
    fracture, 399–402

reduction of nasal fracture, 397–399

reduction of zygomatic fracture, 402–404

repair of syndactyly, 418–420

rhinoplasty, 406–409

rhytidectomy, 412–414

Pneumonectomy, 254–255
video-assisted thoracoscopic, 269–270

Polypectomy, nasal, 448–449

Popliteal (Baker's) cyst, excision of, 341 343

Portasystemic shunt, 283–285

Positioning, 10
pediatric considerations, 520

Posterior and/or anterior colporrhaphy, 166–167

Posterior colpotomy, 174–176

Presacral rectopexy (Ripstein procedure), 153–154

Procidentia (perineal resection of the rectum for complete rectal prolapse), 154–155

Prostate, transurethral resection (TURP), 215–217

Prostatectomy, abdominal, tray, 575

Prostatectomy, open, 217–221

Prosthesis
femoral head replacement, 323–326
humeral head, 316–318

Pseudocyst, drainage of pancreatic, 79–81

Psychologic support of the surgical patient, 3–4

Pterygium, excision of, 509–510

Pulmonary lobectomy, 254

Putti-Platt procedure, 310

Pyelolithotomy, 225–227

Pyloromyotomy for congenital hypertrophic py-

loric stenosis, 537–539

Pyloroplasty and vagotomy, 106–108

Radial keratotomy, 516

Radiation safety for operating room personnel, 21

Radical drainage of the antrum of the maxillary sinuses (Caldwell-Luc procedure), 447–448

Radical mastectomy, 55–57

Radical neck dissection, 467–469

Radiofrequency endometrial ablation, 625

Radius, open reduction of, 303–305

Recovery room staff, psychological support of the patient and, 4

Rectal procedures tray, 567–568

Rectopexy, presacral (Ripstein procedure), 153–154

Rectum, abdominoperineal, resection of, 135–138
laparoscopic-assisted, 142

Rectum, anterior resection of sigmoid colon and, 134

Rectum, perineal resection of for complete prolapse (procidentia), 154–155

Recurrent anterior shoulder dislocation, repair of, 310–312

Reduction
ankle, 348–350
femoral condyle, 333
femoral shaft, 330–332
humeral head, 316–318
humerus, 301–303
mammoplasty, 426–428

Reduction—Continued
    mandibular fracture, 399–402
    nasal fracture, 397–399
    olecranon process fracture, 305–307
    orbital floor fracture, 404–406
    patella, 334
    pediatric intussusception, 542–543
    radius and/or ulna, 303–305
    tibial plateau, 333
    tibial shaft, 346–348
    zygomatic fracture, 402–404
Refractive keratoplasty, 516–517
Regional block(s), 32, 42–43
Restraint strap(s), 10
    pediatric, 519
Retinal detachment/scleral buckling, repair of, 511–513
Retinal procedures tray, 610–611
Reversal of Hartmann's procedure, 141–142
Rhinoplasty, 406–409
Rhinorrhea, cerebrospinal fluid, 368
Rhizotomy, 369, 385
Rhytidectomy, 412–414
Right hemicolectomy, 130–131
    laparoscopic-assisted, 142
Rigid sigmoidoscopy, 99–101
    basic tray for, 566–567
Ripstein procedure (presacral rectopexy), 153–154

Safety for operating room personnel
    body mechanics, 20–21
    chemical hazards, 22–23
    fatigue factors, 21
    infection control, 22
    in-service education, 20
    radiation safety, 21
Salpingo-oophorectomy, 172–174
    laparoscopic hysterectomy and laparoscopic-assisted vaginal hysterectomy with or without, 176–180
Saphenous vein, greater, ligation and stripping of, 281–283
Saturated steam under pressure sterilization, 16–17
Scleral buckling/retinal detachment, repair of, 510–513
Scoliosis, procedure for correction of, 360–363
Scrub person
    abdominal extraintestinal surgery and, 83, 90, 94
    cardiovascular surgery and, 283, 294–295
    gastrointestinal surgery and, 132, 138, 147
    genitourinary surgery and, 210, 224
    gynecologic and obstetric surgery and, 158, 161
    neck surgery and, 50–51
    ophthalmic surgery and, 475
    orthopedic surgery and, 340, 353
    otorhinolaryngologic (ENT) surgery and, 437, 459
    thoracic surgery and, 258
Secondary lens implant, 503–505
Segmental resection of lung, 251–253
Sharp counts, 15–16
Shirodkar procedure, 189–190

Shoulder
anterior dislocation of, recurrent, repair of, 310–312
arthroscopy of, 312–316
Shunt, arteriovenous/arteriovenous fistula, 286–288
Shunt, portasystemic, 283–285
Shunt tray, vascular, 581–582
Shunts, ventricular, 381–385
Sigmoid colon and rectum, anterior resection of, 134
Sigmoid resection, laparoscopic-assistred, 140
Sigmoidoscopy, 98–101
basic tray for, 566–567
Simple mastectomy, 55–56
Sinus endoscopy, 451–454
Sinusectomy and pilonidal cystectomy, 149–151
Sinusectomy, branchial cleft, pediatric, 522–524
Small-bowel resection, 119–120
SMR (Submucous resection of nasal septum), 443–444
Spermatocelectomy, 206–207
Spinal, epidural, caudal anesthesia, 40–42
Splenectomy, 89–94
pediatric laparoscopic, 557–558
Sponge count(s), 15
Stapedectomy, 442–443
Stereotactic gamma knife, 369
Sterilization, types of, 16–18
Sterilization, tubal, 5, 174–176
Strabismus, correction of, 490–492
Subcutaneous mastectomy, 55–57

Subdural hematoma, 368
Submaxillary (submandibular) gland, excision of, 461–462
Submucous resection of nasal septum (SMR), 443–444
Subtotal (partial) gastrectomy, 116
Suction curettage, therapeutic abortion, 5, 160–161
Surgical checklist, 6–7
Surgical procedures, 45–558
abdominal extraintestinal surgery, 60–94
breast procedures, 53–59
cardiovascular surgery, 272–295
gastrointestinal surgery, 95–155
genitourinary surgery, 194–245
gynecologic and obstetric surgery, 156–193
neck surgery, 48–52
neurological surgery, 367–392
ophthalmic surgery, 473–517
orthopedic surgery, 296–366
otorhinolaryngologic (ENT) surgery, 435–472
pediatric procedures, 518–558
plastic surgery, 393–434
technical considerations, 47
thoracic procedures, 246–271
Suprapubic laparotomy, 212
Suprasellar tumor, 368
Syndactyly, repair of, 418–420
Synovectomy of the knee, 333–334

T & A (Tonsillectomy and adenoidectomy), 454–456

T & A tray, 600

Tarsorraphy/canthorrhaphy, 478–480

Temporary colostomy, 126

Tendon repair, digital flexor, 420–422

Therapeutic abortion by suction curettage, 5, 160–161

Thiersch procedure, 151–152

Thoracic procedures
  bronchoscopy, 246–249
  correction of pectus excavatum, 259–260
  decortication of lung, 256
  esophagogastromyotomy, video-assisted thoracoscopic, 270–271
  insertion of transvenous endocardial pacemaker, 256–258
  mediastinoscopy, 249–250
  pneumonectomy, 254–255
    video-assisted thoracoscopic, 269–270
  pulmonary lobectomy, 254
  segmental resection of lung, 251–253
  thoracoscopy, 262–268
  thymectomy, 260–262
  wedge resection of lung, 253–254
    thoracoscopic, 268–269

Thoracic trays,
  mediastinoscopy tray, 576–577
  pacemaker tray, 578–579
  thoractomy tray, 577–578

Thoracoscopic wedge resection of the lung, 268–269

Thoracoscopy, 262–268
  pediatric, 556–557

Thoracotomy tray, 577–578
  pediatric, 615

Thymectomy, 260–262

Thyroglossal duct cystectomy, 51–52

Thyroid tray, 564–565

Thyroidectomy, 48–50

Tibial plateau, open reduction of, 333

Tibial shaft, open reduction of, 346–348

Toe, correction of hammer deformity with interphalangeal fusion, 359

Tonsillectomy and adenoidectomy (T & A), 454–456

Tonsillectomy and adenoidectomy (T & A) tray, 600

Topical anesthesia, 35–36, 42–43

Total abdominal hysterectomy, 170–172

Total ankle joint replacement, 354–356

Total gastrectomy, 116

Total hip replacement, 326–330

Total knee replacement, 343–346

Trabeculectomy, 507–509

Tracheostomy, 459–461
  pediatric, 520–522

Tracheostomy tray, 50, 601

Transanal endoscopic microsurgery, 144–147

Transfer procedure, 5, 10

Transplant, corneal/keratoplasty, 497–500

Transsphenoidal hypophysectomy, 378–381

Transurethral resection of lesions of bladder or bladder neck (TURB), 215–217

Transurethral resection of the prostate (TURP), 215–217

Transvenous endocardial pacemaker, insertion of, 256–258

Transverse colectomy, 132–134

Trays. See Instrument trays

Trephination, 367

Trigeminal neuralgia, 369

Triple arthrodesis of ankle, 353–354

Tubal sterilization, 174–176

Tuboplasty of fallopian tubes, 183–186

TURB. See Transurethral resection of lesions of bladder or bladder neck

TURP. See Transurethral resection of the prostate (TURP)

Tympanoplasty, 440–442

Ulcer, perforated, closure of, 113
    laparoscopic (with vagotomy), 113–114

Ulna, open reduction of, 303–305

Ultrasonic lithotripsy, 242–243

Umbilical herniorraphy, 66–67
    pediatric, 529–530

Universal precautions, 11, 22

Upper tract urolithotomy, 225–227

Ureterolithotomy, 225–227

Ureterostomy, cutaneous, 227–228

Urolithotomy, upper tract, 225–227

Uterus
    conization of, 158–159
    curettage of, 156–158

Vaginal hysterectomy, 163–165
    laparoscopic-assisted with or without salpingo-oophorectomy, 176–180

Vaginal hysterectomy tray, 571–572

Vagotomy and pyloroplasty, 106–108

Vagotomy, laparoscopic, 108–114

Vascular procedures tray, 580

Vascular shunt tray, 581–582

Vasectomy, 203–205

Vasectomy tray, 574

Vasotomy, cutaneous, 206

Vasovasotomy, 205–206

Vein ligation and stripping, greater saphenous, 281–283

Ventral herniorraphy. See Incisional (Ventral) herniorraphy

Ventricular shunts, 381–385

Video-assisted thoracoscopic esophagogastromyotomy, 270–271

Video-assisted thoracoscopic pneumonectomy, 269–270

Vitrectomy, 513–516

Wedge resection of lung, 253–254
    thoracoscopic, 268–269

Whipple procedure (pancreaticoduodenectomy), 81–83

Wrist arthroscopy, 307–310

YAG laser, 617–618, 619t

Zygomatic fracture, reduction of, 402–404

ISBN 0-8036-0033-X